The Ulcer Story

The Authoritative Guide to Ulcers, Dyspepsia, and Heartburn

OTHER RECOMMENDED BOOKS BY W. GRANT THOMPSON

The Angry Gut (Plenum Press, New York, New York: 1993)
Gut Reactions (Plenum Press, New York, New York: 1989)
The Irritable Gut (University Park Press, Baltimore, Maryland: 1979)

The Ulcer Story

The Authoritative Guide to Ulcers, Dyspepsia, and Heartburn

W. GRANT THOMPSON, M.D.

PLENUM PRESS • NEW YORK AND LONDON

Library of Congress Cataloging-in-Publication Data

Thompson, W. Grant.
    The ulcer story : the authoritative guide to ulcers, dyspepsia,
and heartburn / W. Grant Thompson.
        p.   cm.
    Includes bibliographical references and index.
    ISBN 0-306-45275-8
    1. Peptic ulcer. 2. Indigestion. 3. Heartburn.   I. Title.
    [DNLM: 1. Peptic Ulcer. 2. Dyspepsia. 3. Heartburn.
    4. Gastroesophageal Reflux. 5. Esophagitis.   WI 350 T478u 1996]
    RC821.T47   1996
    616.3'34--dc20
    DNLM/DLC
    for Library of Congress   96-29022
                                                                   CIP

616.343
T478

The publisher and author disclaim responsibility for any adverse
effects or consequences from the misapplication or injudicious
use of the information contained within this text. Never use any drugs, medical
procedures, or medical products without the consultation and instruction of
your physician. The publisher and author are not endorsing or promoting any
products within the confines of this work.

ISBN 0-306-45275-8

To Sue

Preface

Peptic ulcer is an important twentieth-century disease. Apparently uncommon before 1900, it has caused much disability and even death. Until the 1970s, treatment was very unsatisfactory, and many sufferers required surgery that could be debilitating. Then, in rapid succession, came drugs that first controlled, and then cured, the disease. The 1980s' discovery that most peptic ulcers depend upon an infection revolutionized its management, and now the disease should no longer be debilitating. Just as we learn to control the condition it seems to have become less common. In the West, at least, duodenal ulcer could become rare in the next century.

This book chronicles *The Ulcer Story* for the general reader. While not intended for gastrointestinal specialists, there is much that will interest and challenge physicians. The history of ulcers is a compelling tale and a great medical triumph.

The book is divided into seven parts. The first begins with a review of upper gut anatomy, the stage where the story is enacted. Chapters on physiology and terminology are designed to assist those with a nonmedical background. Throughout, I have tried to employ plain English, but some medical jargon is inevitable. Technical terms and short-forms are redefined at the beginnings of relevant chapters. Next is a brief history of peptic ulcer and gastroesophageal reflux that should interest everyone. Part One ends with a discussion of the epidemiology of ulcers, dyspepsia, and heartburn.

Part Two discusses the causes of peptic ulcer. The disease cannot occur without acid. The anti-arthritis nonsteroidal anti-inflammatory drugs (NSAIDs) and infection of the gastric mucosa with *Helicobacter pylori* are the principal causes of peptic ulcers. The last chapter in Part Two deals with other putative causes laboriously studied for over a century, yet almost eclipsed by recent discoveries.

No book on ulcers should omit a discussion of dyspepsia. Part Three begins with this enigmatic phenomenon. The cardinal symptom of ulcers, dyspepsia more frequently occurs without an ulcer. A brief description of gastric and duodenal ulcers, a review of rare and atypical ulcers, and, finally, a discussion of ulcer complications follow the discussion of dyspepsia.

Part Four shifts the focus to gastroesophageal reflux, the mechanism underlying heartburn and esophagitis. This is relevant to a book about ulcers since heartburn is often confused with dyspepsia, both ulcers and esophagitis depend upon gastric acid, and both diseases are healed with anti-ulcer drugs.

Part Five addresses related subjects—subplots to the ulcer story. The flip side of ulcer dyspepsia is non-ulcer dyspepsia. Lacking the benefits of breakthroughs seen in the treatment of peptic ulcer disease, functional dyspepsia will likely continue to elude definition, explanation, or therapy well into the next century. Abdominal bloating and noncardiac chest pain are sometimes confused with dyspepsia or heartburn. Finally, gastric and esophageal cancers are important here, and not just because at an early state they may resemble ulcers or esophagitis. Gastric cancer has been blamed on *H. pylori*, and esophageal cancer may result from long-standing esophagitis.

In Part Six the drugs prescribed and operations performed for peptic ulcers or gastroesophageal reflux disease are reviewed. This material is for information only. Physicians should supervise treatment, especially since new information is becoming steadily available.

Part Seven describes the tools of discovery. Many treatments for ulcer, heartburn, dyspepsia, and other symptoms have no supporting scientific data. Chapter Thirty discusses why this is so and how costly misapprehensions can be avoided through the proper use and interpretation of clinical trials. The last chapter briefly describes tests that people suspected to have ulcers or reflux might have to undergo. Knowing what to expect may remove unwarranted fear.

The Ulcer Story has many heroes. Most of these are or were working doctors who put the pieces together to produce a coherent picture. For a profession beleaguered by criticism, the result is an inspiration. While laboratory science makes astonishing medical progress, it can do so only when physician–scientists clearly define clinical problems. Most medical advances are small, and establishment of their usefulness depends upon the skills of clinicians. Interaction between physicians and basic scientists underlies the advances in the control of ulcer disease. Dragstedt saw the importance of Pavlov's work. Hirschowitz turned an arcane discovery at the Imperial College of Science and Technology into the modern gastroscope. The teamwork of Warren and Marshall prompted the climax of *The Ulcer Story*, the discovery of *H. pylori*.

The tale is far from complete. There is much to be done to discover the best means to cure peptic ulcers. How can we counter the effects of NSAIDs? There must be a sensible approach to dyspepsia. Can we prevent peptic ulcers and cancer? Nevertheless, ulcers should never again be the scourge they were in the 1900s.

This book is the current view of one observer who has practiced through the period of the greatest advances in ulcer research. For most patients with peptic ulcers and gastroesophageal reflux, it is a happy story. I hope you enjoy the book as much as I have enjoyed writing it.

W. Grant Thompson

The Barn, Blagdon, North Somerset, England

Acknowledgments

Without the love and support of my wife Sue, this book would not have been attempted. She enthusiastically shared the decision to come to England so that I could do the necessary research. She helped me with the editing. I have been helped by many people but can mention only a few. Dr. Ken Heaton at the University of Bristol challenged me to think more clearly about dyspepsia. Discussions with Nick Talley of the University of Sydney, Doug Drossman from the University of North Carolina, and other members of the Clinical Brain–Gut Research Group have been very stimulating over the years. My hospital chief, Dr. Peter Walker, was very supportive, as were my other Ottawa colleagues. I am indebted to the Royal College of Physicians and Surgeons of Canada, who awarded me a Detweiller Traineeship. The University of Ottawa also provided support. The libraries of the University of Bristol, the Ottawa Civic Hospital, and the Royal Society of Medicine were valuable resources. The drawings are by Mr. James Harbinson of the Audio Visual Department of the Ottawa Civic Hospital. Mr. Rob Ellis of Medical Illustration at the Bristol Royal Infirmary helped me prepare some of the figures. As with my other books, Dr. Hardy Tao of the Division of Radiology at the Ottawa Civic Hospital helped me prepare the X-ray illustrations. Finally, Dr. Maha Guindi of the Division of Anatomical Pathology provided the pathology and histology specimens shown in the book.

Contents

PART ONE

Understanding Ulcers and Heartburn

CHAPTER ONE

The Gut

A Brief Anatomy

This chapter briefly describes the anatomy of the upper gut and its support systems. The symptoms and diseases of the ulcer story originate in the esophagus, stomach, and duodenum.

STRUCTURE OF THE GUT

Overview

At autopsy the human gut is 9 meters (30 feet) from mouth to anus. In the living person the gut muscle tone contracts it to about one-half of that length. Although the mouth and throat are part of the gut, our story will begin at the esophagus (gullet) and will continue through the stomach and small intestine. The esophagus, stomach, small bowel, and colon are arranged within the chest and abdominal cavity as shown in Figure 1-1.

The gut is a hollow, very flexible tube, the wall of which has three layers: an outer coating called the *serosa*, a muscular layer called the *muscularis*, and an inner lining called the *mucosa* (Figure 1-2). It is a dynamic organ that, when a person is awake, is usually on the move. The driving force is the muscle coat that extends the length of the gut. There is an outer, thinner layer that consists of muscle cells or fibers arranged longitudinally. This layer shortens and lengthens the gut as it moves its contents along. The inner,

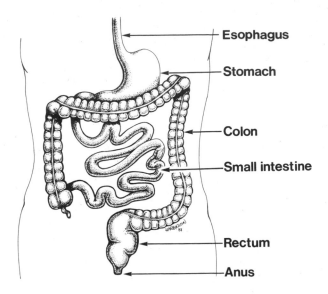

Figure 1-1. The gut. The relationships of the esophagus, stomach, small intestine, and colon within the chest and abdominal cavity are shown.

circular muscle layer becomes thickened or specialized at various points to form one-way valves or sphincters such as the lower esophageal sphincter or the pylorus. Circular muscle contractions coordinate with longitudinal ones to cause ripple-like movements that carry intestinal contents along the gut in a process known as *peristalsis*. Gut muscle from the mid-esophagus to the anus is called *smooth* muscle and is under involuntary control. This distinguishes it from *skeletal*, or *striated*, muscle in the limbs (and throat and upper esophagus) that is under voluntary control.

The innermost gut layer is called the mucosa and is dynamic in a metabolic sense. The *epithelium* is a single layer of cells on the surface of the mucosa that is specialized to handle water, minerals, and nutrients. The epithelium of the esophagus, stomach, and duodenum serves as a barrier to acid or foreign materials. Beneath this cellular layer or epithelium is the mucosa that contains a variety of cells. These handle absorbed nutrients or defend against unwanted invaders such as viruses, bacteria, or toxins.

The gastric (stomach) mucosa produces a fluid so strongly acidic that it will burn other tissues. For example, you may experience burning in the throat when you vomit. This acid (hydrochlo-

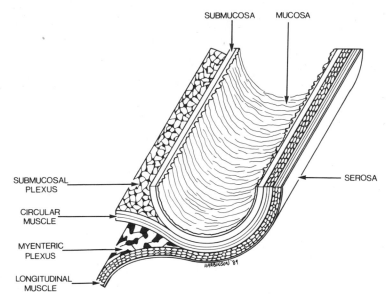

SUBMUCOSA   MUCOSA

SUBMUCOSAL PLEXUS

CIRCULAR MUSCLE

MYENTERIC PLEXUS

LONGITUDINAL MUSCLE

SEROSA

HARBINSON '89

Figure 1-2. The three layers of the intestinal wall. Note also that the submucus nerve plexus (network) lies between the submucosa and the circular muscle. The myenteric plexus lies between the two muscle layers. In the small intestine, semicircular folds shown here increase the mucosal surface, maximizing its contact with the intestinal contents.

ric) is called muriatic acid when used by bricklayers to clean mortar from bricks. Thus, the mucosa of the stomach and upper small intestine must be metabolically tough enough to resist destruction by the acid. Otherwise ulceration occurs.

The small intestinal mucosa is responsible not only for the absorption of most nutrients but also for the daily exchange of about 8 liters of fluid. Along with oral liquid intake, the pancreatic and bile ducts empty pancreatic juice and bile from the pancreas and liver into the upper small intestine. To facilitate this enormous fluid exchange, the small intestinal mucosa is pleated into semicircular folds.

Anatomy of the Upper Gut

Esophagus

The esophagus (or gullet) (Figure 1-3) is a hollow tube 20–22 cm (8–9 inches) long. Its upper end, unlike the intra-abdominal gut,

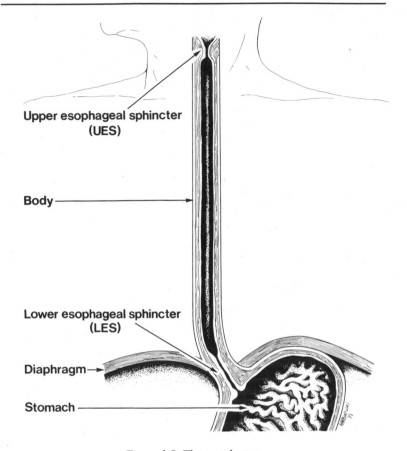

Figure 1-3. The esophagus.

lacks a serosal layer. It begins where the pharynx, or throat, ends,
below and behind the Adam's apple. Here the cricopharyngeous,
a striated muscle under voluntary control, forms the first gut
sphincter, called the upper esophageal sphincter (UES). This muscular valve must relax to admit food into the gullet. The body of
the esophagus is powered by striated muscle in its upper third and
smooth muscle in the remainder. The esophagus is not merely a
passive tube. Through peristalsis driven by esophageal muscle, it
forcefully carries food from the mouth to the stomach. Thus, the
opossum can hang in there without getting up for dinner. At the
lower end there is another valve, the lower esophageal sphincter
(LES), which must relax as food arrives. It normally maintains a

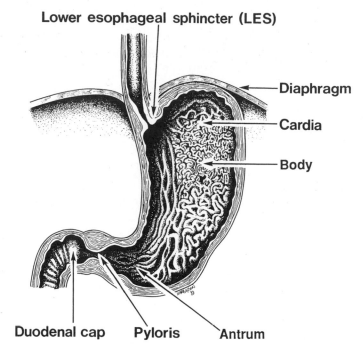

Lower esophageal sphincter (LES)

Diaphragm

Cardia

Body

Duodenal cap   Pyloris   Antrum

Figure 1-4. The stomach.

local increase in pressure that prevents gastric contents from refluxing back into the esophagus. The LES is normally at the diaphragm where the gut enters the abdomen.

The Stomach

> The stomach is the distinguishing part between an animal and a vegetable: for we do not know any vegetable that has a stomach nor any animal without one.
>
> John Hunter, 1728–1793

It is curious that an organ about which so much is written is not essential for life (Figure 1-4). With altered eating habits, nutritional care, and vitamin B_{12} injections, patients with surgically removed stomachs may live for many years. Nonetheless, the stomach stores and mixes a meal, begins the digestive process, and is the putative source of many digestive complaints.

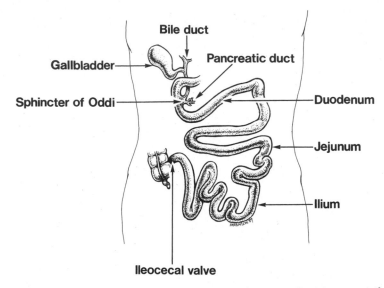

Figure 1-5. The small intestine. The duodenum becomes the jejunum at the ligament of Treitz, a sharp angulation of the gut near the splenic flexure of colon. Note that both pancreatic juice, which contains digestive enzymes, and bile, which contains bile salts, enter the duodenum through the sphincter of Oddi.

The stomach is a variably shaped organ usually resembling a fat reclining "J." It has four parts. The *cardia* is adjacent to the esophageal orifice. The *fundus* is the dome-shaped portion above the cardia against the diaphragm. The *body*, or corpus, is the largest part and extends from the fundus vertically downward. The *antrum* is the foot of the "J" ending at a thickened muscular ring called the pylorus. One should consider the upper stomach as a container, while the antrum has mixing and pumping actions. The pylorus separates the stomach from the duodenum and is the third valve or sphincter that we meet as we travel down the gut.

Small Intestine

The small intestine is the site of absorption of most nutrients (Figure 1-5). It is attached to the posterior wall of the abdomen by the mesentery, a ligament that contains the blood vessels, nerves and lymphatics. The small intestine has three segments: the duodenum, the jejunum, and the ileum. The first part of the duodenum, which is just beyond the pylorus, is called the duodenal *cap*, or *bulb*.

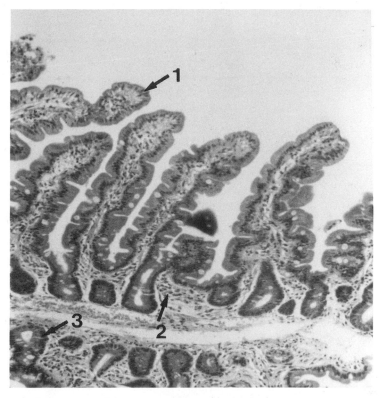

Figure 1-6. Histology of the small intestine. Photomicrograph of the luminal side of small intestinal wall. (1) Epithelium: angle layer of tall columnar, cells lining tall villi that project into the gut lumen. (2) Mucosa: Note the many cell nuclei. These are principally inflammatory or immune-competent cells, essential defenses against foreign invaders. (3) Crypts, where epithelial cell reproduction occurs. (Courtesy of Dr. M. Guindi.)

It is here that duodenal ulcers usually occur. The remainder of the duodenum encircles the head of the pancreas (Figure 1-5) and ends at a sharp angulation called the *ligament of Treitz*. The *common bile duct* and *pancreatic ducts* originate in the liver and pancreas, respectively, and enter the duodenum through the sphincter of Oddi.

The *jejunum* is the longest segment of the small intestine and is the most important site of water, mineral, and nutrient absorption. No feature marks the junction of the jejunum with the ileum. The distal segment of the small intestine is called the *ileum* and is the site

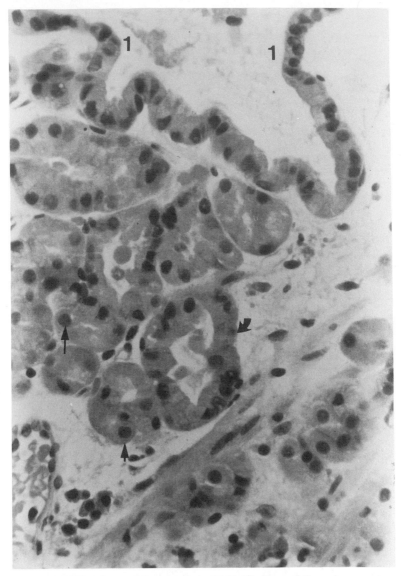

Figure 1-7. Histology of the stomach. (1) Epithelium of the columnar type lines the stomach. Beneath this layer and communicating with it are the gastric glands or crypts, also lined by a single layer of columnar cells. The acid-producing parietal cells are located in this crypt epithelium (straight arrows), and smaller endocrine cells are adjacent (curved arrow). (Courtesy of Dr. M. Guindi.)

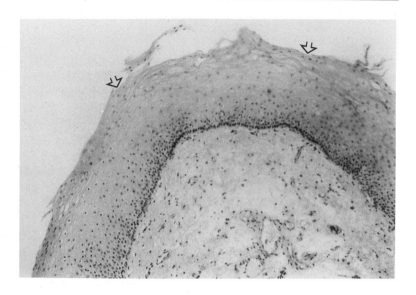

Figure 1-8. Histology of the esophagus. The epithelium lining the esophagus is not a single layer of parietal cells as in the rest of the gut. Rather, it is a stratified squamus epithelium. The arrows point to the surface cells of this epithelium where the cells are now dead and being shed into the lumen of the esophagus. The deeper, darkly stained layer is the germinal layer where cells reproduce and migrate upward through their life cycle. (Courtesy of Dr. M. Guindi.)

of vitamin B_{12} and bile salt absorption. It terminates at the next gut sphincter, the *ileocecal valve*, which guards the entry into the colon.

Peritoneum

Most of the abdominal gut is coiled within a potential space called the peritoneal space. Its peritoneal surface is lined by a thin layer of cells called the serosa (see above). This serosal layer is continuous with the peritoneum so that it becomes a large convoluted envelope that separates the loops of bowel from one another. When the gut perforates, for example as a complication of a peptic ulcer, gut contents soil the normally sterile peritoneal space. If walled off by inflammatory tissue, a local abscess occurs. If not, the result is generalized peritonitis, which is a grave surgical emergency.

Histology of the Gut

Like all living tissue, the gut is made up of cells. The study of cellular tissue is called *histology* and must be conducted through a microscope. Histology of the gut is very complex (Figures 1-6, 1-7, and 1-8). The layer of cells lining the gut is called the *epithelium*. Under this epithelial cell layer are the mucosa and submucosa that contain a variety of cells important in the local immune and chemical reactions to gut injury. These cells include polymorphonuclear leucocytes (many nucleated white blood cells) and mononuclear cells such as lymphocytes, plasma cells, and macrophages, all of which participate in the immune response should any foreign substance invade their territory. Notable among the remaining cells are those of nerve plexes, blood vessels, and chemical-producing cells such as mast cells. Beneath the submucosa are the muscle and serosal layers of the gut. In Figure 1-6 note the tall, fingerlike *villi* that increase the inner surface of the gut to maximize the absorption of nutrients. To further increase the gut's luminal surface, each cell has tiny projections called *microvilli* that can be seen only through the electron microscope.

The stomach lacks villi, but the body of the stomach has deep epithelium-lined caves called crypts or glands. Crypts near the cardia secrete mucus. Seventy-five percent of gastric glands contain the acid-secreting *parietal* cells and the pepsin-secreting *chief* cells (Figure 1-7). These are mainly in the fundus and body of the stomach. The average human stomach has about 1 billion parietal cells. The glands of the antrum, on the other hand, contain neither of these specialized cells. Its mucosa has *antral G* cells, which they can sense lack of acid and release the hormone gastrin. In turn, gastrin stimulates the parietal cells to secrete hydrochloric acid.

Parietal cells lie in the epithelium lining the gastric glands. These cells are unique in many ways. They contain many tiny, energy-producing *mitochondria*. *Tubulovesicles* are other intracellular structures that contain the acid pump, *hydrogen, potassium-ATPase* (H^+, K^+–$ATPase$). This enzyme is capable of transferring hydrogen (H^+) ions across the cell membrane into tiny canals called *canalicula*. When the cell is active, the tubulovesicles invaginate into the canaliculi. The acid pumps then become part of the canaliculi that in turn empty the produced acid into the gastric gland and thence into the stomach. The acid pump itself is a protein chain of 1,034 amino acids looping back and forth across the canalicular membrane. Also in these glands are chief cells that secrete the enzyme *pepsin*, the other digesting component of gastric juice. Small *enterochromaffin* (ECL) cells adjacent to the parietal cells secrete histamine that stimulates the $histamine_2$ (H_2) receptors on the parietal cells.

The histology of the esophagus includes two unique features (Figure 1-8). First, the esophagus is not lined with the tall columnar cells found elsewhere in the gut, but rather with flat squamus cells that resemble those found in skin. This difference reflects the need for the esophageal mucosa to protect rather than to absorb or secrete. The second difference lies in the muscle coat. Most of the gut is powered by smooth muscle that is generally under autonomic, not voluntary, control. Skeletal, or striated, muscles are the voluntarily controlled muscles of the skeleton. Skeletal muscle moves the upper one-third of the esophagus and serves the voluntary act of swallowing.

SUPPORT SYSTEMS

Blood Supply

The gut cannot function on its own. It must communicate with the rest of the body to regulate motility and the transport of nutrients. Three large arteries—the *celiac* and the *superior* and *inferior mesenteric*—arise from the aorta (the main artery coming from the heart) to supply oxygen and other nutrients to the stomach, small intestine and colon (the intra-abdominal gut).

Corresponding veins carry absorbed nutrients and gases away. This process is so efficient that hydrogen gas produced by the action of colon bacteria on ingested intestinal contents appears within seconds in the breath. Besides the blood vessels, tiny vessels called *lymphatics* carry absorbed fats from the small intestine to the circulation.

Gut Regulation

... it still comes as a surprise to most gastroenterologists and neurophysiologists that there are 3 or 4 million enteric neurons in small animals and tens of millions in humans.

M. Costa and S.J.H. Brookes, 1994

The *enteric nervous system* (ENS) regulates the gut. An ever-increasing list of hormones and neurotransmitters have complex effects on gut movement and fluid transport through the mucosa. The ENS is a complex network of nerves and ganglia within the gut wall (Figure 1-2). The nerve network found between the circular and longitudinal muscle layers is called the *myenteric plexus*. That between the muscle and submucosa is called the *submucous plexus*. Through connections to muscle, mucosa, and blood vessels, this gut brain governs our digestion. The ENS communicates with the brain first by the *sympathetic* nerves that pass to and from the gut through transformers called sympathetic ganglia (Figure 1-9). These nerves connect to the spinal cord, and thence to the base of the brain. Second, *parasympathetic* nerves connect the upper gut with the base of the brain through the *vagus* nerve. Each nerve transmission is effected by one of several neurotransmitters or hormones acting upon an appropriate receptor on muscle, ganglion, or other cells. For example, *acetylcholine* released by motor neurons stimulates receptors on gut muscle cells, causing them to contract.

Ganglia are collections of nerve bodies with projections that travel a few millimeters to interact with other ganglia up and down the gut. They receive messages from a sensory organ or send messages to an effector organ such as a muscle or secreting gland. Ganglia in the myenteric plexus supply excitatory and inhibitory impulses to the gut muscle, signaling it to contract and relax. Ganglia in the submucus plexus principally supply the mucosa. Each ganglia has its own neurochemical brew. Neurotransmitter substances in these cells have exotic names such as substance P, vasoactive intestinal polypeptide (VIP), encephalin, neuropeptide Y, tachykinin, and calbindin. Also in these tiny nerve cells are enzymes such as choline acetyl transferase or nitric oxide synthetase, which participate in the dynamic chemical activity of the ENS. Direct or reflex impulses generated or transmitted in and through the ganglia support complex motor functions such as peristalsis. In peristalsis, a relaxed ring of circular gut muscle travels a variable length of gut in a distal direction followed by a ring of contracting muscle. This moves gut contents along. The coordination of reflexes required for such a function is harmonized by the ENS.

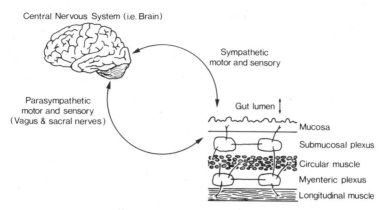

Figure 1-9. The enteric nervous system (ENS). The ENS lies within the gut wall and through the sympathetic and parasympathetic nerves transmits and receives information to and from the brain.

Many of the hormones and neurotransmitters of the ENS are found also in the central nervous system (CNS) (brain and spinal cord). Some drugs act by mimicking neurotransmitters at their receptors. Others inhibit a neurotransmitter by blocking or competing for its receptor on a nerve, a muscle cell, or a secretory cell. It is said that the complexity of the "gut brain" equals that of the CNS, but I would not trust the ENS to drive a car!

From the foregoing one should clearly understand that the brain and the gut are intricately interconnected. Events in the one are unlikely to be ignored by the other! It should also be obvious that that gut function is very complex. For digestion to proceed in a orderly manner, the components of the ENS must be in harmony. Many believe that ENS dysfunction is responsible for functional gastrointestinal symptom complexes such as functional dyspepsia.

Protection

The gut is the body's principal port of entry, and its tortuous anatomy constitutes a vast frontier. If the body is to restrict entry it must have a customs and immigration service; otherwise, the gut would be subject to invasion not only by nutrients but also by all the microbes, toxins, inert substances, and other flotsam that pass its way. Many protective mechanisms are in place. Gastric acid, bile salts, and pancreatic enzymes conspire to destroy most intestinal contents in the stomach and small bowel. A layer of mucous and the sheet of mucosal epithelial cells lining the lumen of the gut provide a natural barrier (Figures 1-6, 1-7, and 1-8). The epithelium has great reparative power and can reconstruct itself within hours. Metabolic transport processes carry only nutrients across the barrier, and those items denied entry are carried away by peristalsis. Despite this, invasive bacteria or damaging toxins can breach the epithelial barrier, permitting entrance of unwanted aliens. It thus falls to the body's immune system to police the frontier and destroy or deport the invaders.

The gut is well equipped to mount an immune defense. There are numerous cells in the mucosa of the gut that possess various immune capabilities (Figure 1-6). Cells with single nuclei, called *mononuclear cells*, may develop in several ways. Some produce antibodies that recognize and attach themselves to foreign proteins, thereby participating in their destruction. Other killer cells, or *killer lymphocytes*, directly attack the foreigners and kill them. Still others ingest invaders. These are called *macrophages* (literally, "big mouths").

The battle between these immune forces and the invaders causes inflammation. Blood vessels in the surrounding tissues dilate, causing local congestion with red blood cells (hemorrhage) and fluid (edema). *Polymorphonuclear* white blood cells act as roving policemen in the blood stream. At the first sign of local trouble the polymorphs gather at the site, in this case the gut. They are important participants in the acute inflammatory response. Nearby mast cells release chemical mediators of inflammation such as histamine, bradykinin, and cytokines.

A lipid substance called *arachadonic acid* is degraded through several steps regulated by the enzymes *cyclo-oxygenase* and *lipoxygenase* to produce the inflammatory mediators prostaglandin and leucotriene. Nonsteroidal antiinflammatory drugs (*NSAIDs*) that are used for arthritis interfere with this mechanism and cause ulcers, or erosions, in the gut.

SUMMARY

The gut is a 9-meter-long muscular organ beginning at the throat and ending at the anus. There is an outer longitudinal muscle layer and an inner circular muscle layer. The coordinated contractions (peristalsis) of these layers move intestinal contents in a manner programmed by the ENS in the gut wall. The ENS in turn is influenced by neurotransmitters, hormones, and connections to the CNS. The mucosa lines the gut lumen and is responsible for the absorption of nutrients and the secretion of acid and enzymes. It is also under ENS control. Numerous natural barriers, including mucus, epithelial cells, and a profound immune capability, guard the gut frontier against invasion by microorganisms and toxins.

The esophagus is an active muscular conduit with upper and lower esophageal sphincters. The proximal stomach is a food container where acid and pepsin are secreted and digestion begins. The distal stomach, the antrum, is a pump that grinds food and injects measured amounts of gastric contents through the pylorus into the duodenum. It is also the production site of gastrin, a hormone that stimulates parietal cells in the gastric crypts or glands to release hydrochloric acid. Ducts from the liver (bile ducts) and pancreas enter the duodenum. That part of the duodenum near the stomach and proximal to the ducts is called the duodenal bulb, or cap. It is the usual site of a duodenal ulcer. The jejunum and ileum absorb nutrients.

CHAPTER TWO

Physiology

How the Gut Works

To eat is human, to digest divine
C. T. Copeland 1860–1952

Once swallowed, a mouthful becomes a *bolus* and is carried by the esophagus to the stomach. Here it is mixed and partly digested into *chyme*. Upon entering the small bowel it becomes intestinal contents that are altered by absorption and secretion through the intestinal mucosa. In the colon, intestinal contents become known as *feces*, or stool. So that these metamorphoses may occur in an orderly fashion, gut smooth muscle must convey luminal contents in a manner consistent with optimal digestion and absorption of nutrients. The ENS and its neurotransmitters govern these processes. They in turn are influenced by hormones and interconnections with the brain (Figures 1-2, and 1-9).

Gut movements are influenced by a variety of reflexes that respond to the concentration, osmolarity, size, and nature of the luminal contents and to events occurring elsewhere in the gut. The ENS also governs the secretion of hydrochloric acid by the stomach and digestive enzymes by the small intestine. Each gut segment accepts food, moves it along, adds digestive juices, and extracts the required water, salts, and nutrients. Normally, this gut activity occurs without our consciousness. This chapter is about how the upper gut works, that is, its physiology.

THE ESOPHAGUS (GULLET) (FIGURE 1-3)

The *upper esophageal sphincter* (UES) is the first one-way valve that food meets as it begins its journey down the gullet. (The mouth might be the first, but it is neither one way nor involuntary.) When an individual swallows food, the UES must relax to allow it to pass into the esophagus. This valve may help prevent food and gastric juice that escapes from the stomach into the esophagus from refluxing back into the throat.

The body of the esophagus is not a simple conduit. Its inner and outer muscular layers coordinate to produce primary peristalsis. A wave of increased intraesophageal pressure preceded by relaxation carries a bolus before it into the stomach in approximately 7 seconds. Distension of the esophagus initiates secondary peristalsis to clear the gullet of foreign bodies or acid refluxed from the stomach. This "housekeeping" function minimizes the consequences of gastroesophageal reflux. With age, peristalsis becomes less reliable, and there may be nonperistaltic (tertiary) contractions.

Anatomists cannot identify any thickening of the muscle layer that they could call the *lower esophageal sphincter* (LES). However, electronic sensors that record intraluminal pressures detect a high-pressure zone about 3 cm long just above the gastroesophageal junction. Normally, LES pressure, as measured by intraluminal sensors, is greater than the intraluminal pressure of the stomach. In response to the arrival of a peristaltic wave, this one-way valve relaxes to allow the esophagus to discharge its contents into the stomach.

Often, part of the stomach herniates (protrudes) through the diaphragm into the chest and creates a *hiatus hernia*. Hiatus hernia and heartburn are both very common and occur together through coincidence. Nevertheless, anatomic relationships are important. The sharp angle where the esophagus enters the stomach serves as a flutter valve. The normal intra-abdominal location of the LES just below the diaphragm helps prevent it from being overwhelmed by increases in abdominal pressure.

STOMACH

Gastric Motility

The proximal stomach, or body, is a storage container that expands to accommodate a meal with little change in intragastric pressure (Figure 1-4). Tonic contractions and relaxations finely adjust gastric capacity. These volume or capacity contractions last about 1 minute and control gastric emptying of liquids.

Electrical slow waves propagate from the proximal stomach to the pylorus. They are responsible for the timing of gastric antral peristalsis. A peristaltic wave begins mid-stomach and spreads as a circumferential band through the antrum to the pylorus. These contractions are of two types. The first are small, weak waves that have a mixing function. Larger, more powerful waves have a propulsive as well as a mixing action. After a meal, conditions are such that each electrical slow wave initiates a peristaltic contraction. These waves occur at the rate of 3–6 per minute. Meanwhile, through tonic contractions of the body, the stomach selectively empties liquids while retaining solids of over 2 mm in size. This capacity to selectively retain, grind, and then empty solids requires the antrum and pylorus to act in concert. The pylorus can be seen radiographically and endoscopically to open and close. Antral contractions regularly propel gastric contents toward the pylorus, through which they squirt small amounts into the duodenum. Larger particles that are unable to pass the pylorus are retropelled into the proximal stomach through the nozzle formed by the advancing peristaltic wave. In this fashion the stomach mixes and grinds a meal into particles small enough for the small intestine to digest.

In contrast to the fed state, the fasting stomach undergoes a three-phase cycle: inactive, irregular contractions, and a terminal intense peristaltic phase that sweeps all before it into the duodenum. This cycle may take 1–2 hours. Thus, the stomach is a receptacle, a mixer, and a grinder. The pylorus, subject to gastroduodenal activity, is the gate keeper of the intestine, controlling the rate that food presents for digestion.

Control of Gastric Emptying

Gastric motor function is very complex. Its role in *The Ulcer Story* is uncertain, but disturbance in motor activity may cause dyspepsia, and often causes symptoms following surgery for ulcer disease. Central to motor control is the ENS or "gut brain." The ENS programs stomach motor activity under the influence of the autonomic nervous system acting through the vagus (cholinergic) and sympathetic (adrenergic) nerves. The brain exerts its influence through these nerves. Vagotomy, for instance, delays the tonic relaxations of the stomach in anticipation of food and impairs antral emptying of gastric contents. Psychic circumstances such as stress can override the autonomy of the ENS and delay emptying of a meal.

Many gut hormones and neurotransmitters influence the ENS. *Motilin* stimulates interdigestive motor activity. *Gastrin, secretin, cholecystokinin (CCK)*, and *gastric inhibitory polypeptide* relax the proximal stomach and inhibit emptying. The nerve cells in the ganglia of the ENS itself influence one another by neurotransmitters passed from cell to cell. Local nonadrenergic, noncholinergic influences include *nitric oxide* and *dopamine*. Many of these naturally occurring substances are mimicked or antagonized by the drugs described in Part 6.

The nature of ingested food is a major determinant of gastric emptying. Liquids empty faster than solids. The larger the solid particles, the slower they empty. Duodenal nerve endings sense the presence of fat, amino acids, glucose, and other substances and reflexively modulate their emptying according to the intestine's ability to assimilate them. Such fine tuning is lost following most ulcer operations. The result may be inappropriate release of insulin, low blood sugar, disturbances in satiety, and malassimilation of calories and other nutrients. Surely,

> Our digestions . . . going sacredly and silently right . . . is the foundation of all poetry?
>
> G. K. Chesterton, 1908

Gastric Secretion

When the parietal cell is stimulated to secrete hydrogen ions, its tiny intracellular tubulovesicles invaginate and fuse with the canaliculi. This increases the secretory membrane area by 75% and exposes the acid pumps to the canalicular surface. From the cell fluid (cytosol), hydrogen ions (H^+) are pumped into the canaliculi in exchange for potassium ions (K^+). This reduces the pH in the canaliculi to about 1, compared to 7.3 in the cell fluid. The membrane also permits chloride ions (Cl^-) to pass into the canaliculi, where they combine with the H^+ ions to form hydrochloric acid. All the associated reactions need not concern us here, but the Cl^- ions passed into the canalicula exchange with bicarbonate ions (HCO_3^-) that are then carried away by the blood. This egress of the alkaline bicarbonate in the gastric veins is called the "alkaline tide."

Many factors stimulate the parietal cell to produce acid. Psychic influences such as the smell of food can, through the vagus nerve, release acetylcholine from cholinergic nerve endings adjacent to the parietal cell. Nearby *enterochromaffin-like cells* (ECL) produce histamine that combines with the histamine (H_2) receptors on the acid-secreting cells. In response to an increase in intragastric pH, the antral G cells release the hormone gastrin. These three mechanisms—cholinergic nerve impulses, H_2 receptor stimulation by histamine, and release of gastrin—have synergistic effects on the parietal cell. Their combined effect is greater than the sum of their individual effects. The exact relationship is unknown, but histamine may be the final pathway. Most anti-ulcer drugs act by interfering in some way with these effects. Antacids neutralize H^+ ions in the stomach lumen, while anticholinergic and H_2-blocking drugs counteract the vagal or histamine effects. Proton pump blockers disable the acid pump itself. (see Chapter 6.)

SMALL INTESTINE

Motility

Local stimulation of the gut produces excitation above and inhibition below the excited spot.

W. M. Bayliss and E. H. Starling, 1899

This is the law of the intestine, expounded by the pioneering physiologists Bayliss and Starling in 1899 to explain how the gut carries along a bolus of food. Besides peristalsis, nonpropulsive contractions occur at adjacent sites in the intestine. These move the gut contents back and forth in pendulum fashion. Contractions are most active following a meal. They mix the intestinal contents and ensure maximal contact with the absorbing surface of the mucosa.

In the period between meals there are cycles of propagating contractions lasting from 2 to 2 ½ hours. These *migrating motor complexes* (MMCs) correspond to small intestinal peristalsis and are moving rings formed by circular muscle contractions preceded by relaxations. The MMCs and peristalsis keep the normally sterile small gut clear of residual food and bacteria. There are also infrequent, powerful, giant migrating contractions originating in the distal small bowel that sweep through the colon into the rectum.

Absorption and Secretion

There is a remarkable exchange of fluids and nutrients across the intestinal mucosa. The small intestine handles up to 8 liters of fluid from ingestion and secretion into the gut by the stomach, intestine, liver, and pancreas. The intestine, especially the jejunum, absorbs most nutrients, vitamins, and minerals. Food ground up by the stomach is exposed to bile and pancreatic enzymes that prepare it for absorption through the mucosa. Some stomach operations divert these juices and impair absorption. Rapid gut transit after vagotomy (surgical interruption of the vagus nerves) may cause diarrhea and malabsorption.

SUMMARY

In response to a swallow, the UES relaxes, allowing passage of the bolus into the esophageal body. The LES relaxes with the arrival of the food bolus, allowing an esophageal peristaltic wave to sweep all before it into the stomach. Impaired LES tone or incomplete peristalsis may permit acid, pepsin, and sometimes bile to reflux into the esophagus. This causes heartburn and sometimes esophagitis.

The body of the stomach adjusts the gastric capacity for food through tonic contractions and relaxations. From the stomach, distally, rhythmic electrical activity determines the timing of gut smooth muscle contractions. Gastric peristalsis begins in mid-body and may sweep through into the duodenum or conclude in a vigorous contraction against a closed pylorus to mix and grind the food. The antrum and pylorus, acting in concert, prevent the reflux of duodenal contents into the stomach. These functions may be disrupted by local disease such as an ulcer, drug side effects, surgery, or a specific disturbance in gastric motility. The parietal cells in the crypts of the upper stomach secrete hydrochloric acid. Chief cells, deep in the crypts, produce an acid-dependent proteolytic enzyme called pepsin. Acid and pepsin begin the process of digestion, but may damage unprotected upper gut mucosa, causing erosions or peptic ulcers. The ENS regulates acid secretion by gastrin from G cells in the gastric antrum, by histamine from adjacent ECL cells, and by local and central nervous inputs.

The small gut absorbs nutrients from the food as peristalsis moves it along. Contractions occurring 4 or 5 cm apart divide the intestine into segments, mixing the contents and maximizing mucosal exposure.

CHAPTER THREE
Terminology

The ill and unfit choice of words wonderfully obstructs the
understanding
Sir Francis Bacon, 1561–1626, *Novum Organum XLIII*

This chapter introduces the reader to some of the frequently used terms in *The Ulcer Story*. They are more fully described in later chapters.

DYSPEPSIA

The most common peptic ulcer symptom is *dyspepsia*, a pain or discomfort in the upper abdomen. Those with dyspepsia who have no ulcer have *non-ulcer*, or *functional*, *dyspepsia*. Dyspepsia defies definition, but there have been many attempts (see Chapter 10). The current international definition is "three months or more of pain or discomfort in the upper abdomen."

Since upper abdominal pain includes many symptom complexes that are not "dyspeptic," it is perhaps more instructive to consider what dyspepsia is not. Heartburn (described below) is not dyspepsia, even if it is experienced in the lower chest. Dyspepsia is not biliary colic (gall bladder attack), pancreatic, cardiac, or skeletal muscle pain. Sometimes, the pain of irritable bowel syndrome (IBS) is in the upper abdomen, but then it is characterized by its relationship with bowel dysfunction (constipation, diarrhea, bloating, etc.). The pain of dyspepsia is sometimes a discomfort or extreme fullness, and may have a relationship with eating. A careful history should enable the physician to distinguish dyspepsia from other upper gut symptoms. The term *indigestion* is even more imprecise than dyspepsia. An international working team has urged that it not be used.

It is impossible by symptoms to distinguish those with dyspepsia who have an ulcer from those who do not. This requires an X ray or endoscopic examination. A useful working definition of dyspepsia, then, is "a chronic, recurrent abdominal pain or discomfort that leads the physician to suspect a peptic ulcer: not heartburn, not IBS, not biliary, pancreatic, cardiac, or skeletal pain." Dyspepsia is an important character in *The Ulcer Story*, as described in Chapters 10 and 18.

OTHER SYMPTOMS

Anorexia is a lack of appetite. *Belching* is the expulsion of gas through the mouth. *Bloating* is a feeling of abdominal distension or fullness. *Borborygmi* are rumbling or gurgling noises from the abdomen, often audible at a distance. *Flatulence* is a euphemism for farting, but, since it is confused with other terms, it should not be used. *Colic* is a pain that repeatedly comes and goes at short intervals. *Early satiety* describes a sensation that the stomach is prematurely full.

PEPTIC ULCER

A *peptic ulcer* is a defect in the mucosa or lining of the stomach or duodenum that extends deep into the gut wall (Figure 3-1). The term *peptic* implies the presence of gastric acid and pepsin. In most cases of peptic ulcer a bacterium called *Helicobacter pylori* infects the stomach lining. In others, there has been chronic use of an NSAID. An *erosion* is a small, shallow loss of epithelium. Erosions are often multiple, but they do not extend deeper than the muscularis mucosa (Figure 3-2). A gastric tumor is a mass or lump in the wall of the stomach. A tumor may prove on biopsy to be a cancer,

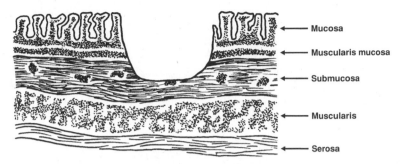

Figure 3-1. Peptic ulcer. The mucosa is destroyed and the ulcer penetrates a variable distance through the muscularis mucosa into the submucosa and even into the muscularis.

but benign tumors do occur. Sometimes a gastric tumor will have an ulcer in it (Figure 3-3).

ULCEROGENIC FACTORS

Acid and Pepsin

Gastric secretion is the production of *hydrochloric acid (HCl)*, the enzyme *pepsin,* and other substances by the epithelial glands of the stomach. Acid secretion by the parietal cells is stimulated by impulses through the *vagus nerve* and by the release of the hormone *gastrin* from the gastric antrum. *Achlorhydria* is a state where the stomach is unable to produce any acid. An *antacid* is an alkaline

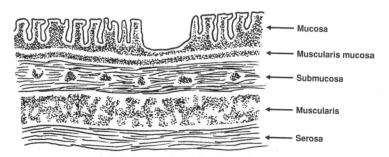

Figure 3-2. Erosion. The mucosa is eroded, but the muscularis of the stomach or duodenum is not penetrated.

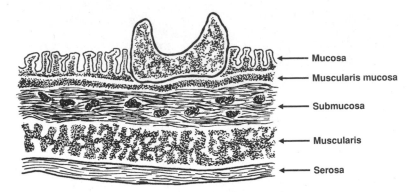

Figure 3-3. A small tumor in the mucosa. If it proves to be malignant, it will soon penetrate in all directions. Acid and pepsin are ulcerating the tumor.

substance such as magnesium hydroxide that, when ingested, neutralizes gastric acid. H_2 *antagonists* and *proton pump inhibitors* are drugs that inhibit gastric secretion.

Nonsteroidal Anti-Inflammatory Drugs (NSAIDs)

NSAIDs are drugs such as aspirin or ibuprofen that have anti-inflammatory properties. They are useful in arthritis. NSAIDs suppress gastric mucosal protective substances called *prostaglandins* and thereby expose the stomach and duodenum to the risk of erosions or ulceration.

Helicobacter pylori

H. pylori is an organism resident in the stomachs of many people, especially those in the Third World and the elderly in Western countries. It is responsible for a chronic inflammation of the stomach called *gastritis*. In some cases this infection and its consequent gastritis permit the development of a gastric or duodenal ulcer. It is the most common cause of peptic ulcer, but most people who harbor the organism never develop an ulcer.

GASTROESOPHAGEAL REFLUX DISEASE (GERD)

The LES functions as a valve that prevents reflux of acid-containing gastric juice into the unprotected lower esophagus. When not acting properly, *gastroesophageal reflux (GER)* occurs. The principal symptom is *heartburn*: a burning retrosternal pain or discomfort aggravated by lying down, bending, straining, or strong emotion. Antacids usually improve heartburn.

If severe, GER may cause inflammation in the lower esophagus, called *esophagitis*. Erosions or ulcers occur in more severe cases. In time, esophagitis may cause bleeding, or a *stricture* (narrowing), so that the patient has difficulty swallowing *(dysphagia)*. *Globus*, the sense of a lump in the throat, is sometimes confused with dysphagia. *Odynophagia* is a pain in the chest as food or drink passes through the esophagus. Chronic exposure to gastric contents is probably responsible for *Barrett's esophagus*. In this condition, the normally squamus esophageal epithelium becomes columnar and resembles that of the stomach or intestines. This process is called *metaplasia*. Barrett's esophagus predisposes the esophagus to cancer. An early warning sign is a further change in the cells called *dysplasia*.

INVESTIGATIONS

An *endoscope* is an instrument through which an examiner may view the interior of an organ, in this case the gut. Modern endoscopes employ fiberoptics or microchips and therefore are flexible. A gastroscope permits one to examine the interiors of the esophagus, stomach, and duodenum (through *gastroesophagoduodenoscopy [EGD]*) (see Figure 31-1). With this instrument, physicians may discover ulcers, erosions, esophagitis or tumors.

X rays turn photographic film black. Passing through the human body, they cause bones and other tissues to project shades of gray onto the film. *Barium* is a radiopaque material that can be swallowed in liquid form to fill the upper gut. Barium blocks X rays, and the barium-filled gut appears white on the film. A *barium swallow* is a test where several X-ray films are taken of the esophagus after barium ingestion. A *barium meal* or *upper GI series* is a similar X-ray film sequence that includes the stomach and duodenum. Ulcers appear on the film as collections or as punched out projections of barium in the stomach or duodenum (see Figure 11-3). Tumors encroach upon the lumen, taking up space.

SUMMARY

This short chapter reviews the terms commonly used when discussing diseases of the upper gastrointestinal tract. Dyspepsia, erosions, ulcers, gastroesophageal reflux, and heartburn are defined. Endoscopy and barium contrast X rays are briefly discussed.

CHAPTER FOUR

The Peptic Ulcer Story

A Brief History

In the continual remembrance of a glorious past individuals and
nations find their noblest inspiration.
Sir William Osler, 1849–1919

The rise and decline of ulcer disease as a major health problem
is fascinating medical history. Gastric ulcer has been known since
antiquity, but its importance was unappreciated until the late 19th
century. Duodenal ulcer seems to be a 20th century disease. It was
an important cause of discomfort, disability, and even death in the
years around World War II, but appears to be declining in Western
countries just as a cure is at hand. Some diseases, like fashions,
emerge and decline by whim or heavenly design.

Just as prevalence of the disease may wax and wane, so too
may its treatments. Some make no sense at all or result from a
misinterpretation of the dim science of the time. Some, like the
bland diet, linger long after benefit is disproven. In the late 19th
century, surgeons first cured perforated ulcers in subjects hitherto
left to die with rest, opium, and no hope. In this century, surgeons
painstakingly devised highly skilled techniques to prevent their
recurrence, only to cast these techniques aside because of the
pharmacological triumphs of the 1980s. Now, even anti-ulcer drugs
that revolutionized the outlook of peptic ulcer patients seem over-

ulcer patients seem overshadowed by the notion that ulcers are, after all, an infection that is curable.

Will infectious peptic ulcer disappear and, like smallpox, become a historical disease, or will it, like tuberculosis, rear its ugly head when we become complacent, careless, and less vigilant? Even now, as the gastric infection causing peptic ulcer seems on the verge of solution, ulcerogenic non-steroidal antiinflammatory drugs (NSAIDs) are becoming the next challenge.

The ulcer story could consume a volume. Here we will briefly survey five periods: the dawn of awareness, 19th century observations, the rise of duodenal ulcer and the acid theorem, the age of surgery, and the movement from control to cure. Since heartburn is part of our story, we will explore its past as well.

THE DAWN OF AWARENESS

Ancient Ulcers

Little was written about peptic ulcers before the 19th century. The relationship of ulcers to dyspepsia is a recent discovery, and in early times ulcers only came to attention if they perforated or bled. About 2600 BC the Chinese described acupuncture sites for stomach bleeding. In 1500 BC, Egyptians recognized gastric hemorrhage from ulcer. Chinese archeologists exhumed the corpse of a man who died in 167 BC from a perforated gastric ulcer. The autopsy showed that death was due to acute, diffuse peritonitis and septic shock.

Since the ancient Greeks disapproved of autopsies, there was little progress in the classical period. Incredible as it may now seem, the Greeks advocated venesection (blood letting) for bleeding ulcers. They also coined the word "dyspepsia," the definition of which troubles us to this day. Pliny the Elder (who perished when Mount Vesuvius crushed Pompeii in 71 AD), discussed dyspepsia in his *Natural History*. He recommended treatment with ground coral, perhaps the first antacid. In the second century, the Roman physician Galen described the first subgrouping of dyspepsia. Dyspepsia meant disordered digestion. Apepsia was no digestion, and bradypepsia was slow digestion. Like the dyspepsia subdivisions proposed today, these had neither proven pathophysiological significance nor clinical usefulness. According to Baron, the Roman scientist Celcus recommended light and glutinous food " . . . if the stomach is infected by an ulcer" everything acrid or acid should be avoided. We know little of what Celsus meant by "ulcer," but his soothing remedies persisted through the middle ages. Galen also described the symptoms of peptic ulcer and noted that black stools meant intestinal bleeding.

Eighteenth Century

In medicine, as in many other disciplines, there was little progress in the Middle Ages. The teachings of Galen were frozen in time, and few dared to challenge even the most incorrect of his theories. Not until 1700, when Bauhin described a young man with melena who perished and whose autopsy showed a gastric ulcer, do we learn more. Four years later, Littre wrote of a man dying after a massive hemorrhage from an ulcer that contained several open vessels at its base. This observation was doubtless inspired by Harvey's description of the circulation of the blood the century before.

Perforation is another way that ulcers came into human consciousness. A surgeon gets credit for the first clinical case report of a perforated ulcer. In 1727, Christopher Rawlinson briefly reported to the Royal Society.

> James Skidmore had complained for Three or Four Years last past, of a violent Pain in his Stomach and Bowels, never being able to rest in his Bed at Night, 'till he had vomited up the greatest Part of what he had eat or drank the Day before. He would often compare his pain to some great Weight laying upon the Region of his Stomach, which he had in some Measure alleviated, by pressing hard with his Hand upon that Part. When he turned himself in bed from one side to the other, he told me, he could plainly perceive that some Fluid or other fell down with Noise to the depending Side; which Fluid he believed to be the occasion of all his misery (pp. 361–362).

The fluid moving about Mr. Skidmore's abdomen was probably a "succussion splash," a sign of excess gastric juice and obstruction of the stomach. The autopsy showed a perforated gastric ulcer with 4 quarts of fluid in the peritoneal space. Rawlinson remarks that it failed to "emit so noisome a smell" as might be expected, possibly because of the sterilizing effect of gastric acid. However, the autopsy also disclosed that the stomach was full of dense matter, even the stone of a prune, and that the pylorus was four times as thick as normal. Based on these findings and the patient's long history of vomiting to relieve symptoms and the succussion splash, there seems little doubt that pyloric stenosis obstructed the stomach many years before Mr. Skidmore's terminal perforation. This appears to be the first coherent peptic ulcer case history in English, and it concisely illustrates two of its complications.

In 1746, Hamberger described in Latin a perforation of what is probably the first recorded duodenal ulcer. Little more was learned about ulcers for nearly a century. There are many reasons for this. Autopsy was the only means of diagnosis, since abdominal surgery was primitive and dangerous and anesthesia nonexistent. More life-threatening illnesses doubtless overshadowed peptic ulcers. When fatal, an ulcer carried off its victim with complications such as infection, anemia, shock, or malnutrition that would direct attention away from peptic ulcers. Since gastric ulcer tends to occur in older people, and duodenal ulcer was rare, few lived long enough for their ulcers to mature.

Early Physiology

The beginnings of gastric physiology were modest. Paracelsus in the 15th century detected acid in animal stomachs, but assumed they had ingested it. An interesting character, Aureolus Theophrastus Bombastus von Hohenheim, was professor of medicine in Basal. He called himself Paracelsus presumably to indicate his equality with the great Roman scientist Celsus with whom he shared a first name. He apparently lived up to his name "Bombastus," as if his parents had predicted his personality. Later commentators suggested that gastric acid originated in the spleen. This probably alludes to the 17th century notion that the spleen was the seat of melancholy, hot temper, and passion.

In 1729 Spallanzani described the solvent action of the fluid secreted by the stomach, but failed to recognize its acid nature. Credit for that observation belongs to de Reaumur, who was assisted by his pet buzzard. Buzzards apparently eject indigestible material, so de Reaumur fed his buzzard sponges. The retrieved sponge was shown to be acidic and to digest meat. When the buzzard died, so apparently did de Reaumur's research.

Baron credits the Belgian Jean Baptiste van Helmont (1577–1644) with the discovery of pepsin. He noticed that, unlike gastric juice, acid alone could not digest food. He reasoned that another factor was necessary. Despite the observations of Reaumur and Van Helmont, few were convinced the stomach produced acid. John Hunter believed it in 1772, but later changed his mind. Others thought gastric juice was lactic, acetic, or phosphoric acid. Studies of gastric fistulas by physiologists in Vienna and Paris about the year 1800 failed to confirm the acid nature of gastric contents. Indeed, the notion that gastric juice was merely saliva persisted well into the next century.

THE NINETEENTH CENTURY

Important developments in gastric physiology and reliable clinical descriptions of ulcers began to appear in 19th century medical literature. With the introductions of anesthesia and antiseptic surgery, ulcer operations became possible by the late 1800s.

Clinical Observations

At the beginning of the century, ulcers were not a hot topic. In 1817, Travers described the first English case of duodenal ulcer. Abercrombie, in an 1830 monograph, described the abdominal pain after eating that clinicians for 150 years (often erroneously) recognized as peptic ulcers as follows:

> the leading peculiarity of the disease of the duodenum, so far as we are acquainted with it seems to be that food is taken with relish, and the first stage of digestion is not impeded before pain begins about the time when the fluid is leaving the stomach, or two to 4 hours after meals (p. 103)

In France, Cruveillier described gastric ulcer in a textbook, and, until 1900, it was sometimes known as Cruveillier's ulcer, despite many prior claims. This was not the first nor the last time that medical immortality was misappropriated. In 1840, James Long, Esq., of Liverpool described 27 patients with severe burns. During postmortem examination, he noted that 19 of them had congestion of the peritoneum, which in modern terms means "peritonitis," or infection in the peritoneum resulting from a perforated bowel. In three of these cases a perforated duodenal ulcer was discovered. Later, this phenomenon became known as *Curling's ulcer*. Curling acknowledged the prior description, but, had Long included ulcer in the title of his own detailed report, he would likely be remembered by *Long's ulcer*.

In 1857, a large autopsy study led to the assumption that about 5% of people suffered a gastric ulcer at some time in their lives. Duodenal ulcer continued to be the subject only of isolated case reports. It was considered very rare by European writers until MacKenzie determined in a 1888 Cambridge MD thesis that it was not so rare after all. It was usually recognized through fatal perforation, and some, but *not all*, had previous dyspepsia. Thus, after the classic descriptions of dyspepsia by Rawlinson and Abercrombie came the realization that an ulcer could be symptomless.

As the century wore on, clinical observations became more astute, permitting premortem diagnosis, logical treatment, and even the hope of cure. In 1867, before Germany and Italy became unified states, a London surgeon accurately described the clinical signs and symptoms in five cases of autopsy-confirmed perforated duodenum. Based on this experience, the surgeon Andrew Clark (671–684) devised a treatment program of rest and abstinence of food and drink "to keep the parts quiet, a pebble in the mouth to allay thirst, and opium." Using these principles and early clinical diagnosis, two of his later cases survived. Here is a fine lesson for modern clinicians that medical advance is not made exclusively in the laboratory.

Early Gastric Surgery

The development of shrewd clinical skill permitted von Rydiger in 1881 to diagnose and successfully operate on a case of perforated duodenal ulcer. In 1894, Morse claimed the first successful closure of a perforated gastric ulcer and emphasized the use of hot water to wash the gastric contents out of the abdominal cavity. As the century closed, several cases of perforated duodenal ulcer were treated with excision, bypass, and eventually closure.

Led by Billroth, great developments in gastric surgery occurred in Germany. They were possible because of the introductions of ether anesthesia in 1840 and aseptic surgery by Lister in 1884. Wolfler successfully treated an unresectable gastric cancer obstructing the pylorus in 1881 by gastroenterostomy. Soon after that, Billroth performed the first partial gastrectomy. In the Billroth I operation, the gastric remnant was joined to the duodenum, maintaining gut continuity (see Figure 29-2). Both operations became popular treatments for peptic ulcer, but ulcer recurrences at the resection margin provoked removal of more stomach. This became possible in 1885 with the Billroth II gastrectomy, where the remaining stomach was joined to the duodenum or jejunum (see Figure 29-1). It was quickly recognized that the greater the resection, the greater the complications. Pyloroplasty was also described by German surgeons in the 1880s, but its purpose then was to widen a pylorus that had become narrowed and scarred by a duodenal ulcer.

It is curious that the early 20th century surgeons Mayo and Moynihan seemed to ignore these great surgical advances. The rational use of vagotomy and gastric resection in peptic ulcer disease had to await the physiological observations of Schwarz, Pavlov, and Dragstedt in this century.

Gastric Physiology

Meanwhile, and in seeming isolation from clinical developments, great discoveries occurred in stomach physiology. In 1823, Prout published "On the nature of the acid and saline matters usually existing in the stomachs of animals" in the *Transactions of the Royal Society*. Applying chemical techniques to animal gastric contents retrieved immediately after death, he proved the acid to be muriatic acid. We know this as the very powerful hydrochloric acid (HCl), which is capable of removing mortar from freshly laid bricks. He also found HCl in "great abundance in the acid fluid ejected from the human stomach in severe cases of dyspepsia." Thus the misleading association of dyspepsia with hyperacidity received the approbation of science.

The story of William Beaumont illustrates the importance of serendipity to medical progress: how, even in the most improbable circumstances, a prepared and alert mind can make an important scientific contribution. Beaumont was a medical officer in the

United States Army. His subject was Alexis St. Martin, a French-Ca-
nadian voyageur. In 1822, St. Martin came into Beaumont's care at
the frontier outpost of Michelemackinac with an accidental gun-
shot wound to the abdomen. No ordinary wound, St. Martin's
became a gastric fistula, that is, an opening of the stomach through
the abdominal wall. This permitted Beaumont to observe gastric
behavior through the fistula. He placed food into the stomach and
retrieved it for examination with a string. Remarkably, the stomach
seemed to function normally. Even more remarkably, St. Martin put
up with Beaumont's experiments over many years. In later years,
he was paid. Oblivious to frontier conditions, Beaumont made
discoveries that are still valid today. He faithfully recorded stomach
movements and secretion in response to meals and emotion.

In 1852, Gunzberg in Germany described secretion of acid
under the influence of the vagus and stated that it was a prereq-
uisite for gastric mucosal destruction. Thus began the debate that
lasted more than a century concerning the role of gastric acid in the
development of peptic ulcer. The notion that gastric secretion was
controlled solely by the vagus persisted through the next 50 or 60
years and was known as *nervism.*

Meanwhile, light microscopy permitted Purkinge to identify
parietal cells in the gastric glands in 1837. In the 1890s, Golgi
confirmed the parietal cell as the source of hydrochloric acid. He
also reported changes in the appearance of these cells when they
were stimulated. Little further progress in gastric physiology was
possible until the development methods to collect stomach contents.

The Gastric Tube

We take the gastric tube for granted, yet it has been clinically
employed for little more than a century. Before 1800, there is little
mention of such a tube. Dutch physicians apparently used flexible
leather catheters soaked in resin, but the how and why is unexplained. A coiled wire and leather catheter were used in the eigh-
teenth century to remove dangerously fermenting fluids and gases
from the ruminant stomachs of cattle. In 1790, John Hunter employed an eel skin supported by a whale bone to feed an incapaci-
tated patient. A bladder fixed to one end injected food and medicine
once the contraption was passed into the stomach.

French physicians dabbled with the idea of a gastric tube, and one even tried the stalk of a leek. One of Bonaparte's generals suffering from a neck injury was fed through a device apparently fitted into the esophagus. In 1800, a Philadelphia physician with the improbable name of Philip Syng Physick advocated the use of a tube and syringe to wash out the stomachs of victims who had swallowed poisoning. He published his first known success in the 1812 *Eclectic Reporting and Analytical Review*. It concerned 3-month-old twins who had accidentally ingested an overdose of the narcotic, laudanum. He apparently saved one by washing out their stomachs with a urethral catheter.

By 1823, various devices for cleansing poisoned stomachs were in use in Britain. We hear little more on the subject until Kussmaul's 1869 paper "Uber die Behandlung der magenweiterung durch eine neue Methode mittelst der Magenpump." This famous physician described the case of Marie Wiener and 12 others who suffered from pyloric obstruction due to peptic ulcer. Using a pump and tube he had acquired in America, he repeatedly emptied and lavaged his 25-year-old patient's stomach and secured her recovery. This technique had a great influence on the understanding and management of complicated peptic ulcer. The early tubes were stiff enough to be forced through the esophagus. Softer, narrower, and more pliable tubes became possible with improved manufacturing, and doctors learned to insert them with relative comfort. Kussmaul is also credited with the first successful gastroscopy, carried out on a sword swallower. Half a century passed before this became a practical procedure in those without special swallowing skills.

Ulcer Therapeutics

Osler's famous *Principles and Practice of Medicine* was published in 1892; nine editions appeared up to 1928. It is a fine text and is interesting and useful reading today. Some of his recommendations now seem illogical and unsubstantiated, yet they were followed for half a century. Osler knew that ulcers often occurred with "hyperacidity." Pathology showed that bleeding blood vessels in the base of an ulcer were aneurysms. However, ulcers were blamed on chlorosis (anemia in young women), rather than the other way around.

Like observers before and since, Osler had great difficulty with the word *dyspepsia*. Under the rubric *neurosis of the stomach*, he places *gastralgia* (or *gastrodynia*) and *nervous dyspepsia*. His notion that these complaints are due to hyperacidity, hypoacidity, anacidity, or gastritis remains unproven. In 1884, Allbutt described dyspepsia as a symptom; a neurosis of the viscera. At that early date he was able to declare, " . . . the diagnosis between ulcer and pure gastralgia is . . . impossible."

Osler recommended many treatments, a good indication that nothing worked well. He admitted that medical measures were of little value in peptic ulcer. Rest and rectal feedings were supplanted by milk and gruel. Gastric lavage was recommended in severe cases. Ironically, bismuth was used, but the rationale was unstated. There was no hint that it might suppress an infection. The desperation of patients in the 1890s is apparent in Osler's use of opium for ulcer pain and the frustration of doctors in his prescription of a *"prolonged sea voyage."*

The Turn of the Century

The century ended with a review of stomach disease by Mayo Robson, a surgeon from Leeds, a small English city that was home to so many famous gastric surgeons. His dissertation to the Royal College of Surgeons and its publication in the *Lancet* in 1900 serves as a contemporary summary of peptic ulcer. Several impressions are outstanding. Mayo Robson's meticulous description of the physical findings in patients with stomach disease represents the highest proficiency attained in that art. There are several reasons for this. Radiology had not yet become practical, and useful endoscopy was not even a gleam in a gastroenterologist's eye. Surgeons, often faced with a life-and-death decision to operate, had to rely on their senses. Almost all the phenomena that a physician or surgeon could expect in an ulcer or cancer patient are described in Robson's lectures. Later physicians, made lazy by technology, could diagnose and take action on gastric disease before such phenomena developed. Furthermore, modern doctors, consulted by so many dyspeptic patients with neither structural disease nor physical findings, have little opportunity to make such observations.

Another feature of Mayo Robson's work is its lack of mention of duodenal ulcer; yet within the next decade, the apparent increase in that disease would be remarkable. Its prevalence would soon outstrip that of gastric ulcer. Another omission was the nonsurgical treatment of gastric ulcer, perhaps because there was none. The principal elements of gastric surgery, save vagotomy, were in place by 1900. What were missing were precise indications for the various operations, a true rationale for their use, and outcome analysis beyond anecdote. These began to fall into place with the great advances in gastric physiology that were about to occur.

THE RISE OF DUODENAL ULCER AND THE
ACID THEOREM (1900-1939)

Gastric Physiology Comes of Age

One such advance was the 1902 discovery of the first hormone, secretin by Bayless and Starling. This gut hormone's principal importance is the stimulation of pancreatic enzyme secretion. Shortly after this, Edkins of St. Bartholomew's Hospital in London demonstrated that an extract of pyloric mucus membrane injected into an animal caused the secretion of gastric juice. He called the active principle gastrin. Secretin and several other gut hormones oppose the actions of gastrin. The work of Bayless and Starling and Edkins challenged the 19th century notion of nervism still held by Pavlov and many others. Some claimed that gastrin was really histamine in the gastric antrum and was not a hormone at all. The controversy was not resolved until Gregory and Tracy finally isolated gastrin 60 years later.

In 1910, Pavlov published his famous work illustrating the role of the vagus nerves in transmitting "psychic" influences to gastric secretion. That year witnessed two paradoxical observations. Hertz (later Hurst, in accord with the anti-German sentiment of wartime Britain) noted that both normal and ulcerated stomachs were insensitive to hydrochloric acid. Meanwhile, in Germany, Schwarz reaffirmed Gunzberg's belief in the dependence of peptic ulcer on the presence of gastric acid. His aphorism "no acid, no ulcer" became the rallying cry of peptic ulcer researchers for most of the century. In 1928, German researchers found that duodenal ulcer patients, but not controls, continue to secrete acid through the night. A decade later, McGill University investigators found histamine to be a powerful stimulant of gastric acid secretion.

Evolution of Gastric Surgery

Surgeons, taking little notice of the great physiological developments around them, entered the century with a great enthusiasm for stomach operations. Bold advocates that they were, some seemed overconfident and rather uncritical of their results. Two figures stand out in the first quarter of the century: Charles Mayo of Rochester, Minnesota, and Sir Berkeley Moynihan of Leeds, England. Their reviews provide a unique insight into the attitudes and practices of the time. Despite the technical advances in Germany three decades earlier, neither of these authors mention Billroth and his colleagues. Could the fear of rising German power have extended to medicine?

There seemed little interest in a rationale for ulcer operations. The early success of gastroenterostomy in the treatment of pyloric obstruction led to its uncritical use for nonobstructing ulcers. Not until the 1930s was this operation abandoned as a treatment for duodenal ulcer. Moynihan seems to have embraced the notion of Arbuthnot Lane that *intestinal stasis* or *chronic appendicitis* might cause ulcers. He recommended that, along with gastric surgery, the appendix be removed and a search be conducted for causative lesions elsewhere in the abdomen.

There is no doubt that peptic ulcer had become a very serious disease. Moynihan speaks of "the great peril to . . . life which the disease undoubtedly threatens." He is contemptuous of medical therapy, which to be truthful, usually amounted to a placebo at best. "The dangers of medical therapy are formidable," thundered Moynihan, and he derided advocates of "triple carbonates." Both authors advocated gastroenterostomy with excision or cautery of the original lesion. By 1923 Moynihan employed gastrectomy for gastric ulcer, but he clung to gastroenterostomy after physiological advances and patient follow-up might have dissuaded him. A late convert to the importance of acid, he did try attaching the stomach to the alkali-containing gallbladder. No ethics committees inhibited surgical experimentation in those days!

Both Mayo and Moynihan emphasized the need for a precise diagnosis and attributed the reported failures of surgery to surgeons who inadvertently operated on normal stomachs. Even then, dyspepsia was the great confounder of ulcer therapy. Mayo noted that "failure to eliminate the neurotic group leads to harmful and unnecessary operation." "By drugs and diet no harm is done to an ulcer which exists only in the mind of the healer," echoed Moynihan (1923); faint praise indeed for medical therapy.

The Rise of Duodenal Ulcer

Mayo seems to be the first to have recognized the increased incidence of duodenal ulcer. In 1906, he reported that 40% of his ulcer cases was duodenal. Two years later, three-fifths of his ulcer collection was in the duodenum. Mayo wondered if imprecise pathologists had previously confused duodenal ulcer with gastric and drew attention to the pyloric vein as a dividing point between the two. It seems likely, however, that the increase in duodenal ulcer prevalence was real.

Surgeons seemed confident of the diagnosis of duodenal ulcer, but according to Moynihan (1923), "No clinical diagnosis is so apt to be fallacious than that of gastric ulcer." Most physicians today would admit they cannot distinguish a gastric from a duodenal ulcer by history, nor indeed can they tell which of their dyspeptic patients have ulcers. How important X rays were soon to become in the management of dyspepsia!

Medical Management

Advances in the nonsurgical treatment of peptic ulcers were also slow in coming. Alkalis in the form of chalk, lime, and soda have been used for centuries. Despite the common experience that they relieved heartburn and ulcer pains, they were not scientifically studied, and their healing powers were merely assumed. Pepsin is inactive unless it is in an acid medium. Sippy reasoned in 1915 that the aim of treatment should be the protection of the ulcer bed from the effects of acid and activated pepsin for as much of the time as possible. He proposed the hourly institution of a milk and cream mixture and the later introduction of eggs and soft foods. Alkalis (later called *antacids*) were employed as well. These were powders of magnesia and carbonate. Bismuth subsalicylate was also used, 80 years before it was known to be active against *Helicobacter pylori*. Despite Moynihan's disdain, the Sippy diet or some variation of it was the mainstay of ulcer treatment until the 1960s and beyond. Even today some cling to the notion that a bland diet is necessary.

Psychophysiology

The failure of medicine created a vacuum exploited by those interested in gastric psychophysiology. Emotion was popularly associated with dyspepsia, and Beaumont noted changes in gastric secretion in response to fear, anger, or impatience. Dr. Hoetzel, a 1920s Chicago physiologist, collected fasting gastric juice by intubating himself each morning. He recorded an increase in gastric acid secretion when his landlady was shot in a robbery. One needed tough viscera to survive in Al Capone's Chicago! New York physiologists Wolf and Wolff, like Beaumont, studied a man with a gastric fistula. In 1942 they described the effects of emotion on his stomach. In 1932, Harvey Cushing described the relationship between some gastric ulcers and brain injury, reinforcing the notion that the brain might be important in ulcer genesis. Cushing's ulcer ought not to be confused with that associated with burns and described by Curling a century before.

These observations and the writings of Alvarez, Palmer, and Alexander led to interest in psychic causes of peptic ulcer. Engel and others developed theories of psychosomatic disease, which received much attention in the period before effective medical therapy. The popular view that peptic ulcers occur in stressed executives is largely due to this interest.

The notion that diseases had finite bodily causes owes much to the 17th century writings of René Descartes. Engel revived the Greek view of the inseparability of mind and body. He eloquently described how mind and body contrive to produce manifestations of disease and how neglect of one or other resulted in incomplete understanding and treatment. Nowhere has this holistic view been more paramount than in gastrointestinal illness. The discovery of *H. pylori* has temporarily eclipsed this view of ulcer disease. Nevertheless, it is not difficult to see how psychosocial factors might alter susceptibility to the disease or influence its manifestations. Holism has a more promising future in functional dyspepsia.

Gastroscopy

An exciting advance during this period was the 1932 development of a usable gastroscope by Schindler. Although German scientists, beginning with Kussmaul 64 years before, had experimented with primitive instruments, they were too dangerous. An earlier model used a platinum flame at the tip of the instrument for light. Contemporary instruments were rigid, very dangerous to use, and revealed little beyond the esophagus. Schindler introduced a series of light-bending prisms along the stomach end of the tube to allow it to bend. This permitted a view of the antrum and lesser curve where most gastric ulcers are visible. Shindler's instrument, and a gastrocamera introduced three years previously, gave new insights into gastric disease and foretold the development of practical endoscopy nearly 30 years later.

Dyspepsia

People scoff at terminology, but fuzzy terminology reflects fuzzy understanding. In no case is this more true than with *dyspepsia*. It has meant many things to many different people and still does. Vaguely related to *indigestion*, it has been attributed to many conditions without foundation. Dyspepsia is one presentation of peptic ulcer. There may be several dyspepsias, but that of peptic ulcer cannot be recognized without a gastroscopy. In 1924, a Harley street physician (Fenwick) wrote a 500-page book entitled *Dyspepsia: Its Varieties and Treatment*. He describes dyspepsias due to hyperacidity, a weak stomach, nervous distress, foreign bodies, and even living creatures in the stomach (*H. pylori* are not mentioned).*

---

*Unnoticed, Deonges in 1939 described the presence of "spirochetes" in the gastric glands of 43% of 242 stomachs examined at autopsy. In 1954, gastrectomy specimens confirmed the finding. Attempts to establish a causal relationship between these spirochetes and non-neoplastic ulcers were unsuccessful. Deonges also noted that in 1896 a German physician had seen these organisms in the stomachs of patients with gastric cancer. How different would have been the ulcer story had the significance of these findings been realized 50, or even 100, years ago!

THE AGE OF ULCER SURGERY (WORLD WAR II TO 1972)

Rational Surgery

The truly rational management of peptic ulcer began with the work of Dragstedt in Chicago. In the 1930s duodenal ulcer patients were found to secrete acid through the night. Remember too that Pavlov had demonstrated vagal transmission of the psychic impulses that stimulate gastric secretion. Dragstedt reasoned that night secretion could be vagally mediated, and he treated two patients with chronic and complicated duodenal ulcers by severing their vagus nerves through a chest incision. Both noted relief of symptoms and had reduced nocturnal acid secretion. This was not the first vagotomy. Laterjet did the operation in the 1920s, but he failed to develop a following.

Vagotomy has since undergone many metamorphoses. Postvagotomy, the stomach often would not empty, so some sort of "drainage" procedure became necessary. The procedure came to be done though an abdominal incision and was combined with a pyloroplasty, gastroenterostomy, or antrectomy to facilitate gastric emptying (see Figures 29-4, and 29-5). Since some vagus nerve fibers supplied only the acid-secreting areas of the stomach, surgeons designed selective and highly selective vagotomies that spared the nerve fibers supplying the pylorus. Highly selective vagotomy seemed to obviate the need for a drainage procedure (see Figure 29-6). Ironically, just as surgeons became skilled at performing these precise operations, the age of ulcer surgery ended.

Acid Secretion

Physiological experiments just before and after World War II taught us many new things about acid and its relation to peptic ulcer. Collection of gastric juice through nasogastric tubes had become so easy that it seemed as if every academic surgeon and gastroenterologist was doing it (or at least having a research fellow do it). We learned that acid damages mucosa, but moreso in company with pepsin. Rapid stomach emptying prevents hourly feeding of milk from adequately neutralizing the stomach, thus undermining the unpopular Sippy diet. Atropine should mimic vagotomy and interrupt psychic stimuli to secretion. However, the drug was ineffective because the effect was uneven and required doses that produced unpleasant side effects.

In general, people with a duodenal ulcer secrete more acid than those without ulcer, and those with gastric ulcer produce less. Meticulous studies showed that this was true for basal (fasting) acid secretion and secretion after stimulation by histamine. To prevent histamine effects beyond the stomach, physicians learned to give the drug in combination with an antihistamine. This experience was important to the development of the histamine H_2-receptor antagonists in the 1970s. Next, Cox demonstrated that patients with duodenal ulcers have larger than normal stomachs mainly because of increased acid-secreting tissue (parietal cell mass).

Armed with this new information, surgeons strove to design better operations. Larger gastrectomies removed more parietal cells. Although such aggressive surgery prevented recurrences, it exacted a heavy price. Crippling postgastrectomy symptoms and malnutrition were too common. Antrectomy removed only gastrin-producing tissue and resulted in parietal cell atrophy. Antrectomy combined with vagotomy greatly amplified the effect.

In the 1960s and 70s physiologists developed the concept of the *gastric mucosal barrier* by which the stomach defended itself from autodigestion. Davenport, in 1964 and later, demonstrated that the barrier could be broken by detergents, bile, and aspirin. This permits hydrogen ions to back-diffuse into the gastric mucosal cells and damage them. He suggested that this hydrogen ion loss explains the lower gastric acid levels in patients with gastric ulcer.

Fiberoptic Endoscopy

A very significant development during this period was the introduction of fiberoptic endoscopy. Like so much contemporary technological progress, fiberoptics were invented by the British, developed for practical use by the Americans, and successfully marketed by the Japanese. In 1927 J. L. Blair registered with the British Patent Office the idea that an image might be transmitted along a flexible axis through an aligned bundle of glass fibers. Twenty-seven years later, Hopkins and Kapany of the Department of Physics at the Imperial College of Science and Technology constructed such a bundle. In *Nature* (1954) they described the 4-inch-long bundle that, when " . . . curved into a quadrantal arc of a circle visually the image appeared to be of good contrast and well defined." Having made such a momentous discovery, the authors presumably went on to other things.

Basil Hirschowitz, a young South African gastroenterologist training in London, took the idea to a new posting in Ann Arbor, Michigan, where, with the help of physicists, he developed a prototype of the fiberoptic gastroscope. At the 1957 meeting of The American Gastroscopy Society he described how he was able to visualize the esophagus, stomach, and duodenum. I wonder if those attending that presentation had any idea of the impact that this discovery was to have on the practice of medicine? Japanese-manufactured fiberoptic instruments were soon available worldwide. They permitted physicians to view the once-forbidden interiors of the gut, the bladder, the peritoneum, and even the knee joint.

Medical Management

Meanwhile, medical treatment of peptic ulcers continued to flounder. New anticholinergic drugs mimicked atropine, but, like the original, they caused unpleasant effects and failed to improve healing. Antacids remained helpful in relieving symptoms. The bland diet replaced the Sippy, but long-overdue trials by Doll and Lennard-Jones in 1956 and 1965 found both ineffective.

Such was the desperation for ulcer relief that the first drug of proven benefit was stilboestrol, a synthetic estrogen. Doubtless inspired by the relative rarity of duodenal ulcer among women, this feminizing drug had an unlikely future in ulcer therapy. Few men were prepared to exchange their gender for ulcer relief. Liquorice extract was a folk medicine for ulcers. In 1962 Doll showed that it healed gastric, but not duodenal, ulcers. Side effects limited its use and the commercial preparation, carbenoxalone, disappeared with the arrival of cimetidine.

Having begun my career during this period, I now look back in amazement. Peptic ulcer was one of the most common and feared diseases faced by gastroenterologists. Endoscopy was primitive at first, so clinical diagnosis was still paramount. There certainly was no thought of doing anything with an ulcer when we saw it through the instrument. We used the discredited bland diet and antacids.

When things got bad, we admitted the patient, sedated him, and fed him milk and antacid through a nasogastric tube. This clumsy milk-alkali drip was used into the 1970s, when cimetidine made it obsolete (see Figure 4-1). The only recourse was to call a surgeon and then contend with the frequent complications of surgery. No wonder physicians tried drugs such as estrogen and licorice. That this scourge should be first controlled, then cured, in one career span is incredible.

Miscellany

In 1955, Zollinger and Ellison described a syndrome that consists of a pancreatic adenoma, gastric acid hypersecretion, and severe peptic ulcer disease. They hypothesized that the adenoma produced a hormone that stimulates gastric secretion. A rare disease, the ZE syndrome has taught us much about gastric physiology. Five years later, Gregory and Tracy identified the hormone as gastrin and in 1964 worked out the chemical structures of two gastrin molecules.

Also in 1964, John Fry, an exceptional observer, described the natural history of peptic ulcer among patients in his British general practice. Coming as it did on the eve of ulcer control, it has served as a model of untreated disease.

FROM CONTROL TO CURE (1972 TO PRESENT)

The last 24 years have witnessed the most remarkable advances. The concept of peptic ulcer etiology has been radically altered. We can now cure the disease and are on the way to preventing it. Only a brief outline of these developments will be presented here, since the details are discussed later in this book.

Gastric Antihistamines

Earlier, we learned that histamine stimulated the production of gastric acid and that the standard antihistamines failed to block this effect. James Black of the University of Liverpool and others reasoned that there must be a second receptor (histamine 2 or H_2

receptor) and in 1964 began testing about 700 compounds with a chemical structure similar to histamine. Ten years later, Black and Bimblecombe published in *Nature* that a drug, *burimamide*, could specifically block the secretory effect of histamine on the gastric parietal cell, with insignificant effects elsewhere. Despite an alarm when another prototype called *metiamide* caused bone marrow damage in two patients, this discovery led to a great pharmaceutical success story.

Cimetidine came into clinical practice in the late 1970s, followed by several similar drugs. For the first time, physicians were able to dramatically help their ulcer patients. James Black was knighted and received the 1988 Nobel Prize for Medicine, largely for this work. Ironically, even as the H$_2$ antagonists became the largest-selling prescription drugs ever, they were doomed to eventual decline because of a rapid succession of new developments.

Blocking the Proton Pump

In 1973, Ganzer and Forte studied the acid-secreting cells of the lowly bullfrog and discovered the final pathway of acid secretion. These American investigators described the enzyme *hydrogen potassium adenosine triphosphatase* (H$^+$ K$^+$-ATPase), which we now know as the proton, or acid, pump. This is the enzyme blocked by the drug omeprazole and its successors. This proton pump inhibitor (PPI), if given in sufficient dose, can completely inhibit acid secretion and safely permit the healing of virtually any peptic ulcer or peptic esophagitis.

Ulcers an Infectious Disease? Never!

These momentous discoveries now seem dwarfed by the 1983 report by Warren in the *Lancet* on "Unidentified curved bacilli on gastric epithelium in active chronic gastritis." By 1984 he and Dr. Marshall, a gastroenterologist in training, had reported an association of this organism with peptic ulcer, heralding the most important discovery of *The Ulcer Story*. First called *Campylobacter pylori* by its Australian discoverers, it was later renamed *Helicobacter pylori*.

An example of a phenomenon awaiting the notice of a pre-pared mind, Warren's observations had been made as much as 100 years earlier by other pathologists. So indoctrinated were physi-cians of the inherent sterility of the acid stomach that they took no serious notice. Warren's enthusiasm and teamwork with Marshall, the clinician, led to the realization of its significance. And signifi-cant it is! Not only is it the underlying cause of most peptic ulcers that can now be cured by antibiotics, but it also appears to be a cause of gastric cancer. Early reports even suggest a rare form of gastric lymphoma can be cured by killing the organisms—the first cancer cure with antibiotics. As if this is not revolutionary enough, cardiologists, noting the association of ulcer to coronary artery disease, now wonder if the organism has a role in the etiology of that disease.

Many clinical scientists are impatient with the slow acceptance of this discovery by the medical community. Even today, some scientists express reasoned doubts. Frustrating as this may be, there are very good reasons for such conservatism. Too many unsubstan-tiated cures come and go for doctors to immediately alter their thinking and their practices. Nevertheless, this discovery was en-dorsed by a United States National Institutes of Health panel in 1994. The panel recommended that physicians heal the ulcer with antisecretory drugs and at the same time attempt to cure the disease by killing the organisms. The panel did not recommend therapy for those with functional dyspepsia or to prevent cancer. Such recom-mendations would require much more research.

Other Therapeutic Developments

During this era many other treatments were developed for peptic ulcer. Prostaglandins, sucralfate, muscarinic antagonists, intensive antacid therapy, and even highly selective vagotomy have all had their brief place in the sun. If they had been around a decade or two earlier, they would have been very important thera-pies rather than footnotes. Of these, only prostaglandins may have an enduring role—in the prophylaxis of NSAID-induced ulcers.

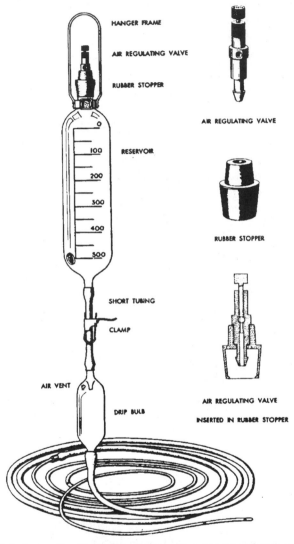

Figure 4-1. Apparatus for delivering a continuous drip of milk and antacid into the stomach of a person with peptic ulcer (circa 1940). This treatment was designed to neutralize all gastric acid, and was often the last resort before gastric surgery. The "milk drip" was a common feature of medical wards through the 1960s and right up to the introduction of cimetidine.

Invasive Endoscopy

While pharmacologists and pathologists made their discoveries, endoscopists gained confidence as well. In 1976, bleeding blood vessels in ulcers were coagulated by a laser beamed through a gastroscope. This technique proved to be unwieldy, expensive, and a little dangerous. Next, heater probes, electrocautery, and injection of the bleeding site appeared in rapid succession. Balloons could now be introduced to dilate a pyloric obstruction. These therapeutic techniques have led to greater nonsurgical control of ulcer complications, saving not only lives but also money. Fiberoptic technology is giving way to the microchip. The gut can be viewed on video, recorded, stored, or transmitted. Some surgical procedures are done through a *laproscope*. Even some cancers can be reduced in size through endoscopic treatment.

THE FUTURE

The Ulcer Story is far from finished. How should the bugs be killed? Who should be treated? Who should treat? Can we prevent stomach cancer?

The short term challenges are many. We need a cheap, safe, effective antibiotic to kill *H. pylori*. We also must have cheap, quick, reliable, and noninvasive means of detecting the organisms and of confirming their death. Before millions are unnecessarily subjected to antibiotics, the importance of this organism in functional dyspepsia must be clarified. With or without the organism, how can this enigmatic condition be managed?

In the long term, we need strategies to prevent children from acquiring the infection. These must take into account the large reservoir of infection in the Third World, and its possible role in cancer and coronary artery disease. It is doubtful that we can exterminate *H. pylori* by antibiotics alone. If a relationship of the bacteria with either or both of these terrible diseases can be verified, then a major public health program will be needed. Prevention might be achieved through public measures supplemented with a vaccine.

There remain ulcers apparently unassociated with the organism. As ulcers due to infection become manageable, those due to

NSAIDs are an increasing threat. There is an urgent need for an NSAID that is not ulcerogenic.

A BRIEF HISTORY OF HEARTBURN

Sense of burning or smarting heat usually denominated heartburn
Caleb Parry, 1815

Heartburn is part of our language. It appears in Shakespeare and in 200-year-old medical books. In literature this symptom implies emotion. In *Much Ado About Nothing*, Beatrice is so affronted by the unpleasant Don John that she is "heartburned" by him. It is also a contemporary expression of distress. In W. O. Mitchell's *Jake and the Kid*, an exasperating situation is "enough to give a gopher heartburn." Hollywood even produced a movie called *Heartburn*. The meaning and nature of heartburn are further discussed in Part 4, but here we chronicle developments in the thinking and management of heartburn and gastroesophageal reflux (GER).

Heartburn, Esophagitis, and Hiatus Hernia

Early reports of esophagitis are murky. In 1722, acute pain in the chest that even reached down into the abdomen was described. Others described the pain in themselves, but it was not until 1884 that the first pathological description of esophagitis that caused odynophagia and aphagia was written. His description bears little resemblance to the esophagitis so commonly seen now. Parry and Abercrombie briefly discuss heartburn in their early 19th century monographs.

In 1922, Chevelier Jackson first associated hiatus hernia with GER, a notion that refuses to go away. Endoscopists in 1929 recognized peptic ulcers in the esophagus, relating them to sour regurgitation, retrosternal pain, and heartburn. Six years later, Winkelstein described esophagitis. His eight cases all had a duodenal ulcer, and he noticed that the symptoms improved with ulcer therapy. In the 1920s this included olive oil, ulcer diet, alkali, milk drip, atropine, and, occasionally, gastrectomy.

In the 1940s, Allison connected esophagitis with the presence of a hiatus hernia, and a succession of hiatus hernia repair procedures followed. Allison also noted that severe esophagitis could cause a stricture. The relationships of hiatus hernia, esophagitis, and gastroesophageal reflux were further explored through the 1950s.

In 1906, a pathologist, Tileston, noted stomach-like epithelium surrounding esophageal ulcers. In 1950, Barrett reported the replacement of the normal squamus esophageal epithelium by columnar cells normally found lower in the gut. He erroneously attributed this phenomenon to a congenitally short esophagus. Subsequent observers recognized an association with hiatus hernia and reflux esophagitis. In the last 45 years it has slowly been appreciated that Barrett's esophagus could result from chronic GER and esophagitis and that the replacing epithelium could be of gastric, intestinal (specialized columnar cells, which include goblet cells), or even colonic type. In some, further changes in the specialized columnar cells, called *dysplasia*, were found to be pre-malignant.

By the 1970s, measurements of LES pressure and esophageal motility convinced many physiologists that the presence or absence of a hiatus hernia is irrelevant to GER. They knew that reflux could occur without a hernia. Nonetheless, surgical repairs of hernias were commonplace even after the introduction of effective antireflux therapy. Ironically, just as hiatus hernia repair became less commonly done, physiologists began to concede that, after all, a hernia could worsen GER.

Peptic Stricture

Bougies, long employed to dilate a narrowed esophagus, provide an interesting footnote to the heartburn story. The name bougie derives from Bougiyah, an Algerian city that was a medieval center for the wax candle trade. Fabricus ab Acquapendante (1537–1616) used a wax taper to dislodge a bolus of food impacted in the esophagus. Ambrose Pare (1510–1590) made leather tubes or wands covered with gut for the same purpose. He also used swan feather quills. Later, a lead instrument with an olive-shaped tip took advantage of gravity.

Willis (1621–1675) was a famous anatomist whose book was illustrated by Sir Christopher Wren. He used a whalebone tipped with a sponge to dilate an esophagus affected by achalasia, a disease in which the LES fails to relax. Whalebone, it seems, has the right combination of rigidity and flexibility for the manufacture of bougies as well as corsets.

X-ray demonstration of an esophageal foreign body occurred only 1 year after Roentgen's discovery in 1895. The first demonstration of a stricture was by bismuth X ray in 1907. In the 1920s and 1930s, Chevelier Jackson, a pioneer ear, nose, and throat surgeon, developed esophagoscopy and designed biopsy instruments. His bougies are prototypes for many of those used today. In 1915, Hurst, borrowing from the lead-weighted instruments, created round-tipped mercury-filled rubber bougies. Later, Maloney developed a tapered version. Both the Hurst and Maloney instruments are available in many sizes and still are used for minor strictures (see Figure 17-5). In 1903, thread was passed through a stricture as a guide. A dilating, stiff bougie could be threaded over this. The technique was the forerunner of guide wire dilatation with bougies or balloons that are now employed for tough or very narrow strictures.

CHAPTER FIVE

Epidemiology of Ulcers, Dyspepsia, and Heartburn

Readers might assume that it is a simple thing to determine how many people have peptic ulcers. Not so! The epidemiology is complex, and data collecting is hampered by incomplete recognition and reporting of the disease. Determining the prevalence of dyspepsia is handicapped by the lack of an agreed-upon definition. Heartburn is universally recognized, but the diagnosis of esophagitis requires an endoscopy. This chapter will define some epidemiological terms and outline the known epidemiology of acid-peptic disease.

DEFINITIONS

Epidemiology is, in part, the study of epidemics. Epidemiologists study the prevalence and incidence of diseases and their coincidence with other diseases. They are also interested in what environmental, genetic, or other factors might influence the existence and course of the disease. *Prevalence* is the proportion of a population with a given disease over a single moment, period, or lifetime. The *point prevalence* of peptic ulcer, that is, the existence of an ulcer crater at a given time, is very much less than the lifetime prevalence, because many people have inactive ulcers. *Incidence* is the occurrence of new cases per population over a period. It is often

59

reported as the number of cases per 100,000 per year. This figure should be less even than the point prevalence, since some people will have an active ulcer for many years. Rarely, incidence and prevalence are the same, such as in drowning or traffic fatalities. In the case of perforated peptic ulcer, the two are very close.

PEPTIC ULCER

Difficulties

Patients who suffer a perforated ulcer experience a singular attack of pain and shock. In most cases, life-saving surgery is prompt and the diagnosis is confirmed within hours of onset. A few perforated ulcers in those who are not diagnosed or too ill for surgery would be authenticated at autopsy. Thus for almost 150 years we can cite the incidence of perforated ulcers from hospital records (see Table 5-1). This is not the case with uncomplicated or bleeding ulcers. Many are simply not diagnosed. Some cause no symptoms at all, or what symptoms they do cause may be passed off as indigestion or something else. Equally important, some people may be said to have had an ulcer when actually they did not. Dyspepsia may incorrectly be assumed to be an ulcer, or a radiologist may overcall an X ray. Endoscopy of a random sample of the population might determine the point prevalence of peptic ulcer. However, determination of incidence would require leaving the instrument in place to watch for the appearance of ulcers. True lifetime prevalence might require lifetime observation.

Thus, most of our information about the epidemiology of peptic ulcer is indirectly derived. Hospital records may capture the patients with serious complications of ulcer, but most patients with uncomplicated ulcers are ambulatory. Records from insurance data or from health maintenance groups overrepresent healthy people. Death records or payment forms are not designed with the needs of the epidemiologist in mind and are unreliable indicators.

Confounding factors include the increase in the use of NSAIDs, longer life, the apparent changing epidemiology of *H. pylori*, and the impact of modern treatment. The distinction of gastric from duodenal ulcers, or peptic ulcer from gastritis, duodenitis, and erosions, causes confusion. Meanwhile, there are ongoing changes in the true incidence of ulcers. Thus, except for perforated ulcer, the data are estimates at best. Nonetheless, there is no doubt that over this century peptic ulcer has been a very common and costly disease.

Current Estimates

Prevalence

There have been several attempts to establish point prevalence (see Langman 1985). A Finnish endoscopy survey of 358 normal subjects found duodenal ulcers in 1.4%. Japanese doctors employed a gastrocamera to test 10,605 men over 40 and found an active duodenal ulcer in 2.5%. A United States national health interview survey found the 12-month prevalence of peptic ulcer to be 1.6%, but the investigators had no way of confirming the diagnosis or detecting "silent" ulcers. Several studies indicate a lifetime prevalence of peptic ulcers of about 10% in developed countries, and the point prevalence is about 1–2%. General autopsy series provide evidence of past or present ulcer in about 20% of men and 10% of women. In the 1970s, ulcers accounted for 1% of all deaths.

Incidence

The incidence of peptic ulcer seems to be about 0.1% per annum. Among the 500,000 residents of Copenhagen, Denmark, the yearly incidence of duodenal ulcer as discovered by X ray or operation was 0.15% in men and 0.03% in women. The incidence increased with age, becoming 0.3% by the eighth decade of life. In Yorkshire, the incidence was 0.21% in men and 0.06% in women. Studies of Massachusetts physicians, health maintenance subscribers, and Seventh Day Adventists found an incidence less than this, but the studies were likely biased by the lifestyle and youth of those studied.

Trends

Before barium contrast radiology became readily available in the 1930s, ulcer diagnosis was by autopsy or by surgery. Therefore, little data are available for uncomplicated, nonfatal ulcers. In 1857,

TABLE 5-1
Changes in the Relationships of Age and Sex to Gastric
Ulcer Deaths, 1867 to 1924[a]

	Perforated ulcer, 1867	Ulcer deaths, 1912	Ulcer deaths, 1918	Ulcer deaths, 1926
Age 34 and younger				
Men	18	182	167	151
Women	96	338	214	109
M:F ratio	0.2:1	0.5:1	0.8:1	1.4:1
Age 34 and older				
Men	42	691	900	1219
Women	43	635	713	620
M:F ratio	1.0:1	1.1:1	1.3:1	2.0:1

[a]After Langman, 1985.

after 7,000 autopsies, Brinton estimated the lifetime prevalence of gastric ulcers to be 5%. Langman (1985) has shown how gastric ulcers evolved over the next 70 years from an uncommon, fatal disease of young women to a common disease of older men and women (Table 5-1).

Duodenal ulcers were rare before 1900. As late as 1894, Collin of Paris was only able to collect 257 cases from the literature. Mayo pointed out that many reported gastric ulcers were actually in the duodenum (see Chapter 4). Over the next 15 years, he observed a rapid increase in the prevalence of duodenal ulcers at the Mayo Clinic. By World War II it was a very common cause of invalidism in the Army. Duodenal ulcer was much more common than gastric ulcer and was a disease of young men.

There is evidence that duodenal ulcer prevalence is declining. Since 1960, hospitalizations, operations, and deaths from duodenal ulcer have decreased. Gastric ulcer has also become less common. Ironically, the decline in ulcer incidence preceded the arrival of effective medication. Despite this, hospitalization rates for ulcer hemorrhage or perforation have remained steady.

Sex and Age

The increase in gastric ulcers in older women may be due to their greater life expectancy and increasing use of NSAIDS. The very high prevalence of duodenal ulcer in men has decreased, so that, like wages, its prevalence in men and women is approaching equality. In 1970 the male to female ratio for duodenal ulcer hospitalizations and mortality were 1.8:1 and 2.4:1, respectively. By 1983 both ratios had fallen to 1.3:1. Duodenal ulcers occur in older people as the population ages. This may parallel the increase in *H. pylori* prevalence with age. As sanitation and housing improve, the prevalence of *H. pylori* infection among children declines. As a result, younger generations are less likely to acquire ulcers. This phenomenon is also occuring in Japan. The epidemiology of *H. pylori* and its relationship with peptic ulcers are discussed in Chapter 8.

Other Countries, Other Races

Within Western countries, there are little data to support any suggestion of different racial susceptibilities. Ulcers are very prevalent in Japan, perhaps because of the very high prevalence of *H. pylori* in that country. Surveys of working people attending periodic health examinations found lifetime prevalences of peptic ulcers of 19% and 17% in men and women, respectively, in Japan and 5% and 0% in Holland.

In the Third World, despite a very high rate of *H. pylori* infection, the prevalence of peptic ulcer is variable. In India and Africa, ulcers are common in the south and rare in the north, yet the organism is common throughout. Australian aborigines have very low prevalences of both the organism and peptic ulcer.

Other Factors

One of the great 20th century myths has been the popular notion that peptic ulcer is a disease of busy executives. Actually, it is a disease of the poor, and it has an inverse relationship with income. This phenomenon may be directly related to the spread of *H. pylori* in conditions where there are overcrowding and poor hygiene. Smoking not only increases the likelihood of ulcer disease and ulcer death, but continued smoking also provokes recurrence of the disease, even when the patient is taking protective H_2 antagonists. Coffee and cola drinks may be blameworthy as well.

Experienced gastroenterologists in temperate climates note a tendency of peptic ulcers to manifest or develop complications in the spring and autumn. (Some would even attribute an effect to the full moon!) Scientific data on these subjects are absent or conflicting.

Ulcer disease is familial, and of great interest to geneticists. While genetic factors are important, it seems likely that the familial clustering is largely due to the acquisition of *H. pylori* in youth.

Clinical associations of ulcers with other diseases are a traditional exercise for medical students in hospitals. Ulcers are said to occur with greater frequency in people suffering from chronic lung disease, cirrhosis, polycythemia, and renal failure. However, there is a notorious confluence of diseases in hospitalized patients where poverty, debility, smoking, drug use, and poor hygiene also come together. True associations are difficult to prove. However, it does appear that ulcers *do not* occur in those diseases that include achlorhydria, such as pernicious anemia or Addison's disease (adrenal gland failure).

The New Confounders

The epidemiology of peptic ulcer requires a complete reassessment that considers important new developments. The most important of these is the discovery of *H. pylori*. The apparent decline in uncomplicated peptic ulcers may parallel the decline in youthful infection. The notion that peptic ulcer is usually an infectious disease is novel. We need to adjust to this radical departure from conventional wisdom, for the discovery undercuts much that we have been persuaded about stress, psychosomatics, genetics, and acid secretion. The susceptibility of the aging population to ulcer causing drugs shifts ulcer prevalence to elderly females.

Smoking and entry into the work force may account for the relative increase in duodenal ulcers among young women. Changes in the social and economic status of women may subject them to the environmental stresses long thought important in males with the disease. Whether this is true or not, the face of peptic ulcer disease will be very different in the 21st century.

Natural History of Peptic Ulcer

We have been so successful in controlling peptic ulcer disease that its natural history is now difficult to determine. The most quoted study is that of John Fry, a general practitioner who faithfully recorded the fate of his 265 ulcer patients (212 duodenal and 53 gastric) from 1948 to 1957. The annual incidence in the 6,385 people in his east London practice was 420 per 100,000 and the prevalence was 1,600 per 100,000. Of 198 patients followed 5 years, 98% continued to have symptoms. At 10 years, 40% of 166 patients had symptoms. He concluded that disease activity peaked at about 8 years and remained active over about 15 years. Sixteen percent required surgery.

A 1977 Danish study (Greibe *et al.*) found that, after 13 years, 63% of X ray-diagnosed duodenal ulcer patients were either symptomatic or had surgery. By 1986, Porro and Petrillo from Italy were able to report on how much H_2 antagonists had improved the ulcer patients' quality of life. However, since the ulcers usually recurred after treatment, the underlying natural history of the disease was little altered. As recently as 1994, Lindell *et al.* reported that, despite the availability of treatment, over half of a cohort of peptic ulcer patients remained symptomatic after 10 years. They estimated the annual risk of death from peptic ulcer to be 0.6%. The advent of anti-*H. pylori* therapy to cure peptic ulcers means that now we can significantly, and perhaps finally, alter the natural history of ulcer disease

DYSPEPSIA

It is difficult to determine the prevalence and incidence of peptic ulcer, even with its observable defect in the mucosa. Imagine how much more difficult it is to acquire accurate figures for functional dyspepsia, given its lack of any physical marker! This task is doubly handicapped by lack of agreement on a definition of dyspepsia. Dyspepsia, like other functional disorders, may be recognized only by its symptoms. A 1980 estimate by Thompson and Heaton that focused on epigastric pain or discomfort (that was not heartburn or IBS) found a prevalence of about 6%. The transient nature of dyspepsia adds further to the challenge. While the prevalence in a community is stable from year to year, in some the symptoms disappear while others become dyspeptic and take their place (see Talley 1994).

A large survey of British general practice lists found a prevalence of about 30%. However, this figure included those with heartburn, a common and totally different symptom from dyspepsia that poses different investigational and therapeutic challenges. In the Japan–Holland study of workers having regular health checks (Schlemper *et al.* 1993), the prevalence of dyspepsia was 13% in both countries. Using the restrictive Rome criteria, dyspepsia was found in only 2.7% of American householders (66% of these relatively affluent people responded to the questionnaire). Therefore, at least 6 million Americans have dyspepsia, and the true figure is likely higher. All of these population studies include patients with and without peptic ulcers. Among dyspeptic *patients* referred to specialist endoscopy clinics, roughly one-half have ulcers.

GASTROESOPHAGEAL REFLUX DISEASE

Determination of the prevalence and incidence of gastroesophageal reflux also presents problems. Heartburn is the most identifiable manifestation of gastroesophageal reflux disease (GERD), and therefore may give some idea of its occurrence. However, physiologists have demonstrated that most people reflux from time to time, usually with no complaint. On the other hand, esophagitis and its complications are relatively uncommon and may even occur without heartburn. Studies in Western countries indicate that one-third of adults have heartburn at least once a year. About 3% have daily heartburn. These figures hold for adults of both sexes and all ages (Table 5-2).

Population studies of esophagitis do not exist. The prevalences of esophagitis and its complications seen by doctors seem to increase with age. One complication, Barrett's esophagus, may be a precancerous condition, so determination of those at risk is an important subject for research.

SUMMARY

In the developed world, peptic ulcer, especially duodenal ulcer, seems to be a 20th century disease. This may parallel a rise and fall in the prevalence of *H. pylori*, which now seems to be the principal cause. NSAID has shifted the prevalence of ulcers toward older women made susceptible by longer life and coexisting

TABLE 5-2
Prevalence of Heartburn

Author and year	Participants	At least once per year	At least once per month	Daily
Nebel et al., 1976[a]	282		36%	7% (M = F)
Thompson and Heaton, 1982[b]	301	33.6%	21.3%	4% (all
		M = 33.6%		female)
		F = 33.5%		
Drossman et el., 1993[c]	5430	30.1%		
		M = 30.5%		
		F = 29.7%		

[a]Hospital staff.
[b]Unselected subjects with no hospital connection.
[c]66% of a random sample of U.S. householders.

chronic illnesses. Smoking and the increasing professional responsibilities of women may account for the decreasing dominance of males among duodenal ulcer patients. Certainly, the large reservoir of *H. pylori* infection in the Third World, its slow decline in our world, and the continued use of ulcerogenic drugs, tobacco, and less than optimal antibiotic treatments ensure that ulcers will continue to employ physicians for some time to come. Furthermore, there has been no parallel decline in the incidence of serious ulcer complications such as perforation and bleeding, suggesting that those who get ulcers now have more severe disease.

No data support a decline in functional dyspepsia, the prevalence of which does not parallel that of ulcers. While harboring none of the sinister overtones of an ulcer, nonulcer dyspepsia will continue to generate health costs until we find a cause and cure.

Gastroesophageal reflux is very common, but its principal manifestation, heartburn, occurs in only one-third of adults. Only about 3% suffer from it daily. The complications of GERD, such as esophagitis and Barrett's esophagus, are of unknown prevalence and are not necessarily accompanied by heartburn.

PART TWO
Causes of Ulcer Disease

CHAPTER SIX

Gastric Secretion

No acid, no ulcer
K. Schwarz, 1910

Gastric secretion has fascinated physiologists and clinicians since the spectacular observations of Beaumont over 150 years ago. According to Schwarz, acid secretion by the stomach was the reason ulcers existed. Schwarz was right, of course. Peptic ulcers do not occur in the achlorhydric gut, and for most of this century medical and surgical treatment endeavored to control gastric acid. However, acid by itself does not cause peptic ulcers. Despite daily acid exposure, most stomachs enjoy a lifetime without ulcers. Something must damage or alter the upper gut mucosa so that its digestive powers are turned against itself. The two most important candidates are NSAIDs and *H. pylori*. Nevertheless, an understanding of gastric secretion is important to the ulcer story. Whatever the mucosal damage, peptic ulcers do not occur without acid.

Gastric juice contains more than acid. The stomach's production of pepsin, mucus, bicarbonate, and intrinsic factor is also important.

ACID SECRETION

The first question to ask about gastric acid is, "Why is it there?" Nature goes to a great deal of trouble to produce and regulate acid

71

secretion, yet its role in digestion is marginal. It is necessary to make pepsinogen active, since it digests protein only at an acid pH. The stomach's acid interior kills most ingested organisms so they do not cause mischief lower down in the gut. Yet, most people rendered achlorhydric with a drug seem to have little difficulty with gut infections. Acid also assists the absorption of iron and probably calcium in the duodenum. However, in some respects, nature has failed to keep up with the times. Acid secretion, like the appendix, has become a vestigial curiosity more prone to mischief than human preservation.

Stimulation of Acid Secretion

Enterochromaffin-like (ECL) cells release histamine in the gastric gland epithelium. It diffuses to adjacent parietal cells and attaches to the H$_2$ receptors (Figure 6-1). The stimulated H$_2$ receptor makes the enzyme *adenyl cyclase* active to convert *adenosine triphosphate (ATP)* to *cyclic adenosine monophosphate (c-AMP)*. c-AMP starts the acid pump.

Vagus nerve impulses from central or local sources release *acetylcholine* from nerve endings (Figure 6-1). This neurotransmitter attaches to parietal cell *cholinergic* receptors of the *muscarinic* type. In this way the thought, smell, and taste of food can trigger acid secretion. Also, distension of the body of the stomach by food can provoke the parietal cell through local vagal reflexes.

G cells in the antral and duodenal mucosa release the hormone *gastrin* into the blood. Stimulants for gastrin release include ingested amino acids, distension of the stomach, and a rise in the pH of gastric contents over 2.5–3. Gastrin release is signaled by the vagus and transmitter substances that may be neurocrine (in nerves), paracrine (local), or endocrine (hormonal). Gastrin has a receptor on the parietal cell, but its release of histamine from the ECL cells may be its most important activity.

The Acid Pump

The complex interrelationships of these three parietal cell stimulants control the switching on of the acid pump. *H$^+$, K+-ATPase*

HISTAMINE

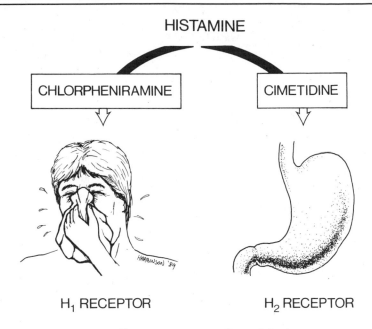

| CHLORPHENIRAMINE | CIMETIDINE |

H$_1$ RECEPTOR   H$_2$ RECEPTOR

Figure 6-1. Histamine affects many tissues through histamine receptors. Standard antihistamines such as chlorpheniramine (Chlor Tripolon™) or diphenhydramine (Benedryl™) compete with histamine for the H$_1$ receptors in the nose or skin, which contribute to allergic rhinitis (hay fever) or urticaria (hives). They have no effect on gastric acid secretion. The H$_2$ receptor antagonists, on the other hand, are specific for the H$_2$ receptors on the gastric parietal cell, and therefore competitively inhibit acid secretion.

mediates the secretion of hydrochloric acid (HCl) through the canalicula into the gastric glands (Figure 6-2). This enzyme is a long protein that straddles the canalicular membrane. Hydrogen (H$^+$) ions from water in the cell fluid exchange for potassium (K$^+$) ions in the glands against a transmembrane concentration gradient of 2,000,000:1. Meanwhile, hydroxyl (OH$^-$) ions also from cell water combine with carbon dioxide (CO$_2$) through the actions of another enzyme *carbonic anhydrase* to produce bicarbonate (HCO$_3^-$) ions. This alkaline product in the parietal cell exchanges for chloride (Cl$^-$) ions delivered to the cell by the blood. Combining with K$^+$ ions, the now intracellular Cl$^-$ transfers into the canalicula. There, through the acid pump, the K$^+$ moves back into the cell in exchange for H$^+$, and the remaining Cl$^-$ combines with the hydrogen as the

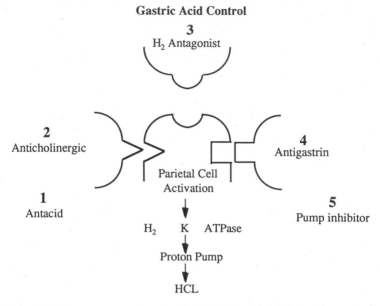

Figure 6-2. Some means of controlling gastric acid. (1) Antacids neutralize it in the lumen after it is produced by the parietal cells. (2) Acetylcholine, released from vagal nerve endings, stimulates the parietal cell through cholinergic receptors. (3) Histamine, released by nearby ECL cells, stimulates the histamine H_2 receptor on the parietal cell. (4) The circulating hormone gastrin acts on the gastrin receptor. These receptors may be blocked by anticholinergic drugs (atropine, propantheline), histamine H_2 antagonists (cimetidine, ranitidine), or antigastrin (commercially unavailable). (5) The proton pump in the parietal cell produces hydrogen ions. Proton pump inhibitors (omeprazole, lansoprazole) block this "final pathway" of acid production.

powerful acid, HCl. The secreted acid has a pH of as low as 1, compared to intracellular pH, which is 7.3.

Omeprazole and lansoprazol are pro-drugs and weak bases that concentrate in the acidic parietal cell, where they are converted to an active sulphenamide (see Chapter 24). This product combines with the H^+, K^+-ATPase and irreversibly inactivates it. Recovery of acid secretion after such proton pump inhibition awaits the generation of new parietal cells.

A stimulated parietal cell changes its appearance. The tiny tubulovesicles, plentiful in the resting state, merge with the secretory canalicula and bring the acid pumps to bear on the secreting membrane. Interestingly, omeprazole does not arrest this physical change, yet the less potent H_2 antagonists do prevent it.

Natural Inhibition of Gastric Acid Secretion

A meal or a psychic impulse stimulates gastrin release from the antrum, but, when the pH of gastric contents falls to 3 or less, gastrin switches off (negative feedback). The duodenum releases secretin, an inhibitor of acid secretion, in response to acid and some nutrients. Naturally occurring gastric prostaglandins, especially prostaglandin E_2 (PGE2), are more potent inhibitors of gastric acid secretion than the H_2 antagonists (see Chapter 23). The parietal cell appears to have a receptor for prostaglandins as well. Removal of a large segment of intestine increases gastric acid production. This is evidence that there is hormonal feedback control of acid secretion as the intestine digests the food presented to it by the stomach. The actual hormone is unknown. Many gut hormones such as secretin, glucagon, GIP, somatostatin, and others inhibit acid secretion when given intravenously, but it is uncertain if these are important in real life.

Measuring Gastric Acid Secretion

Acid secretion is measured by collecting and analyzing gastric contents through a nasogastric tube. The tip is placed through the nose into the most dependent part of the stomach using a fluoroscope (X-ray). With the patient lying on his or her right side, suction is applied to the tube for four 15-minute periods. The acid concentration is determined by titration or through a glass electrode. There are several sources of error. Hydrogen ions may be lost into the duodenum or through back-diffusion across the gastric epithelium. Saliva or refluxed duodenal secretions may dilute and neutralize the acid. The hourly basal acid output has a circadian pattern, with the lowest rates from 5 AM to 11 AM and the highest from 2 PM to 11 PM. Even a person's emotional state can alter the rate of basal acid secretion.

To determine the secretory capacity of the stomach, a maximal acid output (MAO) is determined by collecting gastric juice after stimulation of the parietal cells. Obviously the most informative results would be obtained after a meal, but collection from a fed stomach is difficult. A subcutaneous injection of a standard dose of histamine stimulates the H_2 receptors on the parietal cell. Gastric juice is collected for 1 hour thereafter. Prior injection of an H_1 antihistamine such as chlorpheniramine (Chlor Tripolon™) or diphenhydramine (Benedryl™) prevents the many effects of histamine throughout the body. H_2 receptors are unaffected by these drugs so that the parietal cells are "maximally" stimulated by histamine. Pentagastrin is a 5-amino acid, synthetic gastrin analogue that accomplishes the same thing with fewer side effects and no need for an antihistamine.

The MAO is the sum of the four 15-minute collections expressed as millimoles of H^+ ions per hour. The peak acid output (PAO) is a refinement in which the two highest 15-minute collections are added and multiplied by 2. The values of the MAO and PAO, unlike the BAO, vary little over time. They reflect the number of parietal cells in the stomach (the parietal cell mass) and the acid secretory capacity of the stomach. This varies with the sex, age, and weight of the subject. The parietal cell mass and MAO will increase if there is a prolonged excess of gastrin. Thus in a patient with a gastrin-secreting tumor, the MAO increases (Zollinger–Ellison Syndrome). After surgical removal of the gastric antrum the lack of gastrin causes parietal cell atrophy and a reduced MAO. By removing the psychic stimulation to the parietal cells, vagotomy also greatly reduces acid secretion. This is the surgical justification for antrectomy and vagotomy.

WHY DO A GASTRIC ANALYSIS?

The reader may rightly ask, "What is the use of an acid secretion test." "Practically none" should be the answer. Outside the research lab, its only use might be to help identify a rare hypersecretory state, but even here the need is dubious. However, such was the interest in acid as the cause of ulcers that no gastroenterology trainee in the 1960s could avoid the chore of putting patients through these tests. It seemed certain that the clue to an ulcer patient's optimal treatment lay in his or her pattern of acid secretion. In retrospect this seems fanciful. With the arrival of the

H_2 blocking drugs, physicians abandoned gastric acid measurement as a routine test for peptic ulcer.

Nonetheless, acid secretion is abnormal in many ulcer patients. On average, duodenal ulcer patients have greater BAOs and MAOs than those without ulcers, even when adjusted for age, sex, and weight. However, there is so much overlap that the test cannot discriminate ulcer from nonulcer in an individual, nor do its results correlate with the clinical course of the ulcer. The lower than normal BAO and MAO in gastric ulcer patients are probably due to back-diffusion of H^+ ions through the damaged stomach mucosa, which prevents their collection. Before gastrin could be measured in the blood, acid secretion tests were the most useful means of detecting a rare gastrin-secreting tumor. In this instance, the BAO approaches the MAO in value. In achlorhydric states such as pernicious anemia, gastric analysis assists the diagnosis by registering no BAO or MAO. The Schilling's test has made gastric analysis redundant for this indication as well (see below).

PEPSINOGEN SECRETION

Pepsinogens are a group of at least eight enzymes of similar properties that are secreted by the chief cells at the base of the gastric glands. Their different chemical properties and grouping into pepsinogen I and II need not concern us here. When secreted, acid converts pepsinogen to the protein-digesting enzyme *pepsin*. Pepsin is most active when the pH is between 2 and 3.5. It is inactivated reversibly when the pH rises to 5, but it does not survive neutrality (pH = 7).

Analogous to the parietal cell, the chief cell requires the intracellular mediators, calcium and c-AMP. Control of pepsin secretion parallels that of acid in that it is stimulated by acetylcholine, histamine, and gastrin and inhibited by PGE_2 and somatostatin. There are even BAO, MAO, and PAO measurements to quantify pepsin output. Although pepsin initiates the digestion of dietary protein, its role is minor compared to that of proteases produced by the pancreas. No significant malabsorption results from lack of pepsin.

Other enzymes produced by the stomach are of even less significance. A protease secreted from the gastric surface epithelium accounts for 5% of gastric protein digestion. Gastric lipase digests triglyceride in an acid medium, but would not be missed.

MUCUS AND BICARBONATE SECRETION

Most of the single layer of epithelial cells lining the stomach and gastric glands are surface mucous cells. Near the surface of the cell are granules that discharge mucin, membrane and all, into the stomach lumen. This material is 5% glycoprotein and 95% water. Intact mucus clings to the epithelium, protecting it from hydrogen ions. Pepsin can degrade mucus into subunits that are soluble and can be washed away. The balance between mucus production and degradation determines the thickness of the protective layer. Prostaglandins and sucralfate increase mucus thickness, while NSAIDs and aspirin reduce it.

The surface epithelium secretes bicarbonate ions into the mucus blanket. The bicarbonate neutralizes hydrogen ions near the mucosal surface.

INTRINSIC FACTOR AND VITAMIN B_{12}

As if the parietal cell had not enough to do, it also produces intrinsic factor (IF). It too is stimulated by histamine and inhibited by H_2 blockers. Omeprazole, which so precisely blocks the acid pump, ignores IF production. A glycoprotein, IF plays a vital role in the absorption of vitamin B_{12} in the ileum. Its importance to the ulcer story is that its malabsorption after ulcer surgery may cause vitamin B_{12} deficiency and anemia.

IF's function is complicated. In the stomach a certain "R" protein successfully competes with IF to bind vitamin B_{12} after its release from dietary protein acid by pepsin. However, IF wins out in the end when pancreatic enzymes in the duodenum free vitamin B_{12} from the R protein. The IF–B_{12} complex attaches itself to special receptors on the ileal epithelium, which then absorbs the vitamin.

Several things can go awry. In pernicious anemia there is atrophy of the parietal cells, with achlorhydria and loss of IF. Antibodies to parietal cells and IF circulate in the blood. These are evidence that pernicious anemia is an *autoimmune disease*, where the body's own immune system destroys the acid-secreting and B_{12} secreting tissue. Gastric surgery, if very extensive, may also remove parietal cells. Even antrectomy, by ending gastrin secretion, causes eventual parietal cell atrophy.

If the surgery creates a "blind loop" as in a Billroth II gastrec-tomy, bacteria may overgrow in the loop and consume vitamin B_{12} before it gets to the ileum (see Figure 29-1). Disease or removal of the pancreas or ileum also prevents absorption of this ubiquitous, but essential, vitamin.

Intrinsic factor is seldom totally absent, and body stores of vitamin B_{12} are so large that lack of supply takes many years to cause deficiency. Since B_{12} is vital to the production of hemoglobin for red blood cells, deficiency of the vitamin causes the precursor cells in the bone marrow to become *megaloblastic*. The daughter red cells are large and underfilled with hemoglobin (macrocytes). There are abnormal white cells and platelets as well. Once recognized, the deficiency is easily rectified by regular vitamin B_{12} injections.

Schilling's Test

There are assays that measure vitamin B_{12} in the blood. A *Schilling's test* detects malabsorption. The patient swallows a radio-labeled vitamin B_{12} capsule, and the B_{12} appearing in the urine during a 24-hour collection is an index of absorption. If the amount appearing in the urine is low, the test is repeated with IF added to the vitamin. If the second test is normal, then lack of IF is the problem. This may be the result of pernicious anemia or gastrec-tomy. If both tests are abnormal, the cause of the B_{12} malabsorption is likely to be disease of the pancreas, ileum, or bacterial overgrowth. This test is only useful if the 24-hour urine collection is complete.

SUMMARY

By definition, peptic ulcers do not occur without gastric acid. For many years acid secretion and its control were central to our thinking about the cause of ulcers and their treatment. The acid pump H^+, K^+–ATPase secretes hydrogen ions across the canalicular membrane creating a pH gradient of 7.3:1. Histamine released by nearby ECL cells, acetylcholine from vagal nerve endings, and gastrin from the antrum all stimulate parietal cell activity.

There are other substances in gastric juice. Chief cells secrete pepsinogen under circumstances similar to those of acid. Indeed, pepsinogen requires acid for its activation to pepsin, the enzyme that begins the process of protein digestion. Mucus and bicarbonate secretion by the surface mucous cells help protect the mucosa from acid and pepsin. Parietal cells also produce intrinsic factor, a protein that participates in the absorption of vitamin B_{12}.

CHAPTER SEVEN

NSAIDs

Nonsteroidal Anti-Inflammatory Drugs

Nonsteroidal anti-inflammatory drugs (NSAIDs) are commonly used for rheumatic diseases and other disorders that cause inflammation and pain. They are chemically and pharmacologically distinct from *steroids* such as cortisone or prednisone. Steroids are natural or synthetic hormones that have profound metabolic effects as well as potent anti-inflammatory actions. The term steroid refers to the chemical structure of the drugs and is used imprecisely. Many steroids, such as the sex hormones or anabolic steroids illicitly used by athletes have little or no anti-inflammatory action.

There is no doubt that NSAIDs provide great comfort to many by promoting increased activity and general health, but they cause serious gastrointestinal disease. The most widely used NSAID is aspirin. This ancient painkiller is still a respected treatment for rheumatoid arthritis, headaches, and other inflammatory or painful conditions. Because it inhibits the platelet contribution to blood clotting, a small daily dose of aspirin prevents coronary artery occlusion and strokes. The other NSAIDs are more recent developments. Because they are new, their undesirable effects have been more carefully studied.

USE AND COST OF NSAIDs

NSAIDs account for 100 million prescriptions in the United States every year. Four million aspirin tablets (equal to 20 million pounds) and other NSAIDs such as ibuprofen and naproxin are also sold over the counter. There are 20 million prescriptions for NSAIDs annually in the United Kingdom. In 1984, Britons consumed 6 billion aspirin tablets. In Alberta, Canada, prescriptions are free for citizens over 65. Fully 26% of this vulnerable population received at least one NSAID prescription in 6 months during 1991. There are over 30 varieties of NSAIDs available, and more are in the development stage. Sales in 1995 are expected to exceed $1.5 billion.

In the United States, NSAID gastropathy accounts for at least 7,600 deaths and 76,000 hospitalizations yearly. The annual bill for gastric complications in Americans with arthritis is $4 billion. Deaths from complicated peptic ulcers due to NSAIDs are about 1,200 annually in Britain. Despite this, the absolute death rate is not greater in NSAID users, perhaps because of the life-saving advantages of the drugs in the treatment of arthritis. Nonetheless, NSAID gastropathy and ulcer disease are serious drawbacks. Now that victory over *H. pylori* seems at hand, NSAIDs loom as the next major peptic ulcer challenge.

NSAID MUCOSAL DAMAGE

NSAIDs damage the gut in two ways: through a direct topical action and through an indirect, systemic effect. The first is dramatically observable, but may be relatively unimportant clinically. The second mechanism is complicated and less well understood, but very important.

Topical Effects

Aspirin and most NSAIDs are weak acids. In the acid environment of the stomach they are un-ionized and soluble in lipid (fat). These properties permit the drug to pass through the lipid membrane of the gastric epithelial cells where, in the neutral cellular milieu, they become ionized and lipid insoluble. The negatively charged drug and its matching hydrogen ion are therefore trapped in the cell. Toxic effects occur as they become concentrated there. Within 1 hour of aspirin ingestion, tiny mucosal hemorrhages and erosions can be observed through an endoscope. Occult loss of blood can be detected in the stool and may cause an iron deficiency, anemia. These small lesions seldom result in overt bleeding. The acute mucosal abnormalities reach a peak in three days and, despite continued drug use, usually disappear by four weeks. This *adaptation* does not occur in all subjects, and sometimes the mucosal damage progresses to gastric or duodenal ulcer. White blood cells adhere to the NSAID-damaged tissue and to the endothelium of mucosal blood vessels, impairing blood flow. These developments impair mucus production and repair of the damaged area. Back-diffusion of more hydrogen ions into the mucosa exacerbates the injury.

Systemic Effects (Prostaglandins)

The pro-drug sulindac (Clinoril™) converts into an active NSAID after absorbtion, sparing topical injury to mucosa. Yet this drug still causes peptic ulcers. Even when given by injection or by rectal suppository, NSAIDs provoke ulcers. Similarly, enteric coated aspirin arrives intact in the small intestine, avoiding topical injury to the stomach, but the absorbed aspirin remains ulcerogenic. Moreover, the small gut may be at risk.

Discussion of the systemic effects of NSAIDs requires an understanding of prostaglandin metabolism. *Prostaglandins* owe their name to the prostate gland. In the 1930s a substance was identified in semen that dilated blood vessels and contracted the uterus. Since then, prostaglandins have turned out to be many and varied, with actions throughout the body. They are denominated PGA_1, PGA_2, and so on to PGF. The subscript number indicates how many double bonds are found in the 20-carbon prostaglandin molecule. Our interest here is in the role of PGE prostaglandins in regulating inflammation and protecting the upper gut mucosa. However, some prostaglandins have diverse and often harmful consequences, such as spasm of blood vessels and bronchi, aggregation of blood platelets, and elevation of blood cholesterol.

Research in this area has focused on the metabolism of a cell membrane lipid called *arachadonic acid*. The enzyme *cyclo-oxygenase* (cox) acts on arachadonic acid to initiate a cascade of reactions that produce several inflammatory prostaglandins. However, a separate enzyme, *lipoxygenase*, catalyzes the production of a bewildering array of *leucotrienes* that also have pro-inflammatory activity. NSAIDs inhibit cyclo-oxygenase, an action that may account for their anti-inflammatory activity. Perhaps steroids are more potent anti-inflammatory drugs because they inhibit the production of both prostaglandins *and* leucotrienes. It is uncertain if the arachadonic acid pathway is the only, or the most important, one altered by NSAIDs. Other lipid metabolic pathways produce different prostaglandins and leucotrienes, some of which are themselves anti-inflammatory, so there are both inflammatory and anti-inflammatory varieties.

Many prostaglandins, for example PGE_1 and PGE_3, exert a protective effect on the gastric mucosa. Evidence for this includes: (1) the production of ulcers in animals given antibodies to prostaglandins, (2) the prevention of NSAID ulcers through the coadministration of a synthetic prostaglandin, and (3) the ability of NSAIDs to reduce the prostaglandin concentration in gastric mucosa. Prostaglandins increase mucosal blood flow, inhibit gastric acid secretion, and increase gastric mucus production. NSAIDs, by inhibiting prostaglandin production, reverse these effects and impair the ability of the gastroduodenal mucosa to defend itself. It has become apparent that there are two distinct cyclo-oxygenase molecules: Cox-1 and Cox-2. The first, present in most tissues, is important for cell homeostasis. This implies a protective effect on gut mucosa through the mechanisms described above. In contrast, Cox-2 is found in inflammatory cells and is induced at sites of inflammation by cytokines and other chemical mediators of inflammation. Clearly Cox-2 is the proper target for NSAIDs, since it is the site of inflammation such as an arthritic joint, not the gut, that the drugs are designed to treat. Ironically, currently available NSAIDs have a higher affinity for Cox-1. There is therefore a need for a drug that is selective for Cox-2. Such a drug, if theory holds, could capture most of the $1.5 billion market world-wide.

Other Effects

Aspirin, and to a lesser extent other NSAIDs, impair blood platelet function, thereby reducing the capacity of blood to clot. For this reason, aspirin is used to prevent strokes and heart attacks. Since the effect on each platelet is irreversible, recovery of normal clotting awaits a new generation of platelets, which usually takes about a week. Blood leaking from blood vessels in an NSAID ulcer may fail to clot, in some cases causing significant hemorrhage.

Prostaglandins stimulate the uterus to contract and thus are contraindicated in pregnant women. Through smooth muscle activity they may cause diarrhea, and, not unexpectedly, those taking NSAIDs often complain of constipation.

NSAIDs AND GASTRODUODENAL INJURY

Up to 50% of people on long-term NSAIDs complain of dyspepsia. More than half of these have no ulcer or other upper gut disease. Furthermore, one-third of those with mucosal ulcers have no dyspepsia. Most worrisome, most of those having a complication of an ulcer have no warning dyspepsia. Thus, dyspepsia is an unreliable indicator of NSAID mucosal injury.

Clinically significant gastric NSAID damage to the gastroduodenal mucosa is unpredictable. The small, acute, NSAID-induced hemorrhages and erosions are usually not accompanied by symptoms or important consequences. Despite continued exposure, they usually heal over a few weeks. Not all stomachs adapt in this way, and some may develop an ulcer. However, it seems that most ulcers occur through other means. When subjects taking full doses of NSAIDs for a longer period are endoscoped, up to half will be found to have superficial lesions, 14% will have a gastric ulcer, and 10% will have a duodenal ulcer. It is uncertain what proportion of these are new lesions as opposed to reactivations of previous ulcers.

Endoscopic ulcers are different from *clinical ulcers*. The former may be asymptomatic and are perhaps unimportant, while the latter often make themselves known through bleeding, anemia, or perforation. Clinical ulcers are larger, cause more inflammation, and have a different natural history. While NSAIDs can cause dyspepsia with or without ulcers, it is a disconcerting paradox that many NSAID users may develop bleeding from an ulcer without any preceding dyspepsia. Therefore, dyspepsia cannot be relied upon to warn of impending disaster. To be relevant, clinical trials should study the prevention of *complicated* clinical ulcers. We need not prevent all endoscopically observed NSAID injuries if we can establish which are likely to be dangerous.

Crude statistics such as hospitalization and death rates indicate the prevalence of significant ulcers, but the data exclude patients managed outside of hospitals. Case-control studies compare the presence of ulcers in NSAID users with age and sex-matched controls. They may be biased in that the NSAID users are more readily investigated. Cohort studies follow NSAID-users prospectively and compare them with nonusers. These studies indicate that NSAID use produces a threefold to tenfold increase in risk of bleeding, perforation, and death.

RISK FACTORS

Many factors increase the risk that an NSAID user will develop significant ulcer disease (Table 7-1).

Age and Sex

NSAID complications are particularly numerous among the elderly. This population, however, exhibits the most rheumatic disorders and therefore has the greatest exposure to the drug. There is no proof that the elderly are *individually* more susceptible to NSAID mucosal damage, but many suspect that this is so. In any case, elderly persons who do suffer ulcer complications tolerate them poorly since age and accompanying disease impair compensatory mechanisms.

Duration and Timing of Treatment

Endoscopic and clinical ulcers tend to occur within a month after an individual has begun taking an NSAID. The ulcers may appear as new lesions or as activations of previously existing ulcers. Alternatively, those patients destined to react badly may do so early and stop the drug because of dyspepsia. The remaining lower-risk subjects tolerate chronic use.

There is little scientific evidence to support the recommendation that NSAIDs be taken with food. Mucosal injury is the same

TABLE 7-1
NSAIDs: Risk Factors

Age >60
Female gender
Duration of treatment
Dose
Type of NSAID
Multiple NSAIDs
Steroid use
Previous ulcer

whether the drug is taken with meals or 2 hours before, but ranitidine seems to prevent injury more effectively in the former case.

Dose

Experimental endoscopic studies and clinical studies emphasize that NSAID damage to the mucosa is dose-dependent. Nevertheless, a risk exists at all dosages. In a large project that compared doses of 1g of aspirin daily to placebo for the prevention of myocardial infarction, those taking aspirin had a tenfold increase in risk of hospitalization for peptic ulcer. In other studies, as little as one 325-mg aspirin tablet taken daily to prevent stroke or heart attack increased the risk of bleeding. This may be due in part to aspirin's prolonged inhibition of platelet function.

Type of Drug

All NSAIDs inhibit prostaglandin synthesis, which is an important mechanism for both benefit and grief. It is doubtful that the benefits can be separated from the unwanted effects, but successive NSAIDs have appeared on the market with just that claim. One of the difficulties lies in distinguishing between endoscopically observed damage to the gastroduodenal mucosa during NSAID administration and clinically important ulcers. The pro-drugs sulindac and fenbufen (Lederfen, Bufemid™) that are activated after absorption cause no immediate injury, yet they are no safer than other NSAIDs (Table 7-2). Similarly, enteric coated aspirin offers little protection. Nonacetylated salicylates such as salsalate may inhibit prostaglandins without causing mucosal ulcers, but require more research.

Assessment of the relative safety of NSAIDs is hampered by the variability of the indications, dose, and exposed population. Recently introduced drugs are more closely monitored but have had less time to accumulate adverse events. Indomethacin (Indocid™) and aspirin are old drugs not subject to the strict monitoring imposed on the newer products.

Until recently the prevailing view was that toxicity was similar in all NSAIDs. However, the British Committee on Safety of Medicine's adverse event reporting system ranks the risks of newer NSAIDs (see Table 7-1). Data from the Tennessee Medicaid program suggests that ibuprofen (Motrin™) was the least toxic in elderly enrollees. Two British groups report relative risks of complications that are remarkably consistent with the CSM rankings. The study by Langman *et al.* is of 1,144 patients over 60 years of age hospitalized for peptic ulcer bleeding, compared to suitable hospital and community controls. As expected, peptic ulcer bleeding is very common with all non-aspirin NSAIDs taken within 3 months before admission. There is no such association of ulcer complications with the non-NSAID analgesic acetaminophen (Tylenol™). A second study of 1,457 people of all ages in general practice who developed gastrointestinal bleeding or perforation produced similar results. In 1980 to 1982, billing data from all Medicaid patients in Michigan and Minnesota permitted a cohort study of patients with gastrointestinal bleeding associated with NSAID therapy. Using ibuprofen as a reference drug, the relative risks of several NSAIDs were calculated. Sundilac demonstrated the largest and only significant increase in relative risk compared to ibuprofen. Unlike other studies, indomethacin had the same relative risk as ibuprofen. Piroxicam and several other NSAIDs were unavailable at the time the study was done. In a New Zealand case-control study of 494 patients and 972 controls, the odds ratios of bleeding with several NSAIDs were calculated. Again, ibuprofen had the least relative risk, and piroxicam and indomethacin had the highest. An older study from Barcelona includes only a few of the available NSAIDs. It confirmed the relative toxicity of piroxicam, and the intermediate positions of diclofenac, naproxen and indomethacin (Odds ratios; 7.9, 6.5, and 4.9, respectively).

TABLE 7-2
NSAIDs: Relative Risks of Peptic Ulcer Disease

Drug	CSM ranking[a]	Tennessee elderly[b]	Hospital GI bleed[c]	UK GP STUDY[d]	Medicaid study[e]	New Zealand[f]
Ibuprofen	1	2.3	2.0	2.9	1.0	1.9
Diclofenac	2		4.2	3.9		3.3
Naproxen	3	4.3	9.1	3.1	1.1	5.1
Sulindac		4.2			1.8	3.6
Fenprofen		4.3			1.6	
Ketoprofen	6		23.7	5.4		2.4
Indomethacin		3.8	11.3	6.3	1.0	13.9
Tolmetin		8.5				
Meclofenamate		8.7				
Piroxicam	11		13.7	18		6.4
Azapropazone	12		31.5	23.4		
Overall			4.5	4.7		4.1

[a]United Kingdom Committee on Safety of Medicines (CSM) rank order of serious reports of gut toxicity expressed per million prescriptions in first 5 years of marketing.
[b]Relative risk of ulcer of enrollees in Tennessee Medicaid program 1984-86 (>65 years) (Griffin et al.).
[c] Odds ratio for acute gastrointestinal bleeding in hospital, (Langman et al.).
[d]Odds ratio for GI bleeding or perforation in general practice patients, 1994 (Rodriguez and Jick).
[e]Relative risk of upper abdominal bleeding in Medicaid patients in Minnesota and Michigan in 1982 (Carson et al.). Ibuprofen is reference.
[f]Odds ratio in New Zealand case control study (Savage et al.).

The data suggests comparative safety for ibuprofen, and the highest risks for piroxicam (Feldene™) and azapropazine. One explanation may be that piroxicam has the greatest affinity for cyclo-oxygenase Cox-1, followed by aspirin, sundilac, and indomethacin. However, the studies do not assess efficacy. Nevertheless, it does seem sensible to recommend the apparently safer drug first. No currently available NSAID is completely safe, and we await the production of ideal Cox-2 inhibitors.

OTHER RISK FACTORS

Steroid anti-inflammatory drugs include hydrocortisone and prednisone. Debate about their ulcerogenic capacity is unsettled, mainly because recipients are often very ill, and a steroid effect cannot be separated from that of another drug. However, the coadministration of steroids greatly increases the ulcerogenic potential of NSAIDs, perhaps by a factor of ten.

Ulcers are more likely to occur in long-term NSAID users who are infected with *H. pylori*. Smoking and blood group O all predispose to peptic ulcers, but there is no information on their interaction with NSAID toxicity. An interaction with alcohol is possible but unproven.

PREVENTING NSAID ULCERS

Since they help so many with rheumatic pain and stiffness, NSAIDs are here to stay. However, their harmful effects demand a cautious approach. The indications for the drug must be clear. Their anti-inflammatory effect is of little value in a condition where inflammation is not a major factor. Such is the case with osteoarthritis, a disease caused by wear and tear and degeneration of the joints. Compared to rheumatoid arthritis, inflammation plays a minor role, and pain relief might be achieved with safer drugs such as acetaminophen (e.g. Tylenol™).

The lowest effective dose of NSAID should be sought. Ibuprofen should be tried first, and the more toxic drugs should be avoided. NSAIDs should be introduced cautiously in the elderly and should be monitored, especially during the first month of treatment. Cotreatment with steroids is dangerous. Those with a history of peptic ulcer should not use the drugs without some protection.

New drug designs are being explored to maximize the anti-inflammatory benefits of NSAIDs and to minimize the mucosal damage they cause. The use of pro-drugs seems unhelpful, and enteric coating may simply shift the trouble further down the gut. Topical NSAID creams may help muscle aches and bypass the gut, but they are not effective in joint disease.

Until a perfect NSAID appears, we must be alert to the high risk of clinical ulcers with their use. Some data favor the use of the prostaglandin analogue *misoprostyl* in high-risk patients, but side effects make it unsatisfactory. Therefore, many physicians prefer an H_2 antagonist. While misoprostil can prevent both endoscopic and clinical gastric and duodenal ulcers, so far, H_2 receptor antagonists have proven efficacy in only the former situation (famotidine). The proton pump inhibitors are expensive and have not yet been properly tested for this purpose. Since the administration of anti-ulcer drugs to all NSAID users would be an expensive impracticality, they should only be given to high risk patients or to those with previous ulcers (see Chapter 26).

Recent work suggests that the PGE_2 content of gastric juice is depressed by naproxen. Moreover, the degree of PGE_2 depletion may predict the degree of gastric mucosal damage. If this holds true, it may be possible through gastric juice analysis to predict those NSAID users in need of anti-ulcer drugs.

SUMMARY

NSAIDs damage the gastric and duodenal mucosa in two ways. The first is topical, caused by the concentration of the drug within the cell, and most users adapt within 1 month. The second is systemic and probably relates to the drug's inhibition of cyclooxygenase and the consequent reduction in prostaglandin production. This is probably the most important factor in the development of clinical ulcers. The risks of mucosal ulceration and its complications seem greatest in the elderly, in the first month of therapy, in the company of steroids, and in those with a history of peptic ulcer. Ibuprofen seems to be the safest, but all NSAIDs carry some risk.

The risk increases with the dose, but ulcer hemorrhage sometimes occurs with the daily use of a single aspirin tablet. Although the overall benefits of these widely used drugs justify their use for the proper indications, the risk of dangerous complications is considerable, perhaps 250,000 people in the United States every year.

CHAPTER EIGHT

Helicobacter pylori

Tis time to give 'em physic, their diseases
Are grown so catching.
W. Shakespare, *Henry VIII*, Act I, Scene iii

The climax of the ulcer story is surely the discovery that bacteria are the cause of most non-NSAID peptic ulcers. Clinging to the inhospitable lining of the stomach, *Helicobacter pylori* is a remarkable creature. It is probably the world's most common infection, and it affects most humans. Should claims that it is an important cause of cancer and heart disease prove true, extinction of these bacteria will become a public health priority. Although *H. pylori* was noticed a century ago and again in 1939, nobody believed that any organism could survive in the stomach, let alone do it any harm. Even when Warren and Marshall brought *H. pylori* to public attention in 1983 and 1984, they were ignored. Acid causes ulcer, does it not? The dominance of the acid hypothesis was such that few could grasp the notion that peptic ulcer could be an infectious disease.

Of its importance, little doubt remains. It is perhaps the most important development in the history of gastroenterology—the stuff of which Nobel Prizes are made. New information now floods the medical literature. Between 1988 and 1993, 1,191 scientific articles appeared on *H. pylori* and peptic ulcer disease. Yet there is much to learn about this enigmatic little bug. Why, for example, do all who are infected not have ulcers? How can it survive in a pH of 1? Can it cause symptoms without ulceration? What is its role in cancer?

Who should be treated, and how? This chapter will describe *H. pylori*, its detection and epidemiology, and its relationship to disease.

THE ORGANISM

Originally called a Campylobacter, *Helicobacter pylori* is a small, curved rod that is gram negative. This means that it stains red in a histological specimen. Its presence is best detected by gastric biopsy as described by Warren in 1983 (Figure 8-1). The bacteria do not usually invade the epithelium, but rather cling to mucus-secreting epithelial cells, especially in the antrum and the gastric pits or glands. In the duodenum it appears only in areas of gastric metaplasia. Metaplasia is a transmogrification of duodenal epithelial cells into gastric-like cells, analogous to the esophageal changes that occur in Barrett's esophagus (see Chapter 17). Gastric metaplasia may be due to infection of duodenal mucosa and the presence of acid. *H. pylori* does not attach to stomach epithelium that has undergone atrophy or intestinal metaplasia.

H. pylori produces *urease*, an enzyme that promotes the metabolism of urea to carbon dioxide and ammonia. Scientists have long known about gastric urease, little suspecting it was a bacterial product. The ammonia raises the local pH and may be toxic to epithelial cells. The resulting local alkaline milieu may help explain the organism's ability to survive in the stomach. Whatever its purpose, the release of carbon dioxide by urease is the basis of tests that detect the presence of infection.

Numerous other toxins may cause the tissue damage and inflammation seen with *H. pylori* infection. One toxin damages parietal cells and accounts for the hypochlorhydria reported in the rare observations of acute infection. Another causes vacuoles to form in the surface mucus cells. Others initiate antibody and immune cell reactions. In a misguided attempt at defense, these reactions produce cytokines and other toxins that further damage the mucosa.

H. pylori reproduces slowly and is therefore difficult to culture. For this reason Warren, Marshall, and their colleagues initially had difficulty growing the organism, an essential step in establishing pathogenicity. Growth of the bacteria was observed only after the culture apparatus was inadvertently left over a long weekend. Culture is the preferred means of detection for most bacteria, but

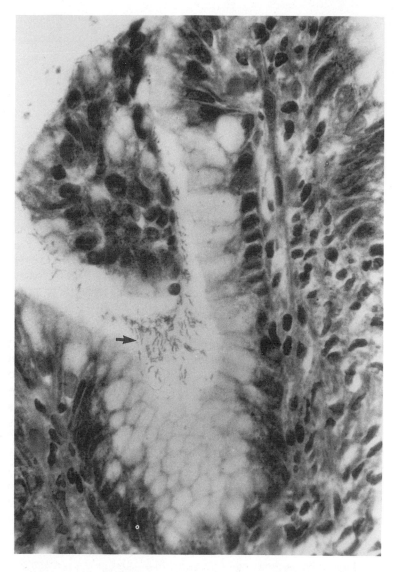

Figure 8-1. *Helicobacter pylori.* The tiny bacterial rods (arrow) nestle in the opening of a gastric gland. Here they cling to the vacuolated surface mucous cells of the mucosal epithelium and, through the release of urease and other toxins, induce the inflammatory response known as chronic active gastritis. (Courtesy of Dr. M. Guindi, Division of Anatomical Pathology, Ottawa Civic Hospital, Ottawa, Ontario, Canada.)

histology from gastric biopsies is more practical for *H. pylori*. A patchy distribution of the organisms in the stomach requires 2–4 specimens of the antrum to avoid a sampling error. There are many strains or subspecies of *H. pylori* that may be identified by DNA fingerprinting. It is too early to be certain, but this may explain some of the differences in peptic ulcer prevalence among carriers. The diverse strains could account for the observed differences in cancer incidence as well. All strains are firmly linked to chronic active gastritis. Its presence in dental plaque may be a source of human to human spread.

DETECTION

Many problems arise when testing for the presence of *H. pylori* in the gastric mucosa. (Tests for detection of *H. pylori* are listed in Table 8-1). Biopsy with histology is the gold standard. Once endoscopy is performed, presumably to establish the presence of an ulcer, it is a simple matter to obtain tissue with forceps introduced through the instrument. However, this is expensive and not always ideal. If the endoscopist discovers a bleeding ulcer, he or she will want to treat it promptly. Histology results take two days or more, and cultures are even slower. A rapid test for the presence of urease is available for this purpose. The biopsy specimen is incubated with urea. If urease is present, ammonia will be released, increasing pH and changing a color indicator. This is accurate and may be positive within 60 minutes. The urease test is cheapest if there is an endoscopy. Histology specimens could be submitted only if it is negative. The absence of chronic antral gastritis most accurately excludes *H. pylori* infection.

None of these options is suitable for screening or for epidemiological study since endoscopies would be required. A serum test for *H. pylori* antibodies has a sensitivity and specificity of over 90%. However, this requires blood-letting, and a positive test may linger several weeks after the bacteria are dead. That makes serology inconvenient to check the adequacy of treatment. A saliva test for antibodies avoids the needle, but not the problem of persistent antibodies.

Breath tests may be an answer. ^{14}Carbon can be incorporated into urea. This is then fed to the individual to be tested. If the stomach is infected, ^{14}carbon dioxide is released and excreted in

TABLE 8-1
Tests for Detecting *H. pylori* Infection

Diagnostic tests	Sensitivity[a]	Specificity	Cost[b]
^{13}C-urea breath test	90–100%	80–90%	unavailable
^{14}C-urea breath test	90–100	80–90	unavailable
Serology	88–96	89–100	13.50
Saliva			16
Culture	77–94	100	24.46
Histology	93–99	95–99	76.44
Rapid urease test	86–97	86–98	3.05

[a]Sensitivity and specificity after D.T. Smoot, presented at U.S. National Institutes of Health Consensus Development Conference, Bethesda, Maryland (February, 1994).
[b]In Canadian dollars. Figures from Ottawa Civic Hospital, 1994, courtesy Dr. D. S. Ooi (for comparison only).

the breath, where it can be collected and measured. The test is highly accurate, but it requires radioactive material and is not available everywhere. Pretreatment with omeprazole increases the intragastric pH and reduces *H. pylori's* urease activity, thereby decreasing the sensitivity of the urea breath test. Nevertheless, the breath test is the most appropriate test for eradication that does not require endoscopy. It must be done after treatment, including omeprazole, is complete. Attempts to substitute the nonradioactive isotope ^{13}carbon have proved expensive. The polymerase chain reaction (PCR) shows some promise.

EPIDEMIOLOGY

Throughout nature, infection without disease is the rule rather than the exception.

Rene Dubos, 1901–

The ubiquity of *H. pylori* is startling. Most humans are infected, yet most experience no symptoms from it. In the developing world, most individuals harbor the organism from childhood. This is not the case in Western countries, where it has become uncommon under the age of 20. In the West, the current prevalence increases with age until 50 or 60, where it levels off at about 50%. This fits old Scandinavian data indicating that gastritis increases with age. Initially it seemed reasonable to conclude that one acquired the disease over the passing years. There is now evidence that this is not so.

In a small western Australian community, serum was stored from men undergoing observations over 20 years for another purpose. In 1990, 141 such cases who were now over 40 years of age were randomly selected. Retrospective analysis of their serum stored in 1967–1970, when they were 20–40 years old, found that 39% had *H. pylori* antibodies. The 78 subjects who were tested again in 1978 included 40.9% who were seropositive. For 1990, the figure was 34.8%. In 1990, 78% of those who were positive initially were still carrying the organism, while only 7% of the negative cases had acquired it. Acquisition of the infection in healthy adults is unusual, so the observations are best explained by a cohort effect. It now appears that most infected adults acquired the bacteria as children. Since children are less likely to contact the bacteria nowadays, a cohort of young people are maturing with less *H. pylori* infection.

Childhood acquisition of the infection is more likely in overcrowded, deprived, and unhygenic conditions. These are most strikingly encountered in institutions. In the United States *H. pylori* is more common in the black and Latino populations than in the Caucasian population. The rapid post-World War II socioeconomic revolution in Japan produced a later cohort phenomenon, so that now the prevalence *H. pylori* is also declining in young Japanese. It may be this cohort effect that accounts for the apparent decrease in ulcer disease in developed countries. The situation is very different in the underdeveloped world, where 50% of children under 10 and almost 100% of people over 40 have the infection.

Infection with a single strain of *H. pylori* seems to cluster in certain families who doubtless pass it to one another. However, simple transmission may not be the only factor at work. A Scandinavian study of 269 twin pairs disclosed that if one twin were affected, the other was more likely than expected to acquire the organism. This concordance was greater with monozygotic (identical) than dizygotic twins. Although it was greatest if the twins lived together, concordance was still observable in those who were separated from infancy. The effect was greater in the case of identical twins. Inherited traits may account for differences in infection rates.

Other sources of infection are spouses and contaminated water. Gastroenterologists worry that infected gastroscopes might convey the infection to other patients or to staff. Indeed, before the great concern about AIDS and hepatitis, endoscopes were less thoroughly sterilized, and there is a hint that some endoscopists may have acquired the infection.

In Western countries, *H. pylori* occurs commonly in asymptomatic individuals over the age of 50. This will decline as less-exposed generations move up into this age bracket. The infection usually causes chronic active gastritis. It is found in over 90% of cases of non-NSAID duodenal ulcers and in 75% of gastric ulcers. The prevalence of the organisms in non-ulcer dyspepsia is probably similar to that in healthy asymptomatic individuals. In gastric atrophy, intestinal metaplasia, or after gastrectomy, where surface mucous cells have been altered or removed, the likelihood of infection is less.

CHRONIC ACTIVE GASTRITIS

Gastritis means inflammation of the gastric mucosa. There is tissue damage with a gathering of circulating granulocytes and local mononuclear cells in the superficial mucosa. These mononuclear cells are normally present in smaller numbers, but when made active, they proliferate and emit chemical messengers that amplify the tissue damage. Inflammation of the mucosa occurs in Crohn's disease and in other uncommon diseases, but by far the most common inflammation is that of chronic active gastritis, for which *H. pylori* is the specific cause. The organism usually clings to the surface mucus cells and emits urease and other toxins that initiate the inflammatory response. Some inflammation exists in almost all cases of *H. pylori* infection. Gastritis is usually not visible to the endoscopist, so a biopsy is necessary to detect it. In children there is often a nodular appearance to the mucosa that disappears with treatment. Indeed, killing the bacteria cures the gastritis.

Two research workers deliberately swallowed the organisms and sustained acute gastric injury. (One volunteer was Marshall himself.) One case was self-limited, while the other infection continued for 966 days, during which several single drug courses failed to kill the organisms. Eventually triple therapy cured the disease with no recurrence 2 years later. Before *H. pylori* was recognized there were two mini-epidemics in research volunteers being tested for gastric secretion. Gastritis and prolonged hypochlorhydria were features of this self-limited illness that, in retrospect, appears to have been due to *H. pylori* that the subjects acquired during the project. The acute infection paradoxically appears to transiently suppress acid secretion. During Marshall's self-induced infection he vomited and noted the lack of acid burn in his throat.

Four features fulfill Robert Koch's (1843–1910) postulates, which are necessary to establish an organism as a cause of disease. These include the strong concordance of *H. pylori* and gastritis, the healing that occurs with eradication of the bacteria, the self-inoculation experiments, and the specificity of the organism for gastritis. Koch's postulates are fulfilled for acute, but not for chronic, gastritis.

PEPTIC ULCER

Koch's postulates have not established *H. pylori* as a cause of peptic ulcers, and there are skeptics still. Most people with the infection do not have an ulcer. Nevertheless, the evidence seems overwhelming that this very common bacterial infection must be present before non-NSAID ulcers can occur. One review of 15 studies concludes that 92% of duodenal ulcer patients are infected, and the figure is even higher in children. Infection is present in about 75% of those with gastric ulcers. These infection rates are much greater than those found in the background Western population. Infection and chronic active gastritis does increase the likelihood of an ulcer, as the following data suggest.

In a 10-year study of asymptomatic patients who were examined by endoscopy and biopsy, 1 of 133 patients with a normal gastric mucosa developed a peptic ulcer, while 34 of 321 (11%) patients with gastritis acquired one. In Hawaii, 5,443 Japanese-American men participating in a 20-year heart study had an initial blood test between 1967 and 1970. Of 150 men who developed a gastric ulcer, 93% originally had *H. pylori* antibodies compared to 78% of matched controls (odds ratio 3.2). For duodenal ulcer the figures were 92% and 78% (odds ratio 4.0). Overall, the risk increased with the magnitude of the antibody levels.

How *H. pylori* causes ulcers is unknown, but acid must be present. The sequel to Schwartz's dictum should be, "No acid no ulcer; no *H. pylori* no ulcer." Duodenal ulcer patients tend to have high normal or slightly elevated acid output. The bacteria may block the normal inhibition of gastrin release by the antrum and of acid secretion by parietal cells (Olbe, 1996). This is surprising since transitory hypochlorhydria occurs during an acute infection. Other factors that may interact with the infection to cause ulcers are discussed in the next chapter. The presence of *H. pylori* increases the risk of ulcers in NSAID users. The organism is more difficult to kill in smokers.

FUNCTIONAL DYSPEPSIA

Several studies claim a relationship of *H. pylori* with functional or non-ulcer dyspepsia, but the data are meaningless without controls. Of four controlled studies, two suggest an association. However, the possibility for bias is great, and eradication of the infection has not been shown to cure the dyspepsia.

STOMACH CANCER

Chronic inflammation of the colon (ulcerative colitis) predisposes over many years to colon cancer. It therefore is reasonable to suspect that chronic inflammation of the gastric mucosa could have a similar result. In China and Japan, where *H. pylori* infection is prevalent, gastric cancer is also prominent. A survey of several populations around China suggested that where infection was common, so was gastric cancer. A survey of 17 populations in 13 countries using random blood sampling also showed a relationship between infection rates and cancer mortality for that population.

However, other studies are less conclusive, and there is no evidence that ridding the stomach of infection protects against cancer. In Africa, the great prevalence of infection is not accompanied by an exceptionally high cancer rate. The African enigma is too striking to be explained by inadequate diagnosis of cancer. Studies that show *H. pylori* in stomachs where cancer exists exhibit temporal ambiguity. That is, the cancer could as likely have predisposed to the infection as vice versa. Nevertheless, case control studies suggest that there is a sixfold increase of gastric cancer risk in infected subjects.

MALT LYMPHOMA

Gastric mucosa, like the rest of the gut, is home to many cells important to the body's immune defenses. Most of these cells are mononuclear. That is, they have one nucleus, unlike the multilobed nuclei of circulating granulocytes. These are mainly lymphocytes, and the tissue is sometimes called mucosa-associated lymphoid tissue (MALT). Malignant tumors that occur here are called MALT lymphomas. They are very rare, but occur in company with *H. pylori*. Remarkably, these cancers usually disappear when the bacteria are killed. It is too early to say that the cure is permanent or that all cases will respond to treatment, but this is an important development.

OTHER ASSOCIATIONS

Diverse effects of *H. pylori* have been reported, but few are substantiated. Of great interest is the proposition that there is a connection between the organism and coronary artery disease. An association of peptic ulcer and heart disease has hitherto been blamed on heredity and possession of a type A personality. Now *H. pylori* stands accused. In one cardiac clinic, the presence of the bacteria in coronary artery disease patients far outstripped that in a control population. Much more work is necessary to confirm this exciting possibility. It is likely an epiphenomenon.

The organism is not found in the esophagus unless there is gastric metaplasia, such as in Barrett's esophagus. Perhaps the bacteria are responsible for the higher than normal cancer risk in those with Barrett's esophagus. It may also cause vitamin B_{12} malabsorption. No doubt many suspected associations will surface from time to time. It's presence in dental plaque may be a source of human to human spread. It is the job of slow, plodding, yet careful clinical science to sort fact from fantasy.

TREATMENT

It is curious that killing *H. pylori* has become known as *eradication*, a term employed for the treatment of no other infection. We do not eradicate streptococci or tubercle bacillus. We kill them. Nonetheless, the word has settled into the medical vernacular. Eradication is the inability to detect the organism at least 1 month after cessation of drug treatment.

As long as peptic ulcers are the principal consequence of *H. pylori* infection, the approach should concentrate on their treatment rather than prophylaxis. Killing the bacteria is difficult, but once achieved the risk of reinfection is probably less than 1% per year. Single drugs such as bismuth, tetracycline, or metronidazole achieve a cure in 20% of cases, but when all three are given for 1 or 2 weeks, the cure rate is over 80%. Triple therapy is therefore the treatment of choice. An H_2-blocking drug such as ranitidine is added to heal the ulcer.

Another popular regimen is Omeprazole, 40 mg per day with amoxacillin four times a day for 2 weeks. The former heals the ulcer and, by raising the pH, increases the killing efficiency of the amoxacillin. The cure rate appears to be somewhat less than with triple therapy, but the number of pills and side effects are fewer. Subsequent experience with this simple drug regimen has been disappointing. A consensus conference at the National Institutes of Health at Bethesda endorsed these treatment schedules in February 1994 (see Table 8-2).

Other varieties of double and triple therapy are discussed in Chapter 27. In some parts of the world, *H. pylori* strains are resistant to metronidazole, so another antibiotic is substituted. There is no indication for treating functional dyspepsia. Cancers other than MALT lymphomas will not respond either. There is little chance of exterminating this infection worldwide with antibiotics. The cost in dollars, side effects, and the development of antibiotic resistance is too high a price to pay in such a futile gesture.

PREVENTION

If *H. pylori* turns out to be a major cause of such killers as cancer or coronary artery disease, we will need a prophylactic approach. This could not be a matter for doctors and patients, but one of public policy. Governments would need to improve conditions for the world's children, since childhood is when the organism gains entry into human stomachs. Perhaps the bacteria should be killed in

TABLE 8-2
National Institutes of Health Consensus
Development Conference Statement[a]:
Guidelines for Antimicrobial Treatment of
H. pylori Infection

Patient status	H. pylori negative	H. pylori positive
Asymptomatic (no ulcer)	no	no
Non-ulcer dyspepsia	no	no
Gastric ulcer	no	yes
Duodenal ulcer	no	yes

[a]Bethesda, Maryland, February 7–9, 1994.

expectant parents. Such measures would constitute a major public health effort in the developed world but are clearly impossible in underdeveloped countries. More effective prevention might be accomplished by a vaccine to immunize all infants against H. pylori. Such a vaccine does not exist outside laboratories, and its distribution to the children of 5 billion people is a daunting prospect.

SUMMARY

The discovery that Helicobacter pylori plays a necessary and permissive role in the pathogenesis of non-NSAID ulcers has completely changed the outlook for patients. With discovery of an ulcer and the organism, cure of the infection and of the ulcer disease are possible. While this bacterium clings to the gastric surface epithelial cells and almost invariably causes chronic active gastritis, most carriers never acquire an ulcer. This is merciful since 50% of those over 50 years old in developed countries are carriers, and in underdeveloped countries almost all adults are infected. The factors that lead from H. pylori infection to ulcer are unknown. Because antibacterial treatment is complicated, expensive, and fraught with side effects and antibiotic resistance, only those infected persons with a confirmed ulcer should be treated. Eradication of the organism has no proven value in functional dyspepsia. There appears to be a sixfold risk of gastric cancer in lifetime carriers, but prevention of cancer and other H. pylori-related diseases would require a major public health effort.

CHAPTER NINE

Other Causes

Genetics, Lifestyle, and Stress

Within a generation we have learned three important facts about peptic ulcers: (1) duodenal ulcer patients tend to have increased gastric acid secretion, (2) most peptic ulcers are associated with chronic active gastritis and infection with *H. pylori*, and (3) most of the remainder are attributable to NSAIDs. So important are these facts that we may overlook a legacy of other ulcer information gathered over the last half century. Much was written about the impact of genetics, disturbed physiology, lifestyle, personality, and stress on peptic ulcer. These aspects should not be forgotten, for each makes a contribution to *The Ulcer Story*. After all, they may help explain some of the remaining conundrums. Why do most people with *H. pylori* infection never get an ulcer? Why are only a few of us liable to develop ulcers through NSAIDs? What causes those peptic ulcers that are associated with neither *H. pylori* nor NSAIDs? While they now seem less important than the big three, the other causes of peptic ulcers deserve to be mentioned.

GENETICS

Many believed that the predisposition to develop a peptic ulcer can be inherited. Even now the evidence seems convincing. Twenty to 50% of individuals with a peptic ulcer have affected family members. First-degree relatives of those with gastric or duodenal ulcer have a threefold increase in risk of developing one themselves, and it is usually of the same type. However, the discovery of H. pylori forces us to reexamine this and other genetic evidence. Incomplete concordance of peptic ulcer occurs in identical twins, and the concordance is less in fraternal twins who share fewer genes. At least some of this concordance might be explained by an inherited susceptibility to H. pylori infection.

Duodenal ulcer has several genetic markers. Individuals with blood type O have a 30% greater than normal risk of duodenal ulcer. However, no such relationship exists between blood type and H. pylori infection. Some people secrete the ABO antigens into body fluids such as saliva. Nonsecretors are 50% more likely to have a duodenal ulcer, and the two traits occurring in the same individual increase his or her risk still further. "Inheritance" of increased blood levels of pepsinogen I or gastrin is also likely to be explained by the presence of H. pylori. Rare, inherited, gastrin-secreting tumors are discussed in Chapter 12. Ulcers also have been associated with some very rare inherited diseases, but these have little overall importance to our story. It may be that genes help determine who amongst those infected with H. pylori will develop an ulcer.

PHYSIOLOGIC FACTORS

Anatomy

Anatomical malformations may predispose one to an ulcer. When a surgeon performs a gastroenterostomy, he or she joins the stomach to the jejunum (see Figure 29-1). Since this segment of small bowel is unaccustomed to defending itself from acid and pepsin, ulcers are prone to occur just beyond the anastomosis. In the embryo, the lower small bowel connects to the yolk sac by the vitelline duct. Occasionally it fails to obliterate before birth and persists as a pouch off the ileum known as a Meckel's diverticulum. Most people with a Meckel's pouch are unaware of it, but sometimes it may behave as the appendix and require surgery. Of interest to us here is the presence of acid-secreting parietal cells in the mucosa that can rarely cause a peptic ulcer. Ulcers sometimes occur in Barrett's esophagus, where the lower esophageal epithelium has been replaced by gastric cells (see Chapter 17). The reason the duodenal cap or bulb is the favored site for peptic ulcers is its proximity to the source of acid and pepsin.

Gastrin

Higher than normal serum gastrin levels are common in those infected with *H. pylori*. They return to normal when the bacteria are killed. Since the acid inhibits the antral G cells, hypochlorhydric states result in an elevated serum gastrin. Pernicious anemia is a striking example. The trophic (growth-stimulating) effect of gastrin on gastric mucosa may cause stomach cancer, to which this disease is prone. An elevated serum gastrin also accompanies prolonged gastric acid suppression with a proton pump inhibitor. This explains the temporary rebound increase in gastric acid when the drug is withdrawn.

There are two situations where very high serum gastrin levels directly cause peptic ulcers. *Gastrinomas* are rare, gastrin-secreting tumors of the pancreas. They produce uncontrolled gastrin, and the resulting ulcer disease is known as the Zollinger–Ellison syndrome. Acid production in this syndrome is so intense that ulcers develop even beyond the duodenal cap. Rarely, after a Billroth II gastrectomy for ulcer disease, some antral tissue is inadvertently left attached to the duodenum. Isolated from the rest of the stomach, it is bathed in alkaline duodenal juice. In this environment it secretes gastrin with ulcerogenic results (see Figure 29-1).

Mucosal Factors

Why do *H. pylori* and NSAIDs cause ulcers in only a few exposed persons? Inheritance, lifestyle, and psychosocial factors are important to be sure, but they must somehow act by weakening mucosal resistance to acid and pepsin. *H. pylori* causes gastritis, and NSAIDs damage the gastric mucosa. Natural adaptation permits the mucosa to recover even if NSAID use continues. Many drugs appear to improve the mucosa's ability to resist ulceration. Prostaglandins do so by promoting secretion of mucus and bicarbonate, increasing mucosal blood flow, and modulating acid secretion. Before the discovery of *H. pylori*, mucosal protection was an important line of research, and it should remain so.

LIFESTYLE

We humans are complex. It is difficult to sort the many apparent ulcer associations and folklore from verifiable causes. The dichotomy between ulcers and dyspepsia is confusing. We may have ulcers without dyspepsia and dyspepsia without ulcers. Many associate their ulcer or dyspepsia with a certain food or situation. It does not follow that these are causes. Life experiences with foods or circumstances help determine our future reactions to them, and this may be emotional as well as physiological. Moreover, the overwhelming influence of *H. pylori* and NSAIDs in ulcer disease must dwarf the impact of an errant lifestyle.

Diet

Myths surround diet and ulcers. Despite the common complaint that spices cause or worsen dyspepsia, spicy foods do not cause ulcers. Spice-eating cultures are not at special risk. Conversely, bland diets do not heal ulcers. Coffee and related drinks increase acid secretion and were often prohibited in ulcer treatment protocols. In retrospect, the sudden withdrawal of caffeine probably caused more headaches than ulcer cures. One study demonstrates that coffee causes symptoms in subjects with non-ulcer dyspepsia, but not in those with ulcers.

In South India, where rice consumption is high, duodenal ulcers are common. Northern Indians, with a prevailing unrefined wheat diet, seem protected, but some lost their protection when they emigrated to South Africa. Was this change due to diet, environment, or the stress of dislocation? Low fiber, high sugar, and high salt diets have all been blamed, but, as yet, no specific food has been proven to increase an individual's risk of acquiring an ulcer.

Smoking

Smoking increases an individual's risk of developing a peptic ulcer. The data suggest that the more one smokes, the greater the risk. Smokers are also more likely than nonsmokers to sustain serious ulcer complications such as perforation. The surgical mortality and overall ulcer death rate are also increased by smoking. However, it is uncertain whether the deaths are due to the ulcers or to anesthetic complications of the smokers' heart and lung disease. Once healed, a smoker's ulcer is more likely to recur than that of an abstainer. Indeed, smokers taking regular H_2 antagonist drugs as maintenance therapy are more likely to have their ulcers recur than nonsmokers on placebo. Antibiotics are less effective against *H. pylori* in smokers compared to nonsmokers. Certainly, there are many cogent reasons to quit.

Alcohol

Moderate consumption of alcohol increases gastric acid secretion and stimulates the appetite. Wine and beer are capable of releasing up to 90% of the stomach's maximal acid output. Paradoxically, large doses of alcohol may inhibit gastric secretion. Furthermore, by reducing mucosal protection against hydrogen ions, alcohol also causes acute gastric erosions that occasionally bleed. However, while alcohol undoubtedly provokes dyspepsia and erosions, it is not an important cause of peptic ulcers.

PSYCHOLOGY AND STRESS

Psychology and Personality

Consider not what type of ulcer the person has, but rather what type of person has the ulcer.

Anonymous

The notion that psychological trauma causes ulcers is part of our culture. Without substantiating data, ulcer sufferers are alleged to be tense, aggressive business types. In the 1930s and 1940s, Alexander and others of the psychosomatic school advanced the idea that an ulcer personality included an unconscious dependency/independency conflict. Such persons have a deep need to be loved and cared for and, as adults, this need is accompanied by loss of confidence and shame. Such a person's defenses include aggression, driving ambition, and attempts to demonstrate self-sufficiency.

To test this hypothesis, Mirsky selected, from 200 new United States Army recruits, 63 who were hypersecretors of pepsinogen I and 57 who were hyposecretors. Before training began, each recruit had a barium series and a psychiatric interview by doctors who were unaware of their secretor status. Ten had a high degree of conflict surrounding dependency, and nine of these were hyposecretors. Four of these had a duodenal ulcer at the outset, and three more acquired one during their training. The experiment supports the belief of many that psychodynamic factors in a constitutionally predisposed person may manifest ulcer disease under stress. These data must now be interpreted in the light of new developments. If we knew the rate of *H. pylori* infection in these subjects, we might better understand the manner in which psychodynamic factors interact with the organism to produce an ulcer.

The picture is confused by other studies that associate peptic ulcers with many different personality traits, so that the ulcer population might merely demonstrate a microcosm of the diverse natures that make up humanity. At first glance psychodynamics seem less important now that we are able to cure ulcers. Relieved of their symptoms, ulcer patients seldom look back. However, these issues may be important in those ulcers not caused by infection or NSAIDs. Also, it is tempting to think that personality may do little to cause an ulcer, but rather determines how a person with dyspepsia will behave.

Stress and Psychophysiology

It is the common experience that emotion acutely affects gut function. Who has not experienced a queasy stomach, diarrhea, vomiting, or other gut reaction in response to a stressful situation? Such a situation might be an exam, an interview, a board meeting, a wedding, or any other trying encounter that life brings. It is more difficult to relate stress to chronic digestive complaints such as peptic ulcer or dyspepsia.

Several members of the animal kingdom have given their all to help us understand the role of stress in ulcers. Rats, restrained in the cold, developed gastric erosions. Pairs of monkeys were restrained in chairs and randomly subjected to electric shocks. One of the pair, the executive, could stop a shock by quickly pushing a button. This monkey acquired an ulcer for his responsibility. His partner, apparently resigned to his fate, no doubt suffered in other ways, but his duodenum survived. This is reminiscent of a study of London transport workers, in which drivers of double-decker buses acquired more ulcers than their conductors, who were apparently less bothered by London traffic. Of course, one could argue that it was their "ulcer personality" that made them drivers rather than conductors.

In 1833, Beaumont noted that the gastric mucosa of his gastric fistula subject became pale and produced less gastric juice in response to fear, anger, or impatience. One hundred years later, Hoetzel, a Chicago physiologist who daily collected a morning sample of his own gastric juice, noted that his acid secretion *increased* after his landlady was shot. A high gastric acid secretion might have been a feature of the Chicago of Al Capone, but Hoetzel's reaction was the opposite to that observed by Beaumont. Shay induced increased acid output by stressful interviews, and even conditioned the response so that the mere sight of the interviewer increased acid secretion. In their gastric fistula subject, Tom, Wolf and Wolff found that his stomach flushed and increased its movements and secretion when Tom became hostile, resentful, or anxious. Fear and sadness induced the opposite reactions.

When a balloon was inflated in Tom's flushed stomach, he experienced pain at a lesser than normal degree of inflation. This gut hypersensitivity under stress noted half a century ago predicted much modern research on the functional gastrointestinal disorders. Keep it in mind when we discuss functional dyspepsia and functional abdominal bloating (Part 5).

One experiment demonstrated that young men increase their gastric acid secretion while reading erotic literature. Does this prove that even love has gastric risks? Perhaps the way to a young man's heart is through his stomach after all? Of special interest here is an anticholinergic drug that prevented this vagally mediated secretion. Brain–gut communication from *Playboy* to parietal cell is evidently transmitted via the vagus.

Life Events

Patients often relate their ulcer to a stressful life event such as loss of a job, divorce, or death in the family. In 1944, there was a sharp increase in perforated ulcers in London hospitals after a severe air raid. Physical stress such as brain surgery causes ulcers (Cushing). Long and Curling demonstrated their occurrence after severe burns 150 years ago (see Chapter 4). Nevertheless, the relationship of ulcers to stress is controversial, and other studies fail to support the notion. For example, air traffic controllers, certainly a stressed group, are apparently at no increased risk.

Mind–Gut Conclusions

Our remedies oft in ourselves do lie,
Which we ascribe to Heaven.
W. Shakespeare, *All's Well That Ends Well*, Act 1, Scene i

These observations illustrate the variability of the human response to stress. One author suggested there are 29 kinds of peptic ulcer based on psychobiology. Perhaps genetics or early life experiences program us to respond physiologically in a unique way. The vagus nerve serves as the conduit through which emotions and the brain influence the enteric nervous system and vice versa. The behaviors of the disease and the patient are interdependent. Some bear their ulcer with equanimity approaching indifference, while others cannot cope and permit dyspepsia to consume their daily lives. It is now an easy thing to heal an ulcer, but illness behavior and the stresses of life remain as challenges for some patients, especially those with functional dyspepsia.

SUMMARY

It is now clear that in the presence of gastric acid, *H. pylori* and NSAIDs are the principal causes of most peptic ulcers. However, why most infected persons and NSAID-takers do not have ulcers and why some who have ulcers neither use NSAIDs nor have *H. pylori*, are unexplained phenomena. Many believe that other factors tilt the balance toward ulcer formation. Geneticists point to inherited traits, psychologists to stress and personality, and the Puritans among us to a degenerate lifestyle. Whatever their role in the causation of peptic ulcers, these factors should be remembered when considering the whole patient.

PART THREE

Peptic Ulcers: Diagnosis and Treatment

CHAPTER TEN

Dyspepsia

> The very complexity of the classification and description of gastric neuroses in the text books, the diversity of opinion concerning their causation, and the innumerable modes of treatment suggested by the authors lead us at once to question the supposed facts concerning them. . . . these are disturbances in gastric function, motor, secretory and sensory for which we can, by the minutest examination find no organic basis.
>
> J. B. Deaver, 1909

> Dyspepsia . . . remains a very non-specific term that has been interpreted in many different ways.
>
> N. J. Talley et al., 1991

"Plus ca change, plus c'est la même chose!" Doctors ended the 20th century as they began it, struggling to define and classify dyspepsia. There are many proposed definitions, but none is entirely satisfactory (Table 10-1). We need an understandable concept of dyspepsia to help the primary care physician decide which tests and treatments to choose. Dyspepsia should be defined clearly enough to permit him or her to make rational decisions for the 2–5% of primary care patients who complain of it.

Earlier surveys estimate the prevalence of dyspepsia at from 6–30%. The higher estimate includes individuals with heartburn, which is very common in its own right. Using the more restrictive Rome criteria, a survey of 8,250 householders (66% response) put the prevalence at 2.6%, excluding structural diseases. Thus, omitting those with known peptic ulcers, at least 6 million Americans are dyspeptic, a figure to keep in mind as we consider the manage-

TABLE 10-1
Some Definitions of Dyspepsia[a]

Rhind and Watson (1968)   Epigastric discomfort after meals, a feeling of fullness so that tight clothing is loosened, eructation with temporary relief, and regurgitation of sour fluid into the mouth and heartburn ("flatulent dyspepsia").

Crean et al. (1982)   Any form of episodic or persistent abdominal discomfort or other symptom referable to the alimentary tract, especially jaundice or bleeding.

Thompson (1984)   Chronic, recurrent, often meal-related epigastric discomfort initially suspected to be a peptic ulcer.

Lagarde and Spiro (1984)   Intermittent upper abdominal discomfort.

Talley and Piper (1985)   Pain, discomfort, or nausea referable to the upper alimentary tract that is intermittent or continuous, has been present for a month or more, is not precipitated by exertion nor relieved by rest, and is not associated with jaundice, bleeding, or dysphagia.

Nyren et al. (1987)   Epigastric pain or discomfort a key symptom, in absence of irritable bowel symptoms and organic disease ("epigastric distress syndrome").

Talley and Phillips (1988)   Chronic or recurrent (>3 months) upper abdominal pain or nausea that may or may not be related to meals.

Colin-Jones et al. (1988)   Upper abdominal or retrosternal pain, discomfort, heartburn, nausea, vomiting, or other symptom considered to be referable to the proximal portion of the digestive tract.

Barbara et al. (1989)   Episodic or persistent abdominal symptoms, often related to feeding, that patients or physicians believe to be due to disorders of the proximal portion of the digestive tract.

Heading (1991)   Episodic or persistent abdominal symptoms, which include abdominal pain or discomfort. The term dyspepsia is not applied to patients whose symptoms are thought to be arising from outside the proximal gastrointestinal tract.

Talley et al. (Rome) (1991)   Persistent or recurrent abdominal pain or abdominal discomfort centered in the upper abdomen.

Klauser et al. (1993)   Complaints thought to emanate from the upper gastrointestinal tract, i.e., upper abdominal pain or discomfort, retrosternal pain or discomfort not related to physical activity, heartburn, and nausea and vomiting.

Present definition (1996)   Chronic or recurrent (3 months) epigastric pain or discomfort that suggests peptic ulcer disease; not GERD, IBS, angina, biliary colic, pancreatic, or skeletal pain.

[a]Updated from George et al., 1993.

ment costs of individual cases. This chapter includes a discussion of the definitions of dyspepsia, how dyspepsia differs from other causes of epigastric distress, ulcer versus non-ulcer dyspepsia, and the efficiency of an early diagnosis when compared to a trial of anti-ulcer therapy.

WHAT IS DYSPEPSIA?

Most agree that dyspepsia is a recurrent pain or discomfort in the upper abdomen. Some would add bloating, nausea, and belching. Frequently the symptoms are temporally related to eating. Patients blame what they eat, but specific foods are seldom proved to cause dyspepsia. The difficulty is to distinguish in words what we understand as dyspepsia from other well-characterized structural and functional entities that also cause upper abdominal pain or discomfort. Some translate dyspepsia as *indigestion*. This term is even more confusing, however, and it sometimes refers to diarrhea or constipation. An international panel suggests that it not be used. Since we cannot define dyspepsia well, it is helpful to consider what it is not.

What Is Not Dyspepsia?

The pains associated with cholecystitis and biliary colic are characteristic and readily diagnosed. These consist of acute, severe, unpredictable, self-limited attacks of epigastric or right upper quadrant abdominal pain often felt under the right scapula. This is gall bladder pain, not dyspepsia, and the term "gall bladder dyspepsia" has no pathophysiological basis. Nevertheless, many still believe that the more chronic and recurrent epigastric distress that we call dyspepsia can be caused by gallstones and cured by their removal. This is despite the fact that dyspepsia, defined in various ways, is no more common in those with, than in those without, gallstones (Table 10-2). Certainly, the coincidental presence of dyspepsia with gallstones should not constitute an indication for surgery. Even Deaver, an early 20th century surgeon, cautioned against operation for what he called "gastric neurosis."

Through careful history-taking a physician should identify the exercise-related nature of angina, or the episodic, severe abdominal and back pain of pancreatitis. The irritable bowel syndrome (IBS) may include epigastric pain, but in this case the pain is altered by defecation or followed by a change in the consistency and frequency of stool. Chest or abdominal wall pains are elicited by movement or examination.

TABLE 10-2
Dyspepsia and Gallstones

Author	Study	Dyspepsia and gallstones	Dyspepsia and no gallstones
Price, 1963	147 (women) having gallbladder X ray	12/24 (50%)	63/118 (53%)
Koch, 1964	Hospital patients (fatty food intolerance)	26/27 (28%)	26/47 (35%)
Bainton, 1976	Random sample of 1043 males	5/65 (7%)	88/978 (9%)
Barbara, 1987	70% of Italian town (1936 people)	Bloating (37%)	42%
		Abdominal discomfort (8%)	11%

The term "reflux-like dyspepsia" has been proposed. But, retrosternal or high epigastric burning discomfort provoked by food, chocolate, and large meals; worsened by bending and recumbency; and relieved by antacid is *heartburn*. It is due to gastroesophageal reflux disease (GERD), a syndrome distinct from dyspepsia. Heartburn and GERD present distinct diagnostic and treatment challenges (see Chapter 16). One adult in three suffers heartburn, and one in ten experiences it at least once a month. Thus the clinical distinction of heartburn from dyspepsia is very important.

There remain many people with epigastric pain and discomfort who have dyspepsia. Consensus groups have classified dyspepsia into *ulcer-like* and *motility-like*. This follows the hope that clinical subdivisions might clarify the underlying physiology. Osler and others proposed similar subgroups almost a century ago. Sadly, these subdivisions have no known physiological correlates, and clinically they cannot be distinguished easily from one another. Therefore such distinctions do not help the family doctor.

The real question in the dyspeptic patient is whether there is an ulcer. Thus, in practical terms, dyspepsia is best characterized as epigastric pain or discomfort that suggests peptic ulcer disease. An appropriate 1996 definition might be "chronic or recurrent epigastric pain or discomfort that suggests peptic ulcer disease and is not GERD, not IBS, not angina, not biliary colic, pancreatic or skeletal pain" (Table 10-1).

ULCER OR NON-ULCER?

The principal question raised by a new dyspeptic is "ulcer or non-ulcer?" One has the potential for serious complications, the other not; one is treatable with medication, the other probably not. The discovery that *H. pylori* causes chronic gastritis adds a new urgency to the need to distinguish the two. *H. pylori* also has a strong relationship to peptic ulcer, but it does not follow that there is a relationship between this organism and non-ulcer (functional) dyspepsia. The bacteria are very common in the community and, also by chance, in those with dyspepsia. Yet, most non-ulcer dyspeptics do not harbor the organism. Even if only infected non-ulcer dyspeptics were treated, the costs would be great. So far, attribution of the symptoms of functional dyspepsia to the organism is unconvincing. Clinical trials testing the benefits of eradication are conflicting and flawed. *H. pylori* causes gastritis, but many who have either or both have no symptoms. Older studies fail to associate gastritis with symptoms.

It is important to make the distinction between ulcer and non-ulcer when a patient has severe dyspepsia or has not responded to lifestyle changes and antacids and is at the point where the physician is considering drug therapy. This conclusion assumes that anti-ulcer drug treatment, including eradication of *H. pylori* is ineffective treatment for non-ulcer dyspepsia (Chapter 18).

Are Ulcers and Non-Ulcers the Same Disease?

In 1974, Spiro suggested that ulcer and non-ulcer dyspepsia are the same disease, and that the ulcer is incidental and transient. Both ulcers and non-ulcers have dyspepsia. Both have a chronic remitting natural history. Both seem to be stress-related, affect all ages, and tend to respond to placebos.

However, Spiro's hypothesis predates effective treatment of ulcers and the realization that drug treatment for non-ulcer dyspepsia is no better than placebo. Furthermore, those with functional dyspepsia tend to remain non-ulcer. Unlike ulcer patients, they have acid secretion and genetic profiles similar to normal individuals. *H. pylori* is present in most cases of non-NSAID duodenal ulcer, but it is likely no more common in non-ulcer dyspepsia than in the background population. Non-ulcer dyspepsia is an entity with a different pathogenesis and treatment from peptic ulcer disease.

Can Clinical Examination Distinguish Ulcer from Non-Ulcer?

When, with great confidence, I make the diagnosis of duodenal ulcer from the clinical history alone, I feel wounded and amazed if I prove wrong; whereas when, with a sense of pride in my courage, I make the diagnosis of gastric ulcer, I feel very contented, even a little elated, if I prove right.

B. Moynihan, 1923

Despite Moynihan's confidence with duodenal ulcers, there is no clinical profile that permits the family doctor to determine who among his dyspeptic patients has an ulcer. Of course, a history of previous ulcer or its complications or a strong family history are compelling clues. Nocturnal pain relieved with antacids suggests an ulcer, but not nocturnal pain alone. There are duodenal ulcer patients who describe a typical, Moynihan-like history of pain, food, relief, and pain, but these are exceptional. Other patients with the same history have no ulcer. Even abdominal tenderness is not a sign of an ulcer. Therefore there are no reliable means short of endoscopy or barium contrast radiography to determine which dyspeptic individuals have peptic ulcers.

Among dyspeptic patients endoscoped in specialty clinics, about half have no ulcer or other upper gastrointestinal pathology (Table 10-3). Regrettably, the definition of dyspepsia is unclear in many of these studies. The inclusion of heartburn greatly increases the number of patients entered in the study, which results in an apparent lower prevalence of ulcer. The proportion of non-ulcer to ulcer dyspepsia may be greater in family practice than in specialist centers, and, without diagnosis, the employment of anti-ulcer therapy will be often inappropriate. Consider the cost of providing currently recommended ulcer therapy for the estimated 6 million Americans and 600,000 Canadians with functional dyspepsia! Once a practice of blind therapy becomes established,

TABLE 10-3
Percent of Dyspeptic Patients without Ulcer by
Endoscopy

Study	Participants	No ulcer[a]
Williams, 1988 (UK)	686	49
Mansi, 1990 (Italy)	2086	62
Hallisey, 1990 (Ireland)	2659	32
Möller-Hansen, 1991 (Denmark)	436	59
Bytzcr, 1992 (Denmark)	878	64
Klauser, 1993 (Germany)	220	25
Hu, 1995 (China)	1006	50
	Mean	49%

[a]Or other gross lesion by endoscopy.

many patients with the IBS or GERD will be treated inadvertently for ulcer, especially if we are careless with the definition of dyspepsia.

What Use Is a Trial of Therapy?

If drugs work for ulcers and not for non-ulcers, why not treat every dyspeptic and let the results determine the diagnosis? Oh, that it was that simple! Double blind clinical trials indicate that 30–50% of patients with both conditions experience a symptomatic improvement on placebo (see Table 30-3). Therefore the response of dyspepsia to anti-ulcer medication is of little value in diagnosis.

Furthermore, non-NSAID duodenal ulcers have about a 60% chance of recurring within 1 year of healing. This is true when the drugs are stopped after 1 year of remission maintenance with an H_2 antagonist. It takes at least 5 years of H_2 antagonist therapy to alter the natural history of peptic ulcer. The normal chronic and recurrent course of the disease extends over 10 years or more. Non-ulcer dyspepsia also has a chronic, recurrent course, and, over 2–7 years, 70% of patients continue to have symptoms. Since both types of dyspepsia have a placebo response and both are likely to recur, so will the quandary: ulcer versus non-ulcer.

Is an Initial Diagnosis Necessary?

To 'scope or not to 'scope?
Anonymous

The Best Test

In 1985, the American College of Physicians (ACP), mindful of endoscopy costs, recommended that dyspeptic patients should receive a trial of anti-ulcer therapy. Then, anti-ulcer therapy meant 6–8 weeks of an H_2 antagonist such as ranitidine. Much has changed in the last decade, and it is time to examine whether this policy is the correct one.

If an investigation is to be done, which is the test of choice? Endoscopy is more accurate, cost-effective, and better accepted by patients than barium contrast radiography. Endoscopy is very safe in healthy individuals and permits biopsy to detect gastritis, *H. pylori*, or cancer in suspicious lesions. This procedure is therefore the diagnostic "gold standard." If endoscopy is not available or is too expensive, then an air contrast barium X ray is a less reliable second choice. Other tests are of little value in the investigation of dyspepsia.

Costs

Analysis of the ACP policy must consider not only the initial cost of endoscopy but also the long-term cost of doctor visits, repeated drug therapy, work loss, and poor quality of life of patients with both conditions. Endoscopy is costly in some parts of the United States, but is becoming less so. In Canada, the procedure costs only 60% more than a 2-month course of ranitidine and about the same as 4 weeks of omeprazole (Table 10-4). The cost of an initial, precise endoscopic diagnosis in dyspeptic patients is similar to anti *H. pylori* therapy, perhaps less so if unwanted effects of the drugs are considered.

Most dyspeptics will not need drugs. Those dyspeptics with ulcers cannot be identified by a therapeutic trial, and blind therapy may even obscure the diagnosis. The placebo response will encourage continued use of a drug. Most patients' symptoms will recur within a year. Rarely will a gastric cancer be missed. Therefore, the

TABLE 10-4
Costs of Endoscopy Compared to Ulcer Therapy[a]

Item	Cost	Cure rate	Side effects
Endoscopy and biopsy	117.40		
Dual therapy	107.93	80%	10%
Omeprazole 20 mg twice daily; Amoxacillin 500 mg four times daily for 2 weeks			
Triple therapy	127.57	90%	50%
Bismuth subsalicylate 2 tablets four times daily; Metronidazole 250 mg three times daily; Tetracycline 500 mg four times daily; Ranitidine 300 mg at bedtime each night for 2 weeks[b]			

[a]In Canadian dollars. Ontario rates, 1994.
[b]Ranitidine, a fourth drug, is needed in active disease to relieve symptoms and heal the ulcer.

less obvious costs of the ACP policy may be much greater than those of a precise, initial diagnosis.

Data support this point of view. Four hundred and fourteen Danish patients had "upper dyspepsia" that their general practitioners considered to be eligible for empirical therapy with H_2 antagonists. Investigators compared empirical therapy with prompt endoscopy where those found not to have an ulcer were denied anti-ulcer medication. Although the initial costs were less in the empirical group, 66% of the empirically treated patients required an endoscopy within 1 year because of treatment failure or relapse. Also because of loss of employment and drugs given over the year, the costs in the empiric group were eventually greater.

Moreover, empirical therapy did not improve the case selection for endoscopy, since the ulcer-to-non-ulcer ratio in the repeat endoscopy group was no different from that at the beginning of the trial. Approximately 40% of peptic ulcers were missed in the empiric group after 1 year, and there were two cases of gastric cancer in each group. The trial of therapy clearly failed to identify those at risk, and the outcome was similar for all age groups. The investigators employed "open-access endoscopy," which permits the general practitioner to bypass consultation. Nonetheless, the apparent cost savings of empirical therapy in any system will be greatly diminished if 66% of blindly treated patients require endoscopy within a year.

Australian physicians compared a strategy that required confirmation of an ulcer in dyspeptic patients before H_2 antagonist treatment, with an approach where no diagnosis was made. General practitioners prescribed drugs as they saw fit. The costs of the two strategies were similar over a 6-month period ($392 and $406).

Employing a decision analysis technique, Talley compared the costs of empiric therapy and endoscopy in the management of dyspepsia. As expected, initial empiric therapy was cheaper, but by 1 year, the costs had equalized. Cheaper endoscopy or more expensive drugs would make prompt diagnosis more cost-effective. Expensive new therapies such as omeprazole or *H. pylori* eradication raise the diagnostic stakes. If the policy is to be a trial of therapy, many people without ulcers will be treated. A precise diagnosis may, after all, be the most cost-effective policy.

Fendrick *et al.* employed a decision analysis technique to conclude that a precise diagnosis of dyspepsia was unnecessary, and that testing for *H. pylori*, or blind treatment with antisecretory drugs with or without antibiotics was more cost-effective than any policy involving prompt endoscopy. Decision analysis is an arm chair estimate of the cost of various clinical decisions. Conclusions are based upon assumptions that may or may not be available in the literature. There are several reasons why the conclusions of Fendrick *et al.* cannot be taken at face value. Aside from the uncertainties generated by blind approaches (see below), many of their assumptions may be challenged. For example, the cost of endoscopy plus biopsy is fixed at $1390. In many jurisdictions the costs will be less than a third that amount. The cost of endoscopy is coming down, and open-access endoscopy, where available, is even cheaper. In their sensitivity analysis, Fendrick *et al.* make this point themselves.

Furthermore, the authors put the symptom 1-year recurrence rate in patients with nonulcer dyspepsia at 30% and quote only two of several sources of information. Others see it as twice that rate, and since dyspepsia is a life-long complaint in most, recurrence seems inevitable. Drugs introduced blindly to nonulcer dyspeptics may continue beyond the one year considered in the study. Not mentioned is the accelerated development of bacterial resistance that will result from unwarranted exposure to the few available effective antibiotics. Many would consider the 0.5% incidence of serious antibiotic complications as too optimistic.

Several approaches to dyspepsia are proposed as *The Ulcer Story* goes to press. Greenberg presents data to support endoscopy, eradication therapy in ulcer patients, and no test for *H. pylori*, Fendrick proposes a non-endoscopic approach, while Bytzer prefers prompt endoscopy. Graham and Rabeneck attempt a compromise whereby dyspeptics at risk from complications or other disease should be promptly endoscoped, while the healthy remainder should be tested for the organism. Those who are *H. pylori* positive should receive eradication therapy, while those who are negative should be treated "symptomatically" with an antisecretory drug. Failure of either group to improve in two weeks should prompt an endoscopy. The latter seems destined to forestall few endoscopies in the long run.

Each proponent is greatly influenced by the economic and medical realities of their own community. My bias is clear. A policy where blind therapy of a chronic disease with drugs that have important downsides and costs is substituted for precise, targeted therapy is not merely intellectually unsatisfactory. The uncertainty will have costs that are not easily envisaged from the arm chair. Licentious deployment of drugs will spread to patients with heartburn, or IBS who are not dyspeptic at all. Uncertainty obstructs reassurance and all its healing potential. Eventually, the dyspeptic will insist on the truth, and an endoscopy will be done at the least optimum time.

These economic and social issues cannot be settled in the abstract. Only well-designed studies based in primary care will do. Meanwhile, specialists can do more to improve the access and reduce the cost of evidence-based medicine to the dyspeptic.

Diagnosis as Therapy

However, cost is surely not the only issue here. Many dyspeptics do not seek medical help, but those that do often have psychosocial distress and fear of cancer. Therefore, reassurance becomes a powerful therapeutic tool. One English study demonstrated that nonulcer dyspeptics had only one-fifth the doctor visits or prescriptions in the year following endoscopy compared to the year before. Another study by the Danish group compared non-ulcer dyspeptics 6 months after to 6 months before endoscopy. There were 41% fewer doctor visits, and 72% less drug taking. Fifty-two percent were reassured, and 66% were improved and more productive at work. A second English study produced similar results to the Danish one. The authors concluded that open-access gastroscopy has a major effect on patient management in general practice, and is associated with rationalization of drug therapy, reduced doctor visits, and a low referral rate. The positive results of early diagnosis therefore challenge the stated benefits of a trial of therapy. As Hungin et al. (1994) noted, "A normal endoscopy has as important an impact as an abnormal one."

FACTORS THAT WILL INFLUENCE THE DECISION TO DIAGNOSE DYSPEPSIA

The availability of prompt endoscopy or good quality radiography to the primary care physician is essential to a good diagnostic strategy. An endoscopy service, free of the need for a full consultation, may be cost-effective. Such services are available in Europe. Cheaper and prompter endoscopy may avoid chronic medication and better satisfy patients. To be practical, the service should be used only for the truly dyspetic, and the results of endoscopy should determine the treatment.

Of course, if we believe that the eradication of H. pylori is a desirable end in itself, then diagnosis of an ulcer is less relevant. Screening of the population for the organism and treatment of those infected would involve very many people, with few having dyspepsia. Such a policy would be very expensive, even if the diagnosis were made by serologic means. Not only would the project be futile, but also resistant organisms and antibiotic side effects also seem inevitable.

Once annihilation of H. pylori becomes the objective, overall management would shift from clinics and doctor's offices into the public policy domain. Antibiotics cannot exterminate the bacteria. Only with a worldwide campaign for better sanitation, less crowding, and better child care can we hope to reduce the infection rate. In the future we may have a vaccine, but the enormous reservoirs of infected persons in the developing world make the task of vaccination forbidding and the cost awesome.

Whether eradication of *H. pylori* turns out to alleviate non-ulcer dyspepsia will also influence the decision to diagnose before treating. Here we must insist on clinically significant treatment trial results. Marginal benefits or a chance positive result to one of many symptoms will not do. Even proof that non-ulcer dyspepsia will improve if the organism is killed would still leave unhelped the majority who do not harbor it. As yet that proof is not forthcoming.

A British panel determined that the most common reason for an inappropriate endoscopy was misdiagnosis of IBS. In 1996, it is still best to identify those with dyspepsia through careful history taking. The physician can exclude structural disease through physical examination and can determine if the dyspepsia is ulcer or not by endoscopy or good quality radiography. A United States National Institutes of Health panel recommends combination antibiotic therapy for those patients with peptic ulcer who test positively for *H. pylori* (see Table 8-2). Thus, if an ulcer is found, a test for the organism is indicated (see Table 8-1). Those found not to have an ulcer should avoid drug therapy, at least until subgroups can be identified for which a treatment is beneficial (see Chapter 18).

Case Selection

Blind therapy of dyspeptics is no longer tenable. Curative treatment of non-NSAID peptic ulcers requires diagnosis and detection of *H. pylori*. Is there a way to predict which dyspeptics are likely to have ulcers? A London study concluded that serology for *H. pylori* antibodies was more accurate than symptom questionnaires in selecting ulcer patients from those attending open-access endoscopy. The same group found that a positive salivary test for the organisms predicted all non-NSAID peptic ulcers in dyspeptics under the age of 45. Another study from Northern Ireland produced similar results with serology and calculated that screening could have saved 35% of endoscopies.

Breath tests may prove to be faster and more practical. Once reliable, cheap, noninvasive tests for the organism are available, endoscopy could be restricted to those cases where the organism or where NSAIDS use are present. The remaining dyspeptics likely have no ulcer and require no pharmacotherapy. This ideal may have dollars-and-cents appeal. However, it makes no sense if non-ulcer patients are not reassured and if their physicians are unwilling to withhold anti-ulcer drugs.

SUMMARY

A precise distinction between ulcer and non-ulcer requires endoscopy or high-quality radiology. Its utility depends upon the characterization of dyspepsia as compatible with a peptic ulcer, but not with IBS, GERD, biliary tract disease, or other non-gastric disease, and upon the conviction with which physicians are prepared to withhold unproven drugs in non-ulcer dyspepsia. With these caveats, an initial endoscopic diagnosis is the most cost-effective approach and the most likely to improve the quality of life. Those found to have an ulcer who are infected with *H. pylori* should have the organisms killed by one of the regimens recommended by the NIH consensus development panel.

While a cheap, quick, accurate test for the organism may select those who have ulcers and save endoscopies, two questions remain. Is it safe to manage the others without making a diagnosis? While early studies suggest this is so, how important are the benefits of a negative endoscopy? Until there are better data, an initial, precise diagnosis of dyspepsia is fundamental to rational therapy and should be a sound investment. Cost savings will be greater if drugs become more expensive or if the cost of endoscopy is reduced.

CHAPTER ELEVEN

Peptic Ulcer

Gastric and Duodenal

Gastric and duodenal ulcers have several differences, which are summarized in Table 11-1. Since they both require the presence of acid and since most are associated with either *H. pylori* infection or NSAID ingestion, this chapter will treat them as one disease.

GASTRIC VERSUS DUODENAL ULCERS

Differences

Many regard gastric and duodenal ulcers as separate diseases. Duodenal ulcer was rare in the last century, but much commoner than gastric ulcer in this one. It is most prevalent in young men with blood type O who are not ABO antigen secretors. It tends to occur in people with high or high normal basal and maximum acid secretion.

Gastric ulcers are more common in women, especially older women, and those who have decreased acid secretion. Patients with gastric ulcer are also less likely than those with duodenal ulcer to be infected with *H. pylori*. However, they are more likely than duodenal ulcers to be caused by NSAIDs (Table 11-1).

Similarities

Despite these differences, the similarities between gastric and duodenal ulcers make it convenient to lump them together. They

TABLE 11-1
Comparison of Gastric and Duodenal Ulcers

Duodenal ulcer	Gastric ulcer
Younger men	Older women
Tendency toward blood group O	–
ABO secretors	–
90% H. pylori positive	70% H. pylori positive
Tendency toward acid hypersecretion	Acid secretion normal or low
–	May resemble cancer
Less likely NSAID-related	More commonly NSAID-related

both cause dyspepsia, and their symptoms do not reliably distinguish one from the other. The complications of bleeding, perforation, and obstruction occur in both. The means of diagnosis are the same. Drug treatments for gastric and duodenal ulcers are similar.

The closer a gastric ulcer is to the pylorus, the more it behaves like a duodenal ulcer. Prepyloric and pyloric ulcers tend to be hypersecretors of acid, be of blood type O, and exhibit the pain–food–relief–pain sequence. These observations are of little practical significance, but they emphasize the blurred distinction between gastric and duodenal ulcers.

PATHOLOGY

Ugliness is a point of view: an ulcer is wonderful to a pathologist
Austin O'Malley, 1859–1938

A peptic ulcer results from the destruction of the gastric or duodenal mucosa and excavation to the muscularis mucosa and beyond (see Figures 3-1 and 11-1). For unknown reasons peptic ulcers are usually round and solitary. There is edema and inflammation in the surrounding mucosa, but this may be less marked in NSAID ulcers. The base of the ulcer appears white or gray against the pink of the surrounding mucosa (Figure 11-2). There is necrotic (dead) tissue with inflammatory cells in the ulcer base. In large, chronic ulcers such as that in Figure 11-1, the process undermines the edges and penetrates the muscle coat of the stomach or duodenal wall. Protective inflammation and fibrosis occur, but this ulcer is in danger of penetrating beyond the wall. If it is a posterior ulcer, it may penetrate into the pancreas, causing pancreatitis. If the ulcer

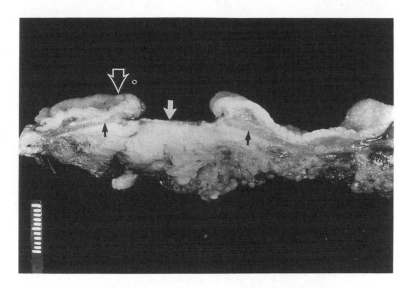

Figure 11-1. Gastric ulcer. A segment of surgically removed stomach wall containing a large gastric ulcer is seen in profile. The solid white arrow indicates the base of the ulcer that has penetrated into and destroyed the muscle layer. (Black arrows indicate the intact muscle area of the stomach that has been destroyed in the ulcer base.) The hollow arrow indicates adjacent inflamed mucosa. Note that there is undermining of the mucosa at the edges of the ulcer.

is on the anterior surface, it may perforate into the peritoneum, requiring emergency surgery.

Acute ulcers and erosions can disappear without a trace. Chronic ulcers go through periods of activity and healing. Since healing includes fibrosis, scarring occurs. This can lead to deformity in the duodenum, a contracted fold opposite a gastric ulcer, or irreversible obstruction at the pylorus.

DIAGNOSIS

History

The leading peculiarity of disease of the duodenum, so far as we are acquainted with it, seems to be that food is taken with relish, and the first stage of digestion is not impeded before pain begins about the time when the fluid is leaving the stomach two to four hours after meals.

John Abercrombie, 1830

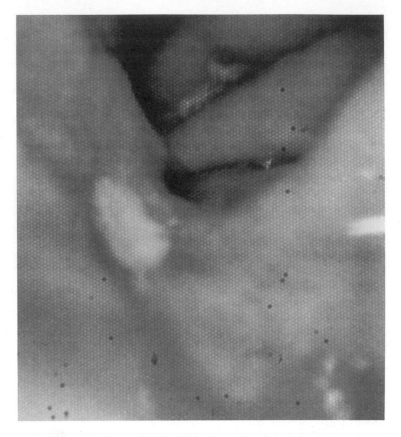

Figure 11-2. A small gastric ulcer seen through a fiberoptic gastroscope. It is circular and solitary, and its white base of destroyed tissue, inflammation, and fibrin formation contrasts with the surrounding pink mucosa. The black dots are caused by broken fiber bundles in the gastroscope.

In exceptional cases, ulcers may become complicated and bring themselves to attention through bleeding, perforation, or obstruction. Here we are concerned with uncomplicated ulcers, the cardinal feature of which is dyspepsia. As explained in the previous chapter, dyspepsia may occur with or without an ulcer; only endoscopy or barium X ray can determine whether or not an ulcer is present.

Moynihan claimed to be able to diagnose a duodenal ulcer by symptoms alone, although he was less confident of gastric ulcer.

This is not the usual case today. Nevertheless, a typical duodenal ulcer history occasionally occurs. The pain is in the upper abdomen and is often burning or gnawing in quality. It occurs with hunger, as the stomach secretes acid in anticipation of a meal. There is relief when food neutralizes and dilutes the acid, but pain returns 1–3 hours after meals, when the neutralizing food leaves the stomach. Much has been made of the significance of nocturnal pain. Certainly, pain that awakes one at night should make one suspicious of an ulcer, but it is not specific for one. Suspicion should be heightened if the awakening pain is promptly relieved by antacids. The pain or discomfort that we call dyspepsia tends to occur regularly and predictably over days and weeks, and then disappear for a time. Many patients report that their ulcer is most active in the spring or autumn.

Regrettably, most ulcers do not fit the textbook pattern. Also, among those with dyspepsia, only half turn out to have an ulcer (see Table 10-3). Nevertheless, a peptic ulcer must be suspected in any dyspeptic patient. Sometimes the pain is to the right or left of the epigastrium (below the breast bone), and it may be felt in the back. Some ulcer patients say the pain has no relation to meals. Indeed, both gastric and duodenal ulcers can occur without dyspepsia and may come to attention because of bleeding or perforation. A family history of peptic ulcer, NSAID ingestion, or evidence of bleeding should increase one's suspicions. Nevertheless, once an ulcer is suspected in a dyspeptic person, its presence or absence can only be determined by endoscopy. The implications of this are often evaded by those who advocate a blind trial of therapy.

Physical Examination

Textbooks describe abdominal tenderness as a feature of peptic ulcers. Tenderness is partly subjective since the examiner must report the patient's reaction or report of discomfort when he or she presses the epigastrium. In a study of dyspeptics attending for endoscopy, two observers tested each patient independently for tenderness. The presence of tenderness did not predict who would have an ulcer. Uncomplicated peptic ulcer has no physical signs.

TESTS

Endoscopy

Endoscopy is the gold standard for ulcer diagnosis (see Figure 31-1). An experienced endoscopist should seldom overlook a peptic ulcer. It is difficult to calculate the exact sensitivity of this procedure, but observer error appears to be small. The endoscopist sees an uncomplicated gastric or duodenal ulcer as a solitary, circular white-gray area against the surrounding pink mucosa (Figure 11-2). It may be 0.5–5 cm in diameter and is rarely larger. Large ulcers may penetrate through the wall of the stomach or duodenum, giving it the craterlike appearance seen in Figure 11-1.

X Ray

After swallowing a suspension of barium, the subject has X-ray pictures taken of various views of the duodenum (Figure 11-3). Barium comes to rest in the ulcer crater and may be seen *en face* as a circular white blob on the X-ray film. In profile it appears as a projection of barium beyond the natural curvature of the stomach or duodenum. There may also be local spasm and eventually scarring. Spasm and scarring of the duodenum deform it, often into a cloverleaf shape. In the stomach, spasm around the ulcer may draw in the opposite wall to form a band or incisura separating the stomach into two parts like an hourglass. Folds radiate from the ulcer, reassuring the radiologist that the adjacent tissue is not malignant.

The quality of barium X-rays of the stomach and duodenum is very dependent on technique. Inexperienced operators sometimes "overcall" collections of barium resting in normal folds, especially in the duodenum (Figure 11-4). Perhaps it is better to err on the side of overcall than to permit a real ulcer to go unnoticed, but the long-term consequences of this can be against the patient's interests. Not only does he or she become committed to unwarranted medication, but having an ulcer diagnosis can also prohibit some types of employment and provoke higher life and health insurance premiums.

Modern radiologists employ an air-contrast technique. The patient swallows gas-forming tablets containing just enough barium to lightly coat the mucosa. Barium in an ulcer stands out in bold relief against the air-filled stomach or duodenum, and the accuracy in all but the smallest lesions approaches that of endoscopy. Where endoscopy is not available or too expensive, radiology must do. However, it is less precise and there are several other disadvantages. If an ulcer is found, biopsies cannot be taken for *H. pylori* or to ensure that a gastric ulcer is not cancer. Esophagitis and small gastric erosions will not be seen. Since the radiologist is not the treating physician, there may be inefficiency between diagnosis, interpretation, and treatment.

Other Tests

Rarely, ulcers are seen by chance using ultrasound or computerized tomography. These are not appropriate investigations for dyspepsia, but they become important when assessing perforation, obstruction, and possible cancer. A blood count is relevant since anemia may result from a slowly bleeding ulcer.

When an ulcer is found and NSAIDs are not implicated, it is expedient to biopsy the antrum to test for *H. pylori*. A rapid urease test is faster and cheaper than histology and culture (see Table 8-1). In the case of a gastric ulcer, where a follow-up is necessary to exclude cancer, a further biopsy will ensure that the bacteria are gone. Otherwise, healthy subjects can be assumed to be cured and should be treated again only if symptoms recur. Complicated or high-risk cases will require proof of eradication, and a serum antibody test several months after therapy is probably most appropriate. However, we urgently need a test that is prompt, cheap, and immediately reliable. Antibodies may linger several months after eradication of the organism, making serology or saliva tests less useful for follow-up. Breath tests are not widely available, so biopsy remains the best option for now.

PROGNOSIS

... although its interruptions to health are numerous, the menace to life of a duodenal ulcer is not great.

J. A. Ryle, 1889–1950

Peptic ulcers have undergone so much medical intervention over the last generation that their natural history is difficult to determine. In the 40-year-old general practice study of John Fry, the disease peaked at about 8 years and remained active for about 15

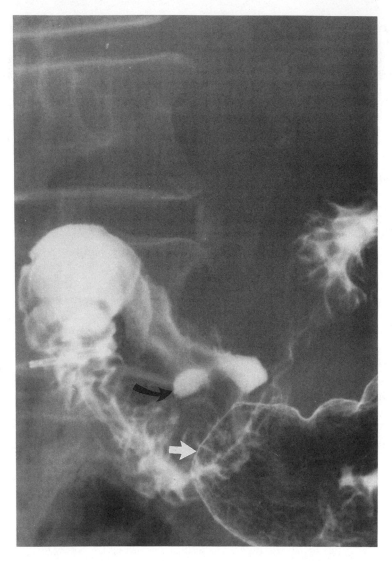

Figure 11-3. Air contrast barium X ray of a duodenal ulcer. The curved arrow points to barium resting in the ulcer crater. Thin bands of barium are seen radiating from the ulcer. These represent crevices between folds thrown up by the inflammation and spasm caused by the ulcer. The white arrow indicates the end of the gastric antrum. Not shown behind the arrow is the narrow pyloric canal joining the antrum to the duodenum. Compare this figure to the normal upper gastrointestinal series shown in Figure 31-2.

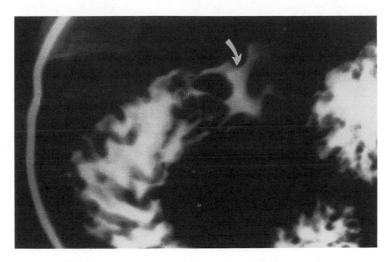

Figure 11-4. Barium contrast X ray of a patient with dyspepsia. The arrow points to barium in a normal duodenal fold that was erroneously called a duodenal ulcer. The consequences of this "overcall" could be years of inappropriate drug therapy, anxiety, and an increase in the patient's life insurance premiums.

years. Over 10 years, about 10% of his patients required surgery, and none died. Even after H_2 antagonists were in use, most continued to be symptomatic after ten years.

Duggan reviewed ten life-table analyses of peptic ulcer and concluded that patients could expect a normal life span. These studies are flawed in that most relied on radiological diagnoses and centered on hospital cases. Duggan claims that modern investigation and therapy have not altered the occurrence of death and complications of ulcers. However, it would be difficult to demonstrate a reduction in a death rate that was not very high in the first place. Moreover, the increased incidence of ulcers and their complications in the aged would obscure any improvement. Much of the earlier mortality was attributed to ulcer surgery, which is less commonly performed now.

The improvement in management of ulcer disease cannot be measured solely by mortality, or even complications. The better quality of life now available to young and middle-aged ulcer patients is obvious and undeniable. No longer are members of this productive sector of the work force submitted to bed rest, obnoxious diets, hospitalizations, or debilitating ulcer surgery. Now, drugs relieve symptoms and most can anticipate cure of their disease. This is the triumph of *The Ulcer Story*.

TREATMENT

General Measures

There was a time not long ago when general measures were the major thrust of medical management. To some they may seem quaint in the face of effective drug therapy, but they are still important. Cessation of smoking should be a primary objective. Irregular meals and excessive alcohol or coffee should be moderated. Those under excessive stress must obtain help to deal with it. Although the ulcer may soon disappear anyway, dyspepsia may persist, and ulcer patients are prone to other diseases, notably coronary artery disease. In our haste to stamp out *H. pylori*, we must not forget the whole person.

Aspirin and NSAIDs should be stopped if possible. Acetaminophen may relieve pain without putting the gut at risk. It is preferable when there is rheumatism without inflammation such as in osteoarthritis. Where it is necessary to continue the NSAID, anti-ulcer medication will heal the ulcer, and continued use will maintain healing.

DRUG THERAPY

The drugs and surgery employed in the treatment of peptic ulcers and their complications are detailed in Part 6. A brief outline follows here.

To Heal the Ulcer

Several drugs will heal most gastric and duodenal ulcers in 4–6 weeks. Since there is little to choose from among them in terms of efficacy, the determinants will be cost, ease of administration, and undesirable effects. On most counts the H_2 antagonists come out on top. Antacids heal ulcers but require seven daily doses. Sucralfate is as effective as ranitidine, but it constipates and requires the patient to swallow large pills four times a day. Misoprostil causes diarrhea and abortions, and proton pump inhibitors (PPIs) are very expensive.

Among the H_2 antagonists, ranitidine combines the best features of long clinical experience, low record of side effects and drug interaction, and ease of administration. Provided that the cost is competitive, either 150 mg twice daily or 300 mg at bedtime should be standard ulcer healing treatment.

Despite the cost, the sheer potency of omeprazole or other PPIs is appealing. A 2-week course is comparable in healing rate and cost with the other agents. However, omeprazole is often used for longer periods or in more than the 20-mg daily dose. It is also used with antibiotics in anti-*H. pylori* protocols.

To Kill *Helicobacter pylori*

Several drug combinations and their costs for the eradication of *H. pylori* are summarized in tables 27-1 and 10-4. A triple drug regimen achieves the best results, but side effects occur in up to 50% of those receiving one. The patient must consume 14 pills daily for 1 or 2 weeks. Recent protocols overcome these difficulties with 7-day and lower dose courses. Others combine an antisecretory agent with two antibiotics. (See Walsh and Peterson for details). Determination of the best protocol requires more work. An antiulcer drug is added if the ulcer is active.

Some have had almost as much success in killing the organisms with a dual therapy protocol employing a PPI and amoxacillin or clarithromycin. Pretreatment with the PPI may make the organism more susceptible to the antibiotic. The double therapy has obvious advantages, but good results are not universal. Different strains and resistance profiles of *H. pylori* may account for regional differences in response. For more details, turn to Chapters 8 and 27.

To Prevent Recurrence

The ultimate means to prevent recurrence is to eliminate the cause. For NSAID ulcers, stop the NSAID. For *H. pylori* ulcers, kill the bacteria. Some ulcers occur without such a cause, and occasionally it may not be convenient or wise to stop the NSAID or use double or triple therapy. Older studies indicate that a maintenance dose of an H_2 antagonist (ranitidine, 150 mg daily) will prevent recurrence of the ulcer once it is healed. However, if H_2 antagonist treatment stops, even after several years, ulcers will recur at a rate as if they had not been given at all.

To Heal NSAID Ulcers

NSAID ulcers will heal rapidly on an H_2 antagonist or PPI, if the NSAID is stopped. However, these anti-inflammatory drugs delay healing. If the NSAID treatment must continue, then twice the dose of the anti-ulcer drug should be used. Misoprostyl offers no advantage here and has unattractive side effects.

To Prevent NSAID Ulcers

Misoprostyl 200ug four times daily can prevent ulcers in patients taking NSAIDs. While ranitidine is equally effective against duodenal ulcers, it is less so against gastric ulcers. It now seems that misoprostyl can prevent serious complications of ulcers in patients taking NSAIDs, but at great cost. Co-administration of misoprostyl to the 15 million Americans taking NSAIDs is clearly impractical. Therefore the drug should be given to high risk patients such as the elderly, those with previous ulcers, and those with cardiovascular disease. There are now combination NSAID-misoprostyl drugs. While convenient and cheaper, they do not avoid the prostaglandin side effects (see Chapter 26).

SUMMARY

Despite their differences, gastric and duodenal ulcers have similar symptoms, complications, and treatments. Usually in company with *H. pylori* or NSAIDs, both types of ulcers result from destruction of the mucosa by acid and pepsin. Most, but not all, ulcers cause dyspepsia, but many dyspeptics have no ulcer. The only reliable means of diagnosis is endoscopy. While they are not often fatal, untreated ulcers cause much misery and disability. Several drugs will promptly heal the ulcers. By employing a suitable protocol to kill *H. pylori* or by stopping NSAIDs the disease is usually curable.

CHAPTER TWELVE

Rare and Atypical Ulcers

H. pylori or NSAIDs participate in the development of most peptic ulcers. A few otherwise typical ulcers have no known associations. There remain a number of peptic ulcers that occur in rare or unusual circumstances (Table 12-1). Some, like the Zollinger–Ellison syndrome, are very rare. Their importance to *The Ulcer Story* is their contribution to our understanding of ulcer pathogenesis. Others, such as stress ulcers, are common problems in certain settings, where prevention becomes a paramount issue. It is curious that so many of these special ulcers bear the name of their discoverer. Why would anyone would want an ulcer disease named after him? Nonetheless, eponyms such as Curling, Ellison, Dieulafoy, and Meckel ensure immortality for some who might otherwise have been forgotten.

ZOLLINGER–ELLISON SYNDROME

The Zollinger–Ellison (ZE) syndrome accounts for less than 0.1% of all peptic ulcers. A practicing gastroenterologist may not see a case during an entire career. Despite this, ZE occupies a whole chapter in texts and is required learning for all medical trainees. Why is there all this attention for such a rare disease? Is it the embodiment of Al Capp's aged superspecialist awaiting his first case!? The surgeons Zollinger and Ellison described the triad of non-beta islet cell pancreatic adenoma, gastric acid hypersecretion,

TABLE 12-1
Rare and Atypical Ulcers

Zollinger–Ellison syndrome
G cell hyperplasia
Antral exclusion
Anastomotic ulcer
Stress ulcer
Curling's ulcer
Cushing's ulcer
Meckel's ulcer
Barrett's ulcer
Dieulafoy's ulcer
Childhood peptic ulcer
Giant peptic ulcer

and severe ulcer disease in 1955. Since then, this rare syndrome has been extensively studied, collected, and classified. Few diseases are so dramatic and have so many measurable variables. Observations in ZE patients have greatly increased our understanding of the physiology of gastrin and the stomach. The original observers predicted that the tumor would be discovered to produce a hormone capable of powerfully stimulating gastric acid secretion. Gregory did just that 5 years later. Ironically, these great discoveries provoked by this rare disease hastened the end of the age of gastric surgery and accelerated the development of effective medical treatments.

Gastrinoma

The tissue from which gastrinomas originate is unknown. They are non-beta islet cell adenomas of the islets of Langerhans in the pancreas. True beta cell tumors secrete insulin. The adenomas are often very tiny, ranging from 0.1 to 2.0 centimeters in diameter. In more than two-thirds of cases they are multiple or malignant. Many lie outside the pancreas, especially in the regional lymph nodes or in the wall of the duodenum, where they are very difficult to locate. In most cases the tumors spread only to the local lymph nodes and progress slowly. Distant metastases or liver tumors carry a greater threat to life and are rare variations of a rare tumor.

Gastrin

The gastrin produced by gastrinomas consists of several peptides somewhat different from the gastrin I and II produced by the antral G cells. In more than 90% of cases, this ectopically produced gastrin causes gastric hypersecretion with a basal acid output (BAO) of at least 15 meq of acid per hour. Because of the trophic (growth-promoting) effect of gastrin, the parietal cell mass may be three to six times greater than normal, so the stimulated acid secretion will be very high. Gastrin increases small intestinal motility. The low pH of the intestinal contents damages the mucosa and inactivates bile salts and pancreatic lipase. The results of these changes are diarrhea and malabsorption.

MEN I

Multiple endocrine neoplasia (MEN I) is an inherited predisposition to develop gastrinomas and adenomas or hyperplasia (increased growth) in several endocrine organs. These, in turn, produce hormones and function outside the usual homeostatic controls. In MEN I the parathyroid glands, the pituitary, and the beta cells of the pancreas are commonly affected. Less commonly, there may be tumor or hyperplasia of the thyroid, or the adrenal cortex. Each of these tumors may secrete several endocrine polypeptides. The most commonly diseased is the parathyroid gland. Excess parathormone causes a high serum calcium, which, among other things, may enhance gastrin release. Beta cell adenomas secrete insulin. Management of these two conditions may dominate the treatment priorities in this rare disease. These other hormonal abnormalities are subjects in themselves, and are not germane to *The Ulcer Story*.

Twenty to sixty percent of gastrinomas occur with MEN I. Therefore, when confronted by a gastrinoma, one should look for other endocrinopathies and examine vulnerable relatives.

Diagnosis

Clinical Presentation

Diarrhea is common and may precede the ulcer disease. The ulcer itself may be no different from any other peptic ulcer. However, the disease is usually more severe, resistant to treatment, and liable to complications. Sometimes, the ulcers are multiple or in atypical locations, such as the distal duodenum or even the jejunum. As might be expected, severe esophagitis is also common, often with a stricture. If gastric surgery is done without recognition of the gastrinoma, a complicated anastomotic ulcer will likely occur subsequently.

Serum Gastrin

Normally, the fasting serum gastrin is under 60 pg/ml; up to 150 pg/ml is acceptable. Gastrinomas produce levels as high as 450,000 pg/ml. In the presence of acid hypersecretion, a serum gastrin of greater than 1,000 pg/ml is sufficient to make the diagnosis. However, achlorhydria is a more common cause of hypergastrinemia than gastrinoma. In pernicious anemia, for example, the lack of gastric acid causes the antral G cells to produce gastrin. Other rare syndromes, such as G cell hyperplasia or retained antrum, also raise the serum gastrin.

If the gastrin level is not conclusive, a secretin test may help. Unlike normal gastrin-secreting cells in the antrum, a gastrinoma will sharply increase gastrin release after injection of the hormone secretin. If such an injection results in an increase in serum gastrin of 300 pg/ml or more than the fasting level, the ZE syndrome is likely.

Gastric Analysis

Gastric analysis is described in Chapter 6. A BAO of greater than 15 meq indicates an exogenous stimulation of basal acid secretion, most commonly gastrin. There is also a high maximal acid output (MAO) because of the increased parietal cell mass. If the BAO approaches the MAO (>65%), a gastrinoma is likely. Before serum gastrin assays were available, gastric analysis was the principal means of diagnosing the ZE syndrome.

X Ray

Besides detecting an ulcer, often at unusual sites, a barium series may show the hypertrophied gastric folds and increased fluid produced by the enlarged parietal cell mass. These phenomena are also evident on computerized tomography (CT), ultrasound, or magnetic resonance imaging (MRI). The challenge is to locate the adenomas. One technique is to inject a radiopaque solution into the arteries supplying the upper gut and pancreas. A tumor may show as a blush on X ray. A combination of CT and angiography may show a tumor of 1.5 cm or larger in less than half of cases. If the surgeon does not see it on an X ray, he or she will have great difficulty in locating the gastrinoma at operation. In some cases it is never found. Ultrasound and MRI have been disappointing. Selective sampling of blood from veins draining the upper gut may detect a source of gastrin production, but the technique is very difficult.

Treatment

Surgical

The ZE syndrome was discovered in the age of gastric surgery. Until the introduction of cimetidine nearly 20 years later, the treatment was surgical, and the principal objective was to control the life-threatening ulcer disease. The tumor was excised if possible. Partial gastrectomy was fraught with the risk of a recurrent ulcer, so the usual procedure was total gastrectomy. No stomach, no acid, no ulcer! In advanced cases, this operation improved the tumor itself. Take away the target organ, and it seems that the gastrinoma loses its purpose. All this has changed. Now that we have antisecretory drugs, total gastrectomy is seldom performed. The operations had nutritional consequences. Only tiny meals could be tolerated, and vitamin B_{12} malabsorption required regular replacement injections. On the whole, the operation was right for the time and was often life-saving.

Gastrinomas are surgically cured in about 30% of cases. Others are too many, metastatic, or not locatable. Over 90% have not spread beyond the lymph nodes and are slow-growing. These seldom kill. Among the remaining 10%, a surgeon might remove a solitary liver gastrinoma, but the prognosis is not so good. Usually the surgeon, after dealing with the adenoma, will perform a proximal (highly selective) vagotomy to reduce the requirement for antiulcer drugs.

Medical Therapy

Anti-ulcer medication can control hypersecretion of gastric acid and the consequent ulcers and diarrhea. However, the required dose is high and therefore expensive. H_2 antagonists control the disease, albeit with seven to ten times the usual dose. In some cases, control deteriorates over time and requires even greater doses or combination with anticholinergics. The proton pump inhibitors are now the drugs of choice. The optimal dose of omeprazole is 40–80 mg per day in divided doses. Some suggest that the dose be titrated to keep the BAO under 10 meq/h. It is important that the patient never stop the drugs because severe ulcer disease will promptly recur. Intravenous ranitidine controls secretion when the patient cannot eat, such as during and after surgery.

Three drugs, singly or in combination, are useful chemotherapy for the gastrinoma itself. They are streptozotocin, 5-FU, and doxorubicin; they are only given for advanced and metastatic disease. These drugs achieve remissions in about 50% of patients.

OTHER HYPERSECRETORY STATES

A number of diseases, even rarer than the ZE syndrome, may cause gastric hypersecretion. In G cell hyperplasia, the gastrin-secreting G cells produce excess gastrin. If a small strip of gastric antrum is inadvertently left attached to the duodenal stump at a Billroth II gastrectomy, gastric hypersecretion may occur (see Figure 29-1). In this unusual situation, the retained antrum is bathed in alkaline duodenal juice and responds by releasing gastrin. Other islet cell tumors cause acid hypersecretion with normal blood gastrin levels. Another hormone is suspected in these rare cases.

The small intestine produces a (so far) unidentified hormone that inhibits gastric secretion. Therefore, gastric hypersecretion and ulcers may complicate a large intestinal resection. The more gut that is removed, the greater the effect. Systemic mastocytosis is a rare disease in which mast cells proliferate unchecked in many tissues. One of the products of these little chemical factories is histamine, which causes gastric hypersecretion. In all of these rare causes of gastric acid hypersecretion, the ulcer disease is best managed with anti-ulcer drugs.

ANASTOMOTIC ULCERS

After an ulcer operation, the site where the stomach surgically attaches to the intestine is an *anastomosis*. In the cases of gastroenterostomy or Billroth II gastrectomy, the stomach is anastomosed to the jejunum (see Figure 29-1). Newly exposed to acid and pepsin, the jejunum is prone to ulcerate. Anastomotic ulcers are sometimes called marginal or stomal ulcers, and these also occur after gastroduodenostomy.

Anastomotic ulcers may be difficult to diagnose and treat. Before anti-ulcer drugs were available, the only effective therapy was another operation and vagotomy with or without revision of the anastomosis. Now drugs readily heal the ulcers. We must next learn if and how NSAIDs and *H. pylori* contribute to these surgical failures.

STRESS ULCERS

Severe physiological stress causes gastroduodenal mucosal damage. Ninety percent of intensive care patients have endoscopic evidence of this damage, but much fewer than 50% have actual gastric or duodenal ulcers. *Curling* noted duodenal ulcers in severely burned patients over 150 years ago (see Chapter 4). *Cushing* (a neurosurgeon) found ulcers among his patients with trauma or surgery to the brain. It is likely that Curling's and Cushing's ulcers are representative of all those found in severely ill patients.

Cause

Fortunately, most gastroduodenal damage in intensive care patients is of little importance, but some ulcers cause life-threatening hemorrhage. It is difficult to sort out the predisposing factors from the many things that happen to a severely ill person in the intensive care unit. There are often other diseases, complications, malnutrition, and many medications. Bad omens include burns covering more than 35% of the body, trauma, head injury, sepsis, need for artificial ventilation, and impaired blood clotting.

Stress ulcers require the presence of acid and are thus peptic ulcers. They are different from the usual ulcer disease in several respects. There is often no previous ulcer and no associated chronic active gastritis. Most commentators believe that the cause of a stress ulcer is impairment of the gastroduodenum's resistance to the aggressive effects of acid and pepsin. Some suggest that this results from reduced blood flow to the mucosa; others claim that impaired nutrition lessens the restorative power of the mucosal cells.

Treatment and Prevention

Once discovered, a stress ulcer is treated with the principles that apply to ordinary peptic ulcers. However, the outcome is much poorer. Coagulation and nutrition must be optimized and offending drugs should be withdrawn. Most agree that a known peptic ulcer or overt bleeding should be treated aggressively. However, the real issue is prevention of ulcers and bleeding in severely ill patients. At this point the agreement ends.

About 2% of patients admitted to an intensive care unit (ICU) can be expected to suffer an important upper gastrointestinal bleed. Although prophylactic treatment reduces bleeding episodes, there is no proof that it improves overall outcome. Prevention programs are expensive and introduce risks of their own (see below). It is important to select those patients who are at the greatest risk of bleeding and who therefore are most likely to benefit from preventative drug therapy. Next, it would be important to know if outcomes such as costs, length of hospital stay, and mortality are influenced by such treatment.

Cook *et al.* appear to have settled the first issue. In a large, prospective Canadian multicenter study, they found that ICU patients with failure of breathing (requiring a ventilator) or blood clotting had a 3.7% risk of an important bleed, while the remainder had a risk of less than 0.5%. We can prevent bleeding in many of these high risk cases, but await proof that prophylactic drugs favorably influence outcome. Once that is established, we must learn which drug is best for the job.

Antacids, H_2-blocking drugs, and sucralfate have been the most extensively studied. All three can reduce overt bleeding, but whether survival is affected is uncertain. There are many disadvantages. Antacids must be given around the clock with regular sampling of gastric pH. There is risk of aspiration of the infused antacid into the lungs, and the additional burden on attending nurses is hard to justify. It appears also that such treatment increases the already high prevalence of lung infection since the antiseptic effect of gastric acid is absent. Intravenous H_2 antagonists may be a sensible alternative, but they are expensive and need further study.

Sucralfate may provide good protection without the risk of infection, but getting the viscus material through a stomach feeding tube is technically difficult. Prostaglandins and pirenzepine have also been used for this purpose but there are even fewer data on these drugs. Routine ulcer prophylaxis with anti-ulcer drugs is not justified in an intensive care unit. We must have better trials to prove the usefulness of prevention in selected cases with burns, brain injuries, trauma, or coagulation disorders.

MECKEL'S ULCER

Occurring in up to 3% of the population, Meckel's diverticu-lum is the most common congenital anomaly of the gastrointestinal tract. In the uterus, the vitelline duct of the fetus communicates through the umbilical cord with the ileum. Normally it seals off at birth, but occasionally the intestinal end persists, resulting in a full thickness pouch of ileum. The mucosa usually resembles the rest of the ileum, but other gut mucosal tissues can be represented. One such mucosa is that of the stomach, complete with parietal cells. Even *H. pylori* can make a home there.

Ulcers occur where the gastric and ileal mucosas meet. Meckel's ulcers account for half of lower gut bleeding in children, but they may be overlooked in adults. Bleeding presents with red blood from the rectum, and faintness, hypotension, and shock follow if untreated. They are best diagnosed by nuclear imaging. Parietal cells take up the isotope technetium-99 m. Given intrave-nously, it collects in the gastric mucosa in the ileum and can be imaged by a gamma camera. This test is not 100% sensitive, and the gastrin analogue pentagastrin sometimes helps by increasing parietal cell activity. A careful small bowel enema may discover a diverticulum among the ileal folds but will not likely demonstrate the ulcer. Although drugs can control the ulcer, the definitive treatment is surgical removal.

BARRETT'S ULCER

In the next part, we shall discuss Barrett's esophagus, a gastrification of the esophageal mucosa. This phenomenon is probably caused by chronic gastroesophageal reflux. As with other columnar epithelial surfaces of the upper gut, Barrett's esophagus is prone to peptic ulcer (see Figure 17-9).

DIEULAFOY'S ULCER

Dieulafoy probably does not belong in the pantheon of ulcer eponyms. His ulcer is likely not peptic at all. However, when this lesion bleeds, it may appear like an ulcer, complete with an endoscopically visible artery. No whitish ulcer base surrounds the bleeding vessel. The defect is a larger than usual artery that penetrates or abuts into the submucosa and mucosa. It is as if a nutrient gastric vessel forgot to trim down before entering the stomach wall. Most such lesions occur in the upper stomach, so acid and pepsin have been blamed. However, similar lesions occur throughout the gut, so the peptic component is doubtful. It remains a mystery why this odd artery bursts and bleeds through the mucosa.

CHILDHOOD PEPTIC ULCER

Fortunately, peptic ulcer—particularly gastric ulcer—is unusual in childhood. There is a strong association of childrens' ulcers with *H. pylori*, which accounts for the frequency that ulcers occur in family members. The treatment is the same as for adult ulcers, including eradication of *H. pylori*.

GIANT GASTRIC ULCERS

Most peptic ulcers are less than 2 cm in diameter. Larger ones pose special problems. In the duodenum, a large, usually posterior ulcer may penetrate into other tissues, such as the pancreas, causing back pain. It may be so large that it conforms to the contour of the duodenum and is not recognized on X-ray. Giant gastric ulcers often appear in NSAID users and older people, where the diagnosis may be delayed. Giant ulcers that previously required surgery can now be healed with omeprazole, but it may take longer.

SUMMARY

Most ulcers result from *H. pylori* infection or NSAIDs. However, there are a number of unusual or atypical ulcers that, while they retain the descriptor "peptic," are unique in their character, location, or circumstances. Of these, stress ulcers are the most important. Ulcers found in the Zollinger–Ellison syndrome are the most studied. The remaining gallery of unusual ulcers, often furnished with an eponym, are certainly important to those who have one.

CHAPTER THIRTEEN

Complications of Peptic Ulcer

Peptic ulcers cause dyspepsia, which can be severe and can impair quality of life. Although the pain is chronic and recurrent, it can now be controlled, and even cured, by drugs. However, if untreated or unrecognized, an ulcer may develop a life-threatening complication. Unlike dyspepsia, these complications are often emergencies requiring urgent action and sometimes prompt surgery. The complications include intractability, hemorrhage, perforation, penetration, and obstruction (Table 13-1).

INTRACTABILITY

During the age of gastric surgery, intractability was the most common indication for an ulcer operation. An intractable ulcer occurred when "medical" treatment failed to relieve symptoms after several weeks in hospital. Surgery was often performed electively in persons for whom repeated attacks of dyspepsia threatened employability and quality of life. Intractability is not a viable concept in ulcer disease today. Once the H_2-blocking drugs became available, physicians could control ulcer disease and the curtain fell on the age of gastric surgery. Sippy diets, milk drips, and hospital rest cures became obsolete, and the need for elective ulcer surgery declined. Proton pump blockers can control almost any ulcer, while a strategy for lasting cure is applied. It must now be the rare case that requires surgery for pain alone.

TABLE 13-1
Complications
of Peptic Ulcer

Intractability
Hemorrhage
Perforation
Penetration
Pyloric obstruction

Indeed, if pain persists despite adequate therapy, there is likely something else afoot. The pain may not be due to an ulcer at all. Early gastric cancer or lymphoma can masquerade as a gastric ulcer, as can Crohn's disease in the duodenum. Giant or penetrating ulcers require prolonged treatment. Severe or multiple ulcers may indicate a gastrinoma. Inadvertently or otherwise, some patients forget to take their pills or to stop taking NSAIDs.

Dyspepsia can occur without an ulcer, and ulcer and non-ulcer can coexist, the latter remaining after ulcer cure. Long-standing pain may become so embedded in the brain that no treatment directed at the stomach will help. Injudicious surgery in such cases sometimes produces miserable gastric crippling.

HEMORRHAGE

Manifestations

Most patients are alerted to ulcer bleeding by black, tarry stools. This is called *melena*. As little as 50 ml of blood can produce a black stool. With severe hemorrhage, red blood passes per rectum *(hematochezia)*. Rapid bleeding may cause the patient to vomit blood *(hematemesis)*.

Mild bleeding produces no symptoms or mere light-headedness. In more severe cases blood pressure falls, especially when the victim is in an upright position. Often the bleeding person feels faint or light-headed when rising from a lying or sitting position. The pulse races as the heart struggles to compensate for the depleted blood volume, and the patient becomes sweaty and anxious. Shock, collapse, and even death may intervene if the bleeding continues or if prompt resuscitation is not instituted. At least 80%

of bleeding ulcers stop spontaneously, but it is impossible to predict those that will not.

The Cause of Bleeding

A gastric or duodenal ulcer may erode into an important artery lying beneath the mucosa. The resulting hemorrhage may be mild or severe and life-threatening, depending on the size of the bleeding artery and the efficacy of blood clotting and other hemostatic mechanisms. It is a matter of chance whether an ulcer lies over an important blood vessel. Death occurs from a bleeding artery over 3.5 mm in diameter, and hemorrhage from an artery larger than 2 mm is difficult to control. Fortunately, ulcers usually erode into smaller blood vessels and cause a slow trickle of blood.

Although overall ulcer prevalence is declining, admissions to the hospital remain constant. This may result from our relative longevity and from the tendency of the elderly to take many ulcer-causing medications, particularly NSAIDs. Anti-arthritis medications not only induce ulcers and impair clotting through inhibition of blood platelet function, but they also increase the likelihood of bleeding from existing ulcers. The risk of bleeding on NSAID therapy is greater if there has been a previous gastrointestinal event.

Many people regularly take aspirin to prevent cardiovascular occlusions. By interfering with blood platelet function, the drug impairs blood clotting. This helps prevent strokes and heart attacks, but it may cause grief in the upper gut. Ingestion of 300 mg per day increases the risk of ulcer bleeding by a factor of eight, and 1,200 mg per day doubles the risk again. Corticosteroid drugs such as prednisone increase the risk in persons taking NSAIDs or aspirin. Some NSAIDs are more dangerous than others. The risk appears to be least with ibuprofen and diclofenac; more with indomethacin, and piroxicam; and greatest with azapropazone and ketoprofen (see Table 7-1). Each drug has a dose-response effect, that is, the more drug, the more bleeding.

Anticoagulants such as warfarin (Coumadin™) or heparin do not cause ulcers. However, if an ulcer exists, anticlotting drugs may convert a minor ooze to a major hemorrhage. Certainly a history of previous ulcer or gastrointestinal bleeding should prompt caution in the use of NSAIDs or anticoagulants.

Treatment of Bleeding

Most patients who bleed from the upper gut should be in the hospital. Those with severe bleeding or shock are best handled in intensive care. Criteria for severe bleeding include low blood pressure, rapid pulse, and faintness. Usually these are worse when the patient in an upright position. The pulse response may be feeble in the elderly or in patients receiving beta-adrenergic drugs such as propanolol for hypertension or heart disease. Signs of shock include cold, clammy skin; faint pulse; collapse; and fading consciousness. Such cases require urgent resuscitation and endoscopy soon afterward. The risks are greatest in an elderly person, especially if he or she is afflicted by another major illness.

Resuscitation begins with the establishment of an intravenous line of sufficient caliber to permit blood transfusions. At the same time a blood sample is drawn for the hemoglobin level and for a cross-match of the patient's blood with that of a potential donor. Blood products digested in the small bowel are metabolized by the liver, and urea is a metabolic by-product. Therefore, an elevated blood urea without kidney disease may indicate upper, rather than lower, gastrointestinal bleeding. Blood tests for kidney or liver disease may be performed if relevant.

Ordinarily, a cross-match takes 1–2 hours. If the blood volume is very low, as indicated by the signs of shock, a rapid cross-match may be done. Of course, this reduces the protection provided by a full match against a transfusion reaction. Usually one can wait for the full cross-match and can temporize by rapidly infusing a salt solution such as normal saline. Oxygen supplied through a nasal catheter helps maintain tissue viability.

The hemoglobin level is not a reliable indicator of the severity of acute bleeding. After loss of 1 or 2 liters, the remaining blood is unchanged so the hemoglobin (or hematocrit) is initially normal. Gradually over several hours the blood volume is made up by fluid entering the blood stream from the tissues or through the intravenous line. The resulting dilution of the blood lowers the hemoglobin concentration. Therefore, in an emergency the decisions of when and how much blood to transfuse must be based on clinical signs alone. In less serious bleeding, these decisions may be delayed 12 hours until the hemoglobin equilibrates. As a rule, it is best to maintain the hemoglobin over 100 mg/dl.

The patient should fast at least until endoscopy. Those with mild to moderate bleeding and a clean ulcer may eat after the procedure and even go home. High-risk patients should remain fasting in the hospital in case further endoscopy or surgery is required. There is no evidence that any drug improves the outcome from an acute ulcer bleed. Therefore, costly intravenous H_2 antagonists are withheld and drug treatment can wait until the patient can eat. Nevertheless, there is no reason to delay oral therapy of the ulcer itself with an H_2 antagonist or proton pump inhibitor. NSAIDs should be stopped. At endoscopy, the physician may take the opportunity to biopsy the gastric antrum for *H. pylori*. In non-NSAID bleeding ulcers one may begin omeprazole, 40 mg/day, and antibiotic therapy for two weeks. If tests for *H. pylori* are negative, the physician can stop the antibiotics. A recent study suggests that 3-day pretreatment with omeprazole may improve the eradication rate.

In any case, omeprazole is continued for 4–6 weeks. Re-endoscopy is generally not necessary. However, in severe or high risk bleeds a second look at the ulcer site and rebiopsy of the antrum is prudent. Some gastric ulcers require a second look to ensure they are not malignant. In elderly or very ill patients it may be safer and more convenient to institute indefinite ulcer prophylaxis with an H_2 antagonist.

Endoscopy

In a series of hospitalized patients, the cause of upper gastrointestinal bleeding was peptic ulcer in 62%, duodenal ulcer in 37%. Since in the remaining 38% the culprit is not a peptic ulcer, patients with significant bleeding should be endoscoped. Even in people with known ulcers, the bleeding is from another disease in one-fourth of cases. Other causes of bleeding include a rent at the gastroesophageal junction (Mallory–Weisz tear), gastric cancer, esophagitis, and gastric or duodenal erosions. Esophageal or gastric varices are large submucosal veins resulting from severe liver disease, usually cirrhosis. The most common cause of cirrhosis is alcoholism. Signs of cirrhosis that cause the doctor to suspect varices include jaundice, ascites (fluid in the abdomen), large liver and spleen, red (liver) palms, and liver spots (spiderlike vascular formations on the skin called spider angiomata). These other causes of bleeding have different treatments from peptic ulcers.

Other reasons for endoscopy are to assess the gravity of the bleeding and to intervene if appropriate. If the ulcer has a clear white base with a little oozing of blood, or a flat pigmented spot, there is little risk of further bleeding. If the physician determines that the risk is low, the patient may eat right away and go home if he or she is young and otherwise healthy. High-risk lesions should be monitored in the hospital for at least three days. The presence of an adherent blood clot increases that risk. If there is a protruding artery or actual spurting of blood, the likelihood of continued or repeated hemorrhage is 50%. Without further action, one-third of these high-risk cases will require surgery. The endoscopist should therefore attempt to stop the bleeding.

Endoscopic Treatment

In those patients with a severe bleed from a protruding or bleeding artery, the risk of surgery is reduced by 60% through endoscopic thermal or injection therapy. A laser is one form of thermal therapy, but it is costly, cumbersome, and too dangerous. More practical is the use of a dipolar electrode or a heater probe to contact and compress the artery while an electric current cauterizes the vessel and coagulates the blood. These generate temperatures of 100° and 250°C, respectively, so the endoscopist must take care not to burn through the base of the ulcer and convert the hemorrhage into a perforation.

Injection of fluid into the bleeding site may stop bleeding by compressing the artery, since several saline injections of 1 or 2 ml are effective. Usually the endoscopist injects a solution of 1:10,000 epinephrine to contract the vessel, or, rarely, a sclerosant such as ethanolamine to damage, inflame, and eventually fibrose the artery. These methods reduce hospital stay, blood transfusions, mortality, and rate of surgery. A physician should not undertake endoscopy if he or she is not prepared to employ one of these measures. The two complications of such interventions, perforation and uncontrollable bleeding, are mercifully rare at 0.5% and 0.3%, respectively. Fortunately, most bleeding ulcers require no such treatment.

Other Treatments

Surgery

If the above measures fail, the principal recourse is surgery. The indications are similar to those of the pre-endoscopic, pre-H_2-blocker period. Continued bleeding under observation is an indication, but timing remains a matter of judgment. As a rule of thumb, one waits no longer if there is evidence of ongoing hemorrhage and transfusion of six or more units of blood. An obviously exsanguinating hemorrhage will tip the surgeon's hand sooner. Rebleeding should also trigger emergency surgery. The endoscopic discovery of a spurting or visible artery at the base of an ulcer means that surgery may be necessary. The endoscopist will attempt to control the bleeding, but obvious failures should go straight to the operating room. Surgery is best done electively, but any ulcer that can wait for elective surgery may not need it after all. Bleeding ulcers seldom kill by exsanguination, but rather weaken the victim so that he or she succumbs to a complicating illness such as sepsis or heart disease. Aspiration of vomited blood is another risk, especially in the elderly or those in shock.

Because of decreasing prevalence and the availability of effective medical and endoscopic therapy, few modern surgeons have much experience with ulcer surgery. Nonetheless, immediate hemostasis is achieved when a surgeon ligates a bleeding vessel. Further surgical treatment is designed to reduce gastric acid and prevent recurrence, not necessarily to remove the ulcer itself. Various operations remove the acid-secreting part of the stomach (subtotal gastrectomy), the gastrin-releasing antrum (antrectomy), or the vagus nerve (vagotomy). Now that there are effective medical treatments, extensive surgery is no longer necessary. It could be argued that the surgeon should stop the bleeding and leave the rest to drugs. However, some would recommend a highly selective vagotomy. Although technically difficult, this is the least likely operation to lead to postoperative complications (see Chapter 29).

Angiography

To catheterize the arteries that supply blood to the upper gut, a fine, flexible tube is passed into the femoral artery in the groin. From there it traverses the aorta into its mesenteric and celiac branches. When radiopaque dye is injected during vigorous bleeding, the material can be seen on a fluoroscope (dynamic X ray) to leak into the gut lumen, accurately locating the offending vessel. With skilled endoscopy, such a procedure is seldom needed for diagnosis, but rather to stop the hemorrhage when all else fails and surgery is too dangerous. Intra-arterial injection of vasopressin causes the bleeding artery to go into spasm, and injection of a solid such as gelfoam blocks the vessel (embolization). There are complications, so this procedure is undertaken only in extremely difficult situations where surgery is not an option.

Prevention of Rebleeding

No effort should be spared to prevent a second ulcer hemorrhage. Ten percent of bleeding ulcers are silent; that is, they have no dyspepsia to warn of an impending bleed. NSAIDs should be withdrawn, or, if that is not possible, they should be accompanied by anti-ulcer drug prophylaxis using misoprostil, an H2-blocker, or a proton pump inhibitor. Those ulcers associated with *H. pylori* must have the organism killed by one of the recommended antibiotic programs. Since no treatment is 100% effective, a repeat endoscopy and biopsy should verify that the ulcer is healed and the organisms are gone. Those bleeding ulcers associated with neither NSAIDs nor *H. pylori* should be treated indefinitely with an H2 antagonist.

PERFORATION

Perforation of a peptic ulcer into the peritoneal space is a life-threatening emergency that usually requires urgent surgery. The rent in the gut is sutured, and the peritoneum cleared of debris. Antibiotics are started lest the *peritonitis* get out of control and cause *septicemia* (blood poisoning).

Cause

The gut wall is only a few millimeters thick. An ulcer that penetrates deeply through the muscle coat is liable to burst into the peritoneum, soiling that cavity with gut contents (Figures 13-1; see also Figure 11-1). The result is catastrophic, with acute pain, prostration, and shock. Without prompt intervention, the infected peritoneum causes general sepsis and death.

Clinical Manifestations

Sometimes a perforation occurs without warning, but usually there is a history of dyspepsia or peptic ulcer. The onset of abdominal pain is so sudden and incapacitating that, long afterward, the patient may recall the exact moment when the attack began. Because of the peritoneal inflammation, it hurts to move, and the patient becomes supine and still. There may be signs of shock: hypotension, weak rapid pulse, sweating, clamminess, collapse, and stupor. The muscles of the abdominal wall tighten up to protect the viscera, resulting in a rigid, boardlike abdomen that is difficult to examine. Any movement—even breathing—hurts, and the entire belly is very tender to touch. Sudden release of the examining hand is sharply painful (*rebound tenderness*). Bowel sounds that are normally audible through a stethoscope are absent. These are signs of peritonitis. Because air has been introduced into the normally collapsed peritoneal sac, it may collect over the liver (Figure 13-2). When the abdomen over the liver is tapped, the normal dullness is absent, and a hollow sound is elicited instead.

Diagnosis and Treatment

The diagnosis is usually made by clinical observation, and surgery is promptly arranged. A perforated viscus is confirmed by X rays of the abdomen. When the patient is upright or on his or her left side, air collects in the peritoneum under the diaphragm or over the liver (Figure 13-2). If a patient with a suspected perforation shows no free air on X ray, the test should be repeated several hours

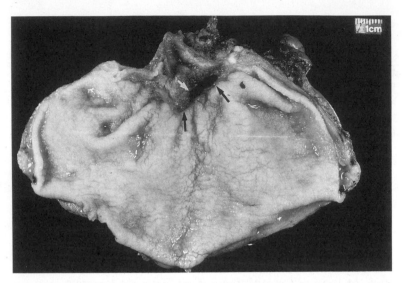

Figure 13-1. Perforated duodenal ulcer. This is a distal stomach, mainly antrum, pylorus and part of duodenum, that has been surgically removed and opened out to show the mucosal surface. The duodenum is seen at the top, and the resection margin is at the bottom. Black arrows point out the pylorus. The white arrow points to the perforated duodenal ulcer immediately distal to the pylorus. (Courtesy of Dr. M. Guindi, Division of Anatomical Pathology, Ottawa Civic Hospital, Ottawa, Canada.)

later. In a difficult case, a water-soluble, nontoxic radiopaque solution called *gastrografin* is used to discover the leak.

The white blood cell count rises sharply. Because intestinal contents spill into the peritoneum and are absorbed, the serum amylase may be elevated. Perforation is difficult to recognize in elderly or immunosuppressed patients. In those taking NSAIDs, there may be no previous dyspepsia to warn of disaster. There are other causes of the "acute abdomen," such as a ruptured appendix, pancreatitis, or cholecystitis. Therefore, a suspected perforation should prompt a surgical evaluation.

The treatment is usually a prompt laparotomy to repair the rent and cleanse the peritoneum. Intravenous antibiotics are necessary for the soiled and infected abdominal cavity. Sometimes an ulcer operation is added to prevent recurrence, but the presence of peritonitis increases mortality. With the new ulcer treatments, simple closure with subsequent drug therapy seems preferable. There

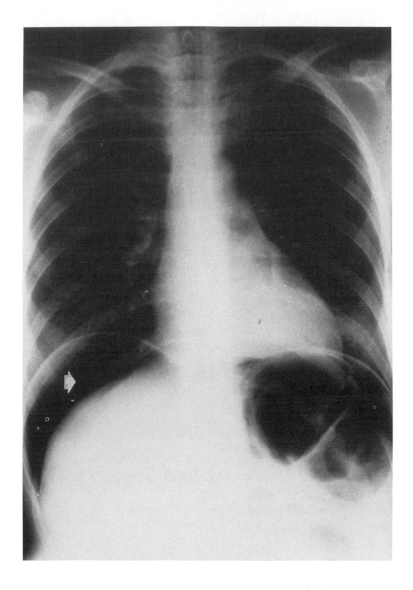

Figure 13-2. Upright plain X ray of the chest and upper abdomen. An ulcer has perforated, permitting air to leak into the normally empty peritoneal space. Air shows as a dark, radiolucent area (arrow), with the diaphragm above and the liver below. Air on the opposite side is located normally within the gut lumen.

is even a revived interest in nonoperative treatment. If the spillage into the peritoneum is small, prolonged suction through a nasogastric tube, antibiotics, and intravenous H_2 antagonists achieve good results. This method is tempting when the surgical risk is high.

PENETRATION

When the ulcer is large or deep, it may penetrate into neighboring pancreas, liver, or omentum. Usually, antiulcer therapy will eventually heal penetrating ulcers, but there are two exceptions. The first is a *gastrocolic fistula*, which occurs when a greater curve gastric or anastomotic ulcer penetrates through the walls of the upper gut and colon, opening a communication between the two organs. Since the small intestine is bypassed, the patient suffers diarrhea and weight loss. Occasionally he or she may vomit fecal material. A barium enema or CT may demonstrate the fistula.

The second exception is penetration of a duodenal ulcer into the bile ducts, called a *choledocoduodenal fistula*. Sometimes this is discovered incidentally when air appears in the bile ducts on X ray. Usually it causes no trouble, but bile duct infection (*cholangitis*) can be severe. Then, as in the case of a gastrocolic fistula, the treatment is surgical.

PYLORIC OBSTRUCTION

Obstruction of the pylorus may complicate a nearby ulcer, causing vomiting, which improves as the ulcer heals. It is sometimes called gastric outlet obstruction. Gastric retention results from obstruction, but it may also occur in an atonic stomach, as in diabetes or with anticholinergic drugs.

Cause

Sometimes a peptic ulcer occurs in the pyloric canal or nearby in the stomach or duodenum. Swelling and inflammation obstruct the narrow pylorus. As the ulcer heals, the obstruction ameliorates. However, repeated or prolonged ulcer attacks may cause scarring of the pylorus, and the obstruction becomes irreversible. A procedure is then required for relief. Peptic ulcer is responsible for at least 90% of pyloric obstructions. Cancer or adult congenital pyloric hypertrophy are less common causes.

Clinical Manifestations

Pyloric stenosis usually occurs in middle age after a long experience with dyspepsia. Symptoms may begin subtly with fullness and nausea after meals. They are sometimes relieved by vomiting partly digested food, often long after the last meal. Later, the vomiting may become a postprandial routine and may be violent and projectile. When recognizable food particles appear 12 hours or more after ingestion, it is difficult not to suspect obstruction. Because little nutrient reaches the small intestine, the patient often loses 20–30 kg in weight.

On examination, the obstructed patient appears dehydrated, wasted, and malnourished. The vomited material is acidic, but recognizable. In an often very thin abdomen, the stomach may bulge under the left rib cage. Peristaltic waves pass from left to right as the stomach tries to empty. There is so much gastric fluid and air that a splash is heard when the patient is shaken. Sometimes, the patient himself is aware of this phenomenon. An upright plain X ray of the abdomen will show a greatly distended stomach full of fluid, with an air–fluid level near the cardia. Endoscopy or barium X ray can resolve doubtful cases.

Gastric retention is worse if a motor dysfunction weakens gastric emptying contractions. This occurs in diabetes mellitus where the visceral nerves are destroyed (*gastroparesis diabetacorum*). Sometimes there are concretions of fiber or other material lodged in the stomach called *bezoars*. If acid production is so low that bacterial overgrowth occurs, hydrogen and carbon dioxide are released. In a letter entitled *Son et lumiere?*, one correspondent describes a patient with pyloric stenosis whose bridge partner offered to light his cigarette. As he leant across the table he felt an undeniable necessity to belch which he discreetly channeled through the nose. "He astonished the company by producing two flame-shaped flames from his nostrils. ' . . . Just like a dragon, doctor.'"

A tube passed into the stomach permits the physician to remove retained food from an obstructed stomach. Retrieval of more than 300 ml of material 4 hr after a meal is good evidence of gastric retention. When the obstruction is due to an ulcer, the removed material should be acidic. Absence of acid suggests an obstructing cancer.

The metabolic consequences of prolonged obstruction are severe. The loss of HCl and water through vomiting causes alkalosis and reduces the blood volume. The kidneys try to conserve sodium at the expense of potassium, so both become depleted. Dehydration reduces blood flow to the kidneys and the urea begins to rise, warning of renal failure. Malnutrition takes many forms, but weight loss and low serum albumin are common. The blood is more coagulable, risking thrombophlebitis or stroke. Impaired consciousness permits aspiration of vomited material into the lungs. Without timely action, shock and death result.

Endoscopy

The obstructed patient needs an endoscopy, but first the stomach must be emptied. This is achieved by the insertion of a large rubber tube through which water can be washed in and fluid contents siphoned out. Endoscopy is attempted when the returning contents are clear. In extreme cases the stomach is large and flaccid. The endoscopist may see a gastric ulcer, or rarely a cancer, but no lesion will be visible if it is in or beyond the narrowed pyloric canal. The pylorus itself is hard to locate. It is very narrow, like a pinhole, and will not admit the endoscope. Sometimes it is necessary to do a barium X ray to see the area properly. However, the usefulness of barium should be weighed against the difficulty of clearing it from the stomach later.

Treatment

Obstructed patients suffer depletion of electrolytes such as sodium, potassium, and chloride and are often alkalotic (high blood pH). If dehydration has been severe and prolonged, there may be renal impairment. Therefore, urea and creatinine levels should be monitored along with the serum electrolytes. Large amounts of saline and potassium must be infused intravenously. Urine output and body weight help determine the amount of fluid replacement. In the elderly or in cardiac patients, too much fluid too fast can precipitate heart failure.

A nasogastric tube attached to an intermittent suction machine decompresses the stomach. Although uncomfortable, this device prevents retching and speeds up the return of gastric tone. Often the above measures are sufficient. In a few days the ulcer begins to heal, local swelling subsides, and the obstruction improves. It used to be said that such relief was temporary and that repeated obstruction is as inevitable as the return of the ulcer itself. This view should change now that there is more effective and curative drug therapy. Aggressive anti-ulcer treatment expedites resolution of the obstruction. At first, H_2 antagonists must be given intravenously, since pills cannot be relied upon to reach their destination.

Hitherto, treatment of pyloric stenosis that failed to resolve with the above measures was surgical. This involved either bypass of the pylorus by joining the stomach to the small bowel (see Figure 29-1) or repair of the pylorus (see Figure 29-4). An ulcer-healing operation such as an antrectomy or subtotal gastrectomy achieved the same end. Vagotomy, unless highly selective, further delayed emptying after the operation and was usually avoided (see Chapter 29).

Surgery is seldom necessary now. The physician can pass a collapsed balloon affixed to the end of a long tube through an endoscope . The tip of the tube is then guided into the pylorus so that the balloon straddles the obstruction. Inflation of the balloon expands the pyloric canal. The procedure may need to be repeated at regular intervals. Nevertheless, this painless outpatient procedure seems quite preferable to surgery, especially in the elderly. It remains to be seen if modern drug therapy will prevent pyloric stenosis and make all invasive procedures unnecessary.

SUMMARY

The three important complications of peptic ulcer are hemorrhage, perforation, and pyloric obstruction. It is likely that modern curative ulcer treatment and the declining prevalence of the disease will make them less common. True intractability has already become unusual. Nevertheless, complications occur as emergencies in people where the ulcer has been hitherto unrecognized, and NSAID use seems destined to continue. Perforation usually requires a surgical repair of the gut wall, but hemorrhage and obstruction are increasingly managed by nonsurgical means, that is, by combined endoscopic intervention and pharmacological healing and cure.

Gastroesophageal Reflux

Heartburn and Esophagitis

CHAPTER FOURTEEN

Gastroesophageal Reflux

Food and gastric contents should not pass from the stomach back into the esophagus. Especially after a meal, gastric contents are rich in acid and pepsin that are capable of tissue damage. The columnar cells that line the stomach save it from self-destruction by this potent brew (see Figure 1-7), but the cells lining the esophagus provide no such protection (see Figure 1-8). Here the surface cells are squamus, like those in the mouth, and are ill-equipped to withstand the digestive effects of gastric juice. When gastroesophageal reflux (GER) occurs, the irritation of the mucosa causes heartburn, and, in severe cases, damages the lower esophagus. The ensuing inflammation is called *esophagitis*. Regurgitated gastric contents that traverse the esophagus burn the throat and potentially damage the larynx and lungs.

This chapter describes the physiological mechanisms that conspire to prevent GER (see Table 14-1), and why they sometimes fail. The most important consequences of GER are heartburn and esophagitis, the subjects of the next two chapters. Esophagitis may cause esophageal stricture, bleeding, or cellular change (see Chapter 17).

RELATIONSHIP OF GER TO HIATUS HERNIA

Relationships between GER, hiatus hernia, and esophagitis are complex. Occasional reflux occurs in all of us. It may be unnoticed, but one-third of people experience heartburn at least once a year, and 10% at least once a month (see Chapter 5). Whether or not a

TABLE 14-1
The Prevention of Reflux

The leading player
    The lower esophageal sphincter
The supporting cast
    1. Anatomic: no hiatus hernia, diaphragm
    2. Motility: esophageal peristalsis (housekeeping), gastric emptying
    3. Diet
    4. Mechanical: low intragastric pressure, gravity
    5. Drugs
    6. Gut hormones
    7. Emotion
    8. Intact pylorus

reflux episode causes heartburn and esophagitis depends the interactions of many factors. Only a few refluxers develop esophagitis,
but many of those report no heartburn. Why GER has such unpredictable and dichotomous consequences is unclear.

A hiatus hernia is a bulging or protrusion of part of the
stomach through the diaphragm up into the chest. This occurs in
about one-third of Western adults by the time they are 60 or 70 years
old. Therefore, it is no surprise that hiatus hernia and heartburn
often occur together. This coincidence led to the erroneous belief
that a hiatus hernia causes heartburn, or even that a hiatus hernia
is heartburn. A patient once referred to her heartburn as "my high
anus hernia." In the 1950s to 1970s, surgeons commonly repaired a
hiatus hernia for reflux symptoms.

There followed a period when clinical scientists declared that
GER and hiatus hernia are merely coincidental. As evidence, they
observed that reflux could occur without a hernia and that many
with a hernia had no heartburn. As often happens, the truth lies
somewhere between these two views. Newer work assures us that
a hiatus hernia may indeed impair lower esophageal sphincter
(LES) activity. Thus a hiatus hernia may be an innocent bystander,
it may contribute to reflux, or it may not even be present. Figure
14-1 summarizes these relationships.

THE LOWER ESOPHAGEAL SPHINCTER

The LES is a special unit of muscle fibers at the lower 2–4 cm
of esophageal muscle (see Figure 1-3). The sphincter contracts to

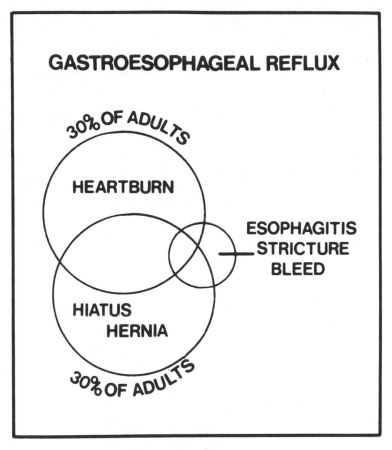

Figure 14-1. The relationships between hiatus hernia, heartburn, and the complications of GER. GER is very common, and is probably universal, yet only about one-third of adults report heartburn. Hiatus hernia is also common. The overlap between these two conditions is largely coincidental, since we know that heartburn commonly occurs without a hiatus hernia and vice versa. The complications of GER are stricture and bleeding, and they may occur with either hiatus hernia or heartburn, neither, or both.

close the esophagus so that reflux cannot occur, and it relaxes in response to a swallow to permit the passage of food. Although this one-way valve cannot be distinguished anatomically from neighboring esophageal muscle, it opens and closes as a unit.

When a subject swallows a barium suspension, its progress through the esophagus can be followed radiographically. The radiologist can observe the LES to relax in response to a swallow. A gamma camera permits similar observations by following a gamma-emitting substance such as technetium-99m through the esophagus. However, the time-honored test of LES function is esophageal motility testing, or esophageal manometry. The subject swallows a tube equipped with pressure sensors, and intraesophageal pressure is recorded and displayed. Withdrawal of sensors through the lower esophagus identifies a high pressure zone known as the resting LES pressure. Sensors are fixed at 5-cm intervals to a tube that is placed in the esophagus, with the lowest sensor in the LES. After a swallow, the upper sensors record the sequential increase in pressure generated by a peristaltic wave. As the wave approaches the LES, it relaxes to permit passage of swallowed material (see Figure 19-1).

A resting LES pressure of 10 cm is sufficient to withstand any tendency of increased gastric pressure to burst open the LES. However, the resting LES pressure is not the most important determinant of GER. Transitory reflux episodes occur unassociated with a swallow, a meal, or esophageal distention. Even small amounts of water in the throat that are insufficient to induce a swallow can transiently relax the sphincter. These episodes are most prone to occur after a meal, especially one containing fat. They permit reflux of gastric contents into the esophagus that may in turn provoke heartburn and esophagitis.

Thus, LES function is the critical factor in determining GER. It is here the battle against reflux is won or lost. However, LES is not enough. Many other factors contribute to LES incompetence and the perception of symptoms (Table 14-2).

FACTORS CONTRIBUTING TO LES FUNCTION

Anatomical

The pinchcock action of the peri-esophageal diaphragmatic structures, especially the sphinctre-like prolongations of the crura, undoubtedly accounts for the fact that man may stand on his head drinking a quart of water, or eating a full meal, without any of the stomach contents gravitating out of the stomach into the esophagus.

C. Jackson, 1922

TABLE 14-2
What Weakens the LES?

Food
  Chocolate
  Fat
  Peppermint
  Alcohol
  Caffeine
Hormones
  Progesterone
  Secretin
  Cholecystokinin
  Somatostatin
  Glucagon
  Vasoactive intestinal polypeptide (VIP)
  Gastric inhibitory polypeptide (GIP)
Drugs
  Calcium channel antagonists
  Anticholinergics
  Tricyclic antidepressants
  Phenothiazines
  Morphine
  Diazepam
  Barbiturates
  Meperidine (demerol)
  Prostaglandin E_2
  Dopamine
  Theophylline
  Beta adrenergics
  Progesterone
  Steroids
  Nitrates
Other
  Smoking
  Stress

The right crus is a muscular part of the diaphragm that hugs the esophagus as it passes through from the chest into the abdomen. This supports and augments the LES. The diaphragm consists of a large sheet of striated muscle that separates the chest from the abdomen (see Figure 1-3). It is enervated by the phrenic, not the vagus, nerve. The crus independently contracts in response to any sudden increase in intra-abdominal pressure that might result from coughing, straining, or even deep inspiration. Furthermore, the intra-abdominal position of the sphincter means that increases in abdominal pressure augment the LES. These mechanisms oppose the tendency of increased pressure within the stomach to force its contents up into the esophagus.

When there is a hiatus hernia, the LES moves up into the chest. The diaphragmatic pinch in response to increased abdominal pressure on the LES is lost. Furthermore, a small hernia can serve as a reservoir of gastric contents that continue to reflux even after the rest of the stomach has emptied.

Motility

The esophagus is more than a passive conduit. In youth and in health, primary peristaltic waves carry a swallowed bolus of food from upper to lower sphincter in about 7 seconds, where LES relaxation permits it to pass. Secondary peristalsis occurs when the body of the esophagus is stretched by food, refluxed material, or experimental intraesophageal inflation of a balloon. This housekeeping function normally sweeps away refluxed material before it does mischief, but in gastroesophageal reflux disease (GERD) there is a defect in the triggering of secondary peristalsis.

With age and disease, esophageal contractions become less vigorous and less orderly. Tertiary contractions are tremulous movements with little propulsive effect. Peristalsis is now inefficient, and this impairs the housekeeper function. This aging phenomenon has been called *presbyesophagus*. In scleroderma, noncontractile fibrous tissue replaces esophageal smooth muscle, so that neither peristalsis nor LES contraction can occur. The result is unopposed reflux of gastric contents and severe esophagitis (Figure 14-2).

Tonic gastric contractions empty fluids into the duodenum. Solids are slowly ground, mixed, and then swept away by antral peristalsis. Any process that interferes with these functions, such as diabetes, pyloric obstruction, or vagotomy, can delay gastric emptying. Gastric retention provides more opportunity for gastric contents to reflux through the transiently relaxing LES. Items that delay gastric emptying include a large meal, fat, hypertonic fluids, exercise, drugs, and even emotion (see also Table 14-2).

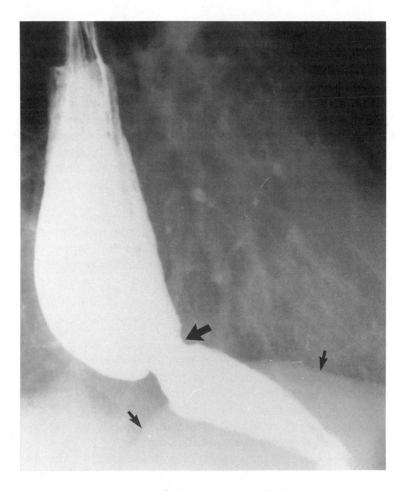

Figure 14-2. Scleroderma of the esophagus. The lower esophagus, its muscle layer replaced by fibrous tissue, is very dilated and atonic. The large arrow points at a stricture caused by reflux of gastric acid and pepsin through the destroyed lower esophageal sphincter. The small arrows indicate the diaphragm. The small amount of stomach above the diaphragm and below the stricture is a hiatus hernia.

Diet

Many foods weaken or inappropriately relax the LES and promote reflux. Some are predictable, and others seem idiosyncratic, that is, they are harmful to only certain individuals. Fat and concentrated salt solutions delay gastric emptying, furthering the opportunity for reflux. Chocolate and fatty or fried foods are notorious among those that directly or indirectly weaken the LES. Peppermint is a smooth muscle relaxant that also weakens the LES. It is ironic that after-dinner mints, presumably given to facilitate a postprandial belch, should also promote GER. So much for "digestives"! Some people notice that onions and garlic give them heartburn. Alcohol, tobacco, and coffee (even "decaf") may adversely affect the LES.

Overeating makes food available to reflux longer and in greater quantity. A full stomach is also more likely to trap food and gastric acid in a hiatus hernia, where it may reflux if given the opportunity. Obesity can crowd the stomach and further encourage reflux.

Mechanical

Obesity, pregnancy, and a tight girdle increase the risk of reflux. Lifting, coughing, and straining intensify intra-abdominal pressure and promote GER. Exercise may cause sudden, unopposed increases in intra-abdominal pressure. Running or violent movements (e.g., squash, tennis) are more likely to cause reflux than a stationary exercise such as bicycling. The reflux potential of exercise is far more consequential after a meal.

Gravity is another important determinant of reflux. The opossum is a favorite animal for LES physiologists to study (or should they be called "refluxologists"?). Known to spend many hours in an inverted position, this curious animal seems remarkable for its antireflux prowess. Humans, it seems, can depend less on the integrity of their LES. Despite the statement by Jackson, few of us can eat upside down. People who tend to reflux do so especially when they bend over or lie down. Reclining after a meal will especially set up reflux in such persons. Just as gravity can provoke heartburn, it can also be used to prevent it. The damage done by reflux at night depends upon whether gas or acid overlies the LES.

Not all of us are anatomically identical, but as a general rule, we are more likely to reflux acid in the right recumbent position. Sufferers learn to favor the upright or left recumbent positions, and even elevate the head of their bed upon retiring.

Drugs

Heartburn in pregnancy often begins while the fetus is still very small. It also occurs more often in the second half of the menstrual cycle. At least some of this reflux is due to impairment of LES function by the hormone progesterone. Similarly, GER is a consequence of hormone therapy and some birth-control pills. Corticosteroid drugs, hormones used as treatment of many medical diseases, cause heartburn. These are often called *steroids* and include the naturally occurring cortisone or the synthetic prednisone.

Anticholinergic drugs, by opposing the effects of acetylcholine in the enteric nervous system, weaken the LES and inhibit esophageal and gastric peristalsis. Drugs such as propantheline (Pro Banthine™) or dicyclomine (Bentylol™, Bentyl™) are less used for gastrointestinal purposes now, but the very commonly used tricyclic antidepressants and phenothiazine tranquilizers have potent anticholinergic effects. For this reason many people cannot tolerate psychoactive drugs such as amitryptaline (Elavil™) or chlorpromazine (Thorazine™, Largactil™).

Drugs with beta-adrenergic activity such as terbutaline, or calcium channel blockers that inhibit smooth muscle contraction, provoke heartburn in some people. Aspirin and NSAIDs may directly irritate the esophagus. Theophylline and many others can also produce troubling reflux symptoms.

Gut Hormones

Many "gut hormones" act in the enteric nervous system, where they greatly influence the integrity of the LES. They are not commercial drugs, but there is interest in agents that might enhance or suppress their activity. Gastrin has a tonic effect on the LES and stimulates stomach emptying. Other hormones that antagonize its actions include somatostatin and cholecystokinin. They favor re-

flux. For the moment gut hormones are of little practical importance in GER, but they may become so in future.

Emotion

In Shakespeare's *Much Ado About Nothing,* the self-confident
Beatrice, regarding the sour Don John, observes to her friends:

> How tartly that gentleman looks!
> I never can see him, but I am
> Heartburned an hour after.
>   II, i

Heartburn has long been linked to emotion. About 60% of patients
who complain to doctors about heartburn recognize stress as a
cause. People in the community who do not report their gut symptoms to a doctor are relatively untroubled. Therefore, it is uncertain
whether emotion generates heartburn or whether it impairs one's
tolerance for heartburn. Undoubtedly both are at work. Some
people with heartburn and no esophagitis are hypersensitive to a
degree of acid reflux that would be unnoticed by others.

There is new evidence that stress, anxiety, and other psychological factors sensitize the individual to perceive heartburn at
lower esophageal acid levels. Poor social support may also sensitize the esophagus. Stress can therefore induce heartburn without
necessarily altering GER. The stressed person may compound
matters by abusing cigarettes, drugs, and alcohol.

Previous Surgery

Gastric surgery is less frequently performed today. Not many
years ago it was a common treatment for peptic ulcer and its
complications. Such surgery might adversely affect antireflux function (see Chapter 29). A vagotomy slows gastric emptying and
impairs esophageal function. To counteract the former, a "drainage" procedure was commonly done. This might be widening the
pylorus, excision of the antrum and pylorus, or a gastroenterostomy, where the stomach is opened into a loop of small bowel.
While these procedures reduce gastric stasis, they sometimes also

permit bile to find its way back into the stomach. Along with gastric juice, bile then may reflux into the esophagus, where the combination of acid, pepsin, and bile salts is particularly noxious.

SUMMARY

In the ongoing struggle to keep noxious gastric contents out of the esophagus, the LES is a key player. Many nerves, hormones, neurotransmitters, and reflexes come into play to permit the LES to respond to a reflux threat, while also allowing it to relax for a meal to pass. Not only is the LES subject to many neural and humoral influences, but it also has a strong anatomic supporting cast. This includes the right crus of the diaphragm that compresses the lower esophagus. In response to increased intra-abdominal pressure, this muscular structure contracts to support the antireflux effort of the LES. The housekeeping effect of the esophagus and the promptness of stomach emptying also help determine the extent of GER. These antireflux forces may be defeated by diseases of the stomach or esophagus, anatomical displacement of the LES by a hiatus hernia, or mechanical forces that overcome the LES such as pregnancy, gluttony, straining, or exercise. Certain foods, drugs, hormones, and nervous impulses weaken the LES or cause it to relax inappropriately. Damaging reflux occurs not only through a weakened sphincter, but also during spontaneous LES relaxations that often follow a meal. The degree of damage depends upon factors addressed in the next chapter.

CHAPTER FIFTEEN

Heartburn and Esophagitis

Heartburn and esophagitis are consequences of GER. Twenty-four-hour esophageal pressure and pH recordings demonstrate that almost everyone has transient relaxations of the LES and reflux, yet only one-third of adults report heartburn. It is likely that esophagitis occurs in less than 5% of people. What factors determine why some, but not all, reflux episodes result in heartburn or esophagitis?

DETERMINANTS OF TISSUE DAMAGE

The causes of GER and impaired esophageal peristalsis were discussed in the last chapter. Most reflux episodes go unnoticed. Tissue damage depends upon conditions in the esophageal lumen and the ability of the esophageal mucosa to resist the noxious effects of the refluxed material.

Luminal Factors

The Refluxed Material

The greater the mucosal exposure to the refluxed material, the greater is the potential for irritation and damage. In chapter 14 the factors that influence reflux were discussed. Esophageal contact is inversely proportional to the efficiency with which peristalsis and gravity clear refluxed gastric contents from the esophagus. In a diseased or elderly esophagus, the weakened esophageal muscle impairs peristaltic housekeeping.

The nature of the refluxate is also important. Hydrogen ions are the most damaging of gastric contents. However, pepsin activated by a low pH may digest mucosa. The corrosive effects of these materials may be appreciated by recalling how the mouth and lips burn after vomiting. If duodenal contents reach the esophagus, trypsin and bile salts may increase the damage. Trypsin, a pancreatic enzyme, is a powerful destroyer of protein. Bile salts are detergents that damage the lipid cell membranes, threatening the integrity of the epithelial cells and permitting the penetration of hydrogen ions.

Ingested Material

Many people relate their heartburn to certain foods. There is great variation in this experience, and what causes heartburn in one person may not trouble another. Ingested material can cause heartburn and inflammation through many mechanisms. It may delay gastric emptying, stimulate gastric acid secretion, favor GER, or "irritate" the mucosa directly. The first three of these have been discussed, and items that relax the LES are listed in Table 14-2.

It is widely assumed that acid provokes heartburn. Infusion of dilute hydrochloric acid through a tube into the acid-sensitive esophagus reproduces heartburn. However, as in all things biological, it is not that simple. Even when the pH of tomato juice is adjusted to neutrality, it evokes heartburn. Coffee, with its pH adjusted to 7, still provokes heartburn in people with a sensitive esophagus. One study determined that fluids caused heartburn in proportion to their osmolality.

Table 15-1 lists fluids likely to directly cause heartburn. These data have scientific limitations, but they can help the heartburn sufferer suspect what to avoid. Investigators analyzed 38 drinks for osmolality, pH, and titratable acid. Titratable acid is a better estimate of total acidity, since other constituents partly buffer or neutralize pH. The researchers then gathered data from 394 subjects known to have heartburn. The percentage of people who identified each of the items as heartburn inducers appears in the last column of the table. Heartburn is graded as follows: 0, absent; 1, occasional; and 2, frequent. The heartburn score for each fluid was calculated by adding the scores and dividing by the number of participants who evaluated the fluid. Possible scores range from 0 to 2 and appear in the second to last column in Table 15-1.

What emerges from this study is that acid, especially titratable acid, is an important instigator of heartburn. Grapefruit, orange, and tomato juices were the most acidic and produced the highest heartburn scores (Table 15-1). These data suggest that osmolality is unimportant. The notion that red wine is more troublesome than white is a myth. Both have acidity values similar to grape juice but induce twice as much heartburn, so alcohol must also be important. Beer causes slightly less trouble, and other alcoholic drinks got a large write-in vote. The heartburn potential of these drinks was not proportional to their alcoholic content, so there must be other factors in wine.

Coffee's effect is not due to caffeine or acidity, yet it reliably causes heartburn in susceptible people. Except for buttermilk, milk is neutral. Its tendency to induce heartburn is proportional to its fat content. Alcohol stimulates acid and loosens the LES. In these cases, it is impossible to be certain that they "irritate" as well as promote reflux. Accidental or suicidal ingestion of lye or strong acid devastates the esophagus. If not immediately fatal, there are inevitably severe complications. Occasionally certain pills (such as tetracycline) lodge in the esophagus and cause a painful "pill" esophagitis.

Neutralization by Saliva

Even when peristalsis or gravity clears the esophagus of gastric contents, the pH of the esophageal mucosa remains low. Bicarbonate in saliva helps neutralize any remaining hydrogen ions. Chewing increases salivation. This provides more salivary bicarbonate, mucus, and other substances that help protect the esophagus against reflux damage. Salivation is inactive at night, worsening the effects of GER when one retires. Patients with scleroderma and some other rheumatic disorders have diminished saliva production (Sjogren's syndrome), further jeopardizing a diseased esophagus. Smokers also produce less saliva, providing yet another reason to quit.

TABLE 15-1
Osmolality, Acidity, and Likelihood of Heartburn of Some
Fluids[a]

Fluid	Osmolality (mOsm/kg)	pH	Titratable acidity (meq/I)	Heartburn score	Reporting heartburn (%)
Water	2	8.61	0	0.22	19.5
Citrus juices					
Grapefruit	532	3.30	155	1.08	73
Orange	622	3.75	109.2	1.00	68.3
Tomato	604	4.19	53.8	0.99	69.5
Pineapple	722	3.56	112.3	0.85	62.4
Cranberry	907	2.72	81.3	0.59	46
Apple	718	3.60	49	0.56	44.2
Grape	1174	3.35	75.2	0.52	39.3
Apricot	973	3.76	53.1	0.38	29.9
Prune	1174	3.81	79.2	0.25	20.8
Soft drinks					
Pepsi	716	2.35	10.2	0.77	56.7
Coke	695	2.35	10.2	0.76	55.2
Diet Pepsi	27	2.95	7.3	0.66	50.8
Diet Coke	29	3.11	8.1	0.65	48.7
Root beer	774	4.19	3.8	0.52	38.4
Sprite	688	3.27	20.4	0.47	34.8
7Up	691	3.15	18.3	0.45	34.7
Alcohol					
Red wine	2428	3.52	64.6	1.05	67.7
White wine	2677	3.32	71.9	0.95	62.7
Beer	1041	4.34	22.5	0.87	60.4
Other					
Coffee	58	5.14	4.6	1.01	78.6
Tea	31	5.80	1.7	0.63	50.7
Whole milk	282	6.73	3.3	0.57	37.6
Low-fat milk	305	6.72	3.8	0.37	27.9
Skim milk	277	6.78	2.7	0.30	22.9
Buttermilk	461	4.51	74.2	0.47	33.3

[a]Adapted from Feldman and Barnet, 1995.

Tissue Resistance

The esophageal mucosa resembles skin in that its epithelium consists of layered squamus cells (see Figure 1-8). The superficial layer consists of dead cells (*stratum corneum*) that protect the deeper, living tissue. In the skin, but not the oral and esophageal mucosa, this layer contains a toughening material called *keratin*.

The *stratum spinosum* is a middle layer of metabolically active cells with tight attachments to one another that act as a barrier to hydrogen ions. In time these become the stratum corneum. The deepest, basal layer of rapidly regenerating cells is destined, in time, to become the other two layers. A few submucus glands secrete bicarbonate as further protection.

Unlike gastric and duodenal mucosa, the esophagus lacks an effective mucus–bicarbonate protective layer. The layered mucosal cells can cope with a low pH only for short periods. The cell membrane, itself, is relatively impermeable to hydrogen ions, as are the "tight junctions" that fuse the cells to one another. With acid exposure, hydrogen ions diffuse into the cells, where phosphates and bicarbonate buffer them to maintain intracellular pH. Bicarbonate is generated by the enzyme carbonic anhydrase or diffuses from the blood in exchange for chloride. A hydrogen–potassium exchanger helps pump hydrochloric acid into the blood, where it quickly disperses. Hydrogen ions also stimulate basal cell reproduction to promptly replace damaged mucosal cells. Basal cell reproductive activity is a hallmark of reflux esophagitis. Hydrogen ions do not easily penetrate these defenses, but if they do, heartburn and esophagitis may ensue.

DETERMINANTS OF HEARTBURN

Most people with heartburn have a normal-appearing esophageal mucosa. Even if a biopsy is examined under the microscope, it too would likely be normal. However, some would have microscopic changes such as epithelial damage, inflammation, and increased basal cell activity. A few patients with heartburn will have overt tissue damage. Conversely, and inexplicably, some people with very severe esophagitis have no heartburn. Since GER is responsible for both heartburn and esophagitis, these facts are difficult to reconcile.

When heartburn occurs, it usually does so in concert with LES relaxation and reflux, as demonstrated by 24-hour recording of intraesophageal pressure and acidity. However, most refluxes—in most people most of the time—are unaccompanied by heartburn. No doubt, luminal and cellular factors protect the esophagus, but the truth is that we do not know how the sensation of heartburn

TABLE 15-2
Grades of Esophagitis

Grade	Endoscopic appearance
Grade 0	Normal appearance (histologic change only)
Grade 1	One or more nonconfluent lesions with erythema or exudate above the gastroesophageal junction
Grade 2	Confluent, noncircumferential, erosive, and exudative lesions
Grade 3	Circumferential erosive and exudative lesions
Grade 4	Chronic mucosal lesions (i.e., ulceration, stricture, or Barrett's epithelium)

occurs. There are no superficial nerve endings to detect acid reflux and send the "heartburn" message to the brain. Probably, acid and other irritating materials penetrate through the tissue barrier deep into the mucosa, where nerve endings do exist. In some people, the esophageal mucosa seems hypersensitive to "normal" refluxes. In other cases, severe esophagitis or Barrett's esophagus destroy these nerve endings, which might explain why some people with esophagitis have no heartburn.

Psychological Considerations

We are becoming aware of the importance of the enteric nervous system and the brain itself in the perception of pain in gastrointestinal disease. Normally, messages from the gut to the brain are suppressed. This suppression may be lessened by stress or emotion. This may be the means by which emotional upset can produce heartburn. In the last chapter we saw that anxiety, stress, and lack of social support increase esophageal sensitivity. Some people perceive heartburn at an esophageal pH of 6, while others feel nothing at a pH of 2.

DETERMINANTS OF ESOPHAGITIS

If the esophagus contains enough acid, pepsin, bile salts, trypsin, or hyperosmolar materials for long enough, mucosal damage will ensue. Under the microscope, the first changes are extensions of papillalike structures normally penetrating into the squamus epithelium from below to 15–75% of its thickness. Inflammation may expose and sensitize the deeper nerve endings. Note that this much change can occur while the endoscopic view remains normal.

Greater exposure to noxious refluxed material produces damage that is visible to the endoscopist. The degree of damage is graded in a variety of ways. One scoring system is outlined in Table 15-2. The earliest abnormality is the appearance of one or more isolated reddened areas above the gastroesophageal junction. As the disease progresses, these lesions become confluent and eroded and develop an exudate (a layer of dead cells and debris). Grades 3 and 4 esophagitis are important because they require more aggressive therapy, and relapse is very likely if therapy is withdrawn. Grade 4 esophagitis includes the complications of ulcer, bleeding, stricture, and Barrett's esophagus, which are discussed in Chapter 17.

SUMMARY

Most adults have spontaneous LES relaxations and gastroesophageal reflux, yet most are unaware of any symptoms. The experience of heartburn and the development of esophagitis depend upon (1) the amount and duration of esophageal exposure to gastric contents, (2) the nature of ingested material, (3) the neutralizing effect of swallowed saliva, and (4) the resistance of the squamus epithelium to the injurious actions of hydrochloric acid and other noxious refluxates. It is uncertain how we perceive heartburn, but it likely results from hydrogen ions and other irritants reaching nerve endings in the deeper layers of the esophageal mucosa. Anxiety and stress sensitize an individual to perceive heartburn at lower acid levels. The apparent independence of heartburn and esophagitis remains unexplained. Esophagitis may be microscopic. Severe esophagitis appears to the endoscopist as an ulcerated, scarred, and deformed lower esophagus, where complications such as bleeding, stricture, or Barrett's metaplasia may be anticipated.

CHAPTER SIXTEEN

Diagnosis and Treatment of Heartburn and Esophagitis

Heartburn is the hallmark of gastroesophageal reflux disease (GERD), even though reflux often occurs without symptoms. The discomfort may be atypical or may occur in circumstances that obscure the diagnosis, but it is usually heartburn that brings the disease to attention. Heartburn is one of the most common human symptoms, and it requires judgment to determine who needs investigation and when to employ expensive drug therapy.

DIAGNOSIS OF GASTROESOPHAGEAL REFLUX DISEASE

History

Heartburn is a burning, hot, or acid sensation behind the breastbone. Sometimes it is felt in the neck or just below the chest. However, people experience and interpret discomfort in many ways. Terms such as *acid indigestion* or *acid regurgitation* usually mean heartburn. More characteristic than the quality of the pain are the circumstances in which it occurs. It frequently begins 1–2 hours after meals, especially if the meals include the items listed in Table 14-2. Onions, spices, fried foods, and chocolates are common provocations. NSAIDs and tobacco also make heartburn worse. Bending over, reclining, or exercise after a meal may elicit heartburn, and many experience it upon retiring. For relief of nocturnal heartburn, sufferers learn to sit on a chair or elevate their upper torso on a pillow. Strong emotions, such as fear or anxiety, may provoke heartburn in susceptible people. The location of the pain and relation to effort may evoke fears of heart disease.

Typically, antacids relieve heartburn. These alkaline, over-the-counter medications represent a billion-dollar industry (see Chapter 22). Home remedies such as baking soda (sodium bicarbonate) may also bring relief. Some foods, even water, relieve heartburn by diluting and washing out refluxed acid and raising intraesophageal pH.

Regurgitation is the effortless appearance of refluxed material into the mouth. This commonly occurs with bending after a meal or at night. It is often, but not always, associated with heartburn. Regurgitation, especially in debilitated people, creates the risk of damage to the larynx or lungs.

Regurgitation is distinct from vomiting, which accompanies nausea and retching. Many people suffering heartburn or other upper gastrointestinal complaint experience a watery material in the mouth. This is a vagus-mediated salivation reflex that when copious is called *water brash*. It has been known to cause some sufferers to foam at the mouth. *Rumination* is an unusual phenomenon that may be mistaken for regurgitation. This is an apparently voluntary act in which the individual swallows a meal and subsequently brings it up for a chew, as a cow chews its cud. This occasions no symptoms but often comes to medical attention when a disgusted family member complains.

Physical Examination

GERD produces no physical findings. The physician's examination concentrates on excluding diseases that may predispose the patient to reflux or that might be mistaken for it. The physician also looks for features that might be important in treatment, such as obesity, nicotine stains, or anxiety. Forced recumbency, as with a fractured hip, may provoke GERD. Patients with scleroderma have tight, shiny skin, especially in the fingers and around the mouth. There may also be calcium deposits in the skin and abnormal skin blood vessels called *telangiectasia*.

In older people, it is important to look for signs of heart disease or high blood pressure. Sometimes a tender breastbone or inflammation of the joints between the ribs and breastbone may cause breast pain. If the patient is diabetic or immunosuppressed, esophageal infections are likely. Candida causes thrush in the mouth and may be a clue to esophageal infection. Discovery of endocrine disease such as hyperparathyroidism in someone with severe reflux symptoms suggests the rare Zollinger–Ellison syndrome.

Investigations

Patients with heartburn seen in primary care need no tests. Simple heartburn unaccompanied by complications usually improves with diet and lifestyle measures. Only those who fail to improve or who develop complications require investigation. Endoscopy is the most useful diagnostic test, but the choice between it and barium swallow may boil down to availability and cost.

Endoscopy

Esophagitis may or may not accompany heartburn. Only endoscopy can reliably detect esophageal mucosal inflammation and ulceration. This procedure is safe and quickly performed (see Chapter 31). The presence of esophagitis helps confirm GERD, but most cases will have a normal mucosa. A system for grading esophagitis as shown in Table 15-2 is helpful in planning therapy. Grades 3 or 4 esophagitis usually means the disease will respond to nothing short of a proton pump inhibitor. Milder grades should improve with H_2 antagonists. If no esophagitis is seen at endoscopy, one should redouble efforts to improve diet and lifestyle and employ drugs sparingly.

Typically, reflux esophagitis is most severe at the gastroesophageal mucosal junction and diminishes proximally. Other patterns should raise suspicion of other diseases. In the immunosuppressed patient, infections such as candidiasis, herpes, or cytomegalovirus are common and a biopsy may help make the distinction. Ordinarily, biopsies are not performed for reflux esophagitis. If the inflammation is not obvious, the finding of microscopic changes will unlikely influence treatment, except under special circumstances. Biopsies increase cost, are of some risk, and require expert interpretation. Cancer of the esophagus usually presents with bleeding, dysphagia, or weight loss. It should be considered in elderly smokers, drinkers, and those of Oriental heritage. Cancer is also a complication of long-standing reflux and Barrett's esophagus (see Chapter 17).

Endoscopy is a poor method of assessing LES function. However, in severe GERD, a lax, noncontracting sphincter may permit free reflux from the stomach during the examination. Unless large, a hiatus hernia is difficult to diagnose through the endoscope, but its presence has little influence on medical therapy.

Barium Swallow

A barium swallow is the preferred first test for GERD only if the patient has dysphagia (see Chapter 17). With careful technique, severe esophagitis or ulceration may be detected, but the test is very insensitive for less than grade 3 esophagitis. This X-ray procedure will show a hiatus hernia or other structural abnormality. Sometimes the radiologist convincingly demonstrates reflux of barium back through a lax sphincter.

Other Tests

Outside of research centers, other tests are seldom required. However, if there is some doubt about the diagnosis, special tests can confirm reflux, measure esophageal motor function, and relate dysfunction or reflux episodes to symptoms. These are especially useful when the origin of chest pain is obscure (see Chapter 19). Before undertaking repair of a weak LES, a surgeon will want to be certain that reflux is indeed the culprit and that there is no underlying motor disorder such as scleroderma.

TREATMENT OF GERD

Treatment of GERD should be undertaken according to the severity of the symptoms and esophagitis and the presence or absence of complications. If one-third of adults has heartburn, it would be a formidable and unnecessary undertaking to recommend drugs for them all. Most will improve with elementary diet and lifestyle changes (see Table 16-1). These measures reduce drug

TABLE 16-1
GERD: Diet and Lifestyle Treatments

Small, low-fat meals
Avoid drugs, foods known to promote reflux
If obese, lose weight
Stop smoking
Drink moderately, no nightcap
No bedtime snacks
Avoid exercise, straining, bending, reclining after meals
Elevate head of bed, or use wedge
Anticipate episodes of heartburn, use antacid
Manage stress

requirements and prevent complications later. In every case, they should be taught and reinforced, since, no matter how severe the GERD, it is a chronic and recurrent disease.

Diet and Lifestyle

Patients should try to identify offending foods, since idiosyncrasies are common. They should be alert to the items in Table 14-2. Chocolate, coffee, fats, and onions are often offenders. The physician should proscribe alcohol and tobacco and review medications to see if they contain ingredients listed in Table 14-2. Overeating is unwise, since a full stomach may force open the LES and prolong the opportunity to reflux. Regular small meals are best, and solids are less likely than liquids to regurgitate. The obese should lose weight and avoid tight clothing. Vigorous exercise, bending, and lifting must not be done until the stomach is empty. Food taken at bedtime is particularly reflux-prone.

If stress is a factor, a stress management program can help. Anxiety and stress increase the perception of heartburn. A relaxation program where muscle groups are alternately tensed and relaxed in time with breathing will reduce anxiety, slow the pulse, and improve heartburn. Relaxed circumstances during meals and deferral of stressful encounters until the stomach is empty are simply common sense.

Position is very important. Bending or reclining after eating encourages reflux (Figure 16-1). For nocturnal heartburn or regurgitation, elevation of the head of the bed on 8-inch (20-cm) blocks is almost as effective as an H_2 antagonist (Figure 16-2). There may be less reflux and better esophageal clearing when the patient lies on his or her left side. Waterbeds are unkind to refluxers, and of course the head cannot be elevated. Pillows are not very effective. A foam wedge purchased at a medical appliance store is better. This device is especially useful when the other partner in the matrimonial bed complains of its elevation. On the subject of matrimony, a report from Glasgow entitled *Reflux Dyspareunia* states that 77 of 100 women suffered heartburn during intercourse. Measures such as weight loss, no stooping, and the "female-superior position" improved 66 of the 77 victims. (Sorry, no illustration!)

Antacids relieve, and even prevent, heartburn (see Chapter 22). Many people can predict when they will get heartburn: after a meal, upon retiring, or at a stressful event. A timely antacid may anticipate and prevent the symptom. Keep in mind that antacids remain in the stomach less than 1 hour, but longer after meals. Liquid antacids disperse better and are most effective, but tablets carried in the pocket or purse are handier for those unexpected episodes that inevitably occur at inconvenient times. Antacids may even reduce reflux, perhaps by improving inflammation. For some, the alginate-antacid preparations Gaviscon™ and Algicon™ are especially helpful. Alginate floats on gastric juice, blocking reflux into the LES. The antacid component of the preparation reduces the mucosal pH.

Drugs

Individual drugs are discussed in Part 6. Here we concentrate on their place in the treatment of heartburn and esophagitis. In principle, systemic drugs should not be employed without an endoscopy. If the situation is important enough to warrant drugs, the severity of esophagitis and risk of complications should guide the choice, dose, and duration of treatment.

In reality, drugs are used for symptoms. Some countries permit over-the-counter sales of H_2 antagonists. Their safety and ease of administration should not beguile us into overlooking the cost and the potential complications that may be temporarily suppressed by inadequate treatment.

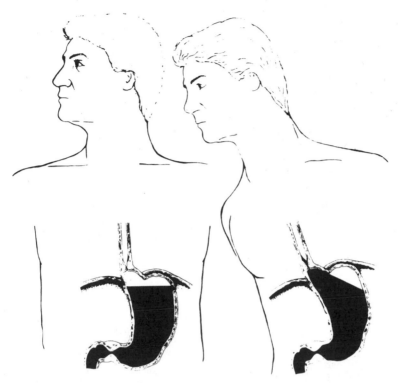

Figure 16-1. Effect of position on gastroesophageal reflux. (Left) Upright position maintains gastric contents in the dependent part of the stomach. (Right) When bending, gastric contents cover the cardia and are poised to reflux through a transiently incompetent LES. (From Thompson, 1989.)

H₂ Antagonists

For grades 1 or 2 esophagitis, H_2 antagonists are the practical choice (see Chapter 23). Many studies support their efficacy in the short term. Table 16-2 indicates their doses and costs. They are more efficient at relieving heartburn than healing esophagitis. When they stop, reflux remains, and so do the conditions favoring recurrence of heartburn and esophagitis. At least 50% of patients so treated relapse within 1 year of stopping the drug. Even a regular but reduced maintenance dose is disappointing. Eight weeks of H_2 antagonist therapy is necessary to heal the esophagitis, so the drug must be continued after the heartburn disappears. Irregular, symp-

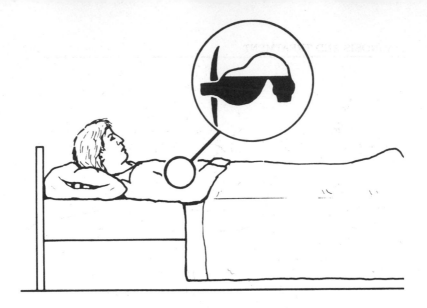

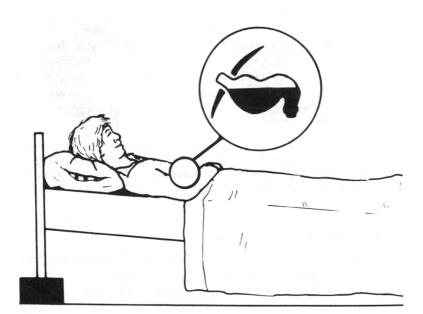

Figure 16-2. Postural treatment of gastroesophageal reflux. (Top) When a subject lies flat in bed, gastric contents overlie the esophagogastric junction. If the LES relaxes, reflux may occur. (Below) Elevation of the head of the bed on 8-inch (20 cm) blocks places the esophagus above the stomach. Gravity maintains gastric contents in the stomach and avoids reflux. (From Thompson, 1989.)

TABLE 16-2
Drugs for GERD: Daily Cost

Drug	Dose[a]	Cost/day[b]
Cimetidine	800 mg daily	2.52
Ranitidine	150 mg twice daily	3.16
Famotidine	20 mg twice daily	2.82
Nizatidine	150 mg twice daily	3.04
Omeprazole	20 mg daily	3.60
Sucralfate	1 g four times a day	2.76
Cisapride	20 mg twice daily	2.72

[a]Very often twice the stated dose is used.
[b]In U.S. Dollars. After Pope, 1994.

tomatic use may control symptoms, but probably does little to prevent complications.

Proton Pump Blockers

Grade 3 or 4 esophagitis and complications require a proton pump blocker such as omeprazole (see Chapter 24). Many cases require twice the recommended dose, that is, 40 mg/day (or 20 mg twice daily). The pump blockers are superior to the H_2 antagonists. They will heal most esophagitis if given long enough and in sufficient doses. These potent drugs are essential for complicated esophagitis and may be used for milder, yet troublesome, cases that fail to respond to lesser therapies.

As with other drugs, the underlying reflux continues when omeprazole is withdrawn, and recurrence is almost inevitable. Maintenance therefore is necessary. Options include symptomatic therapy, pulse therapy, and indefinite maintenance. In symptomatic therapy, heartburn triggers a 2-to 4-week course of the drug on the assumption that the esophagitis has recurred. In pulse therapy, regular treatment courses preempt recurrences. However, severe and complicated esophagitis permit no such compromises and full-dose prophylaxis is required indefinitely. Many patients need 40 mg of omeprazole daily.

About 10% of patients receiving long-term omeprazole have increased serum gastrin (500 ng/L). This fuels earlier concerns about hyperplasia of argyrophil cells in the gastric crypts and reports of carcinoid tumors in animals. Nevertheless, the drug has been used safely for 4 year periods. It is prudent to check the serum gastrin periodically, but the risk in elderly patients must be very small. A more immediate problem is the transient hypersecretion of acid that follows withdrawal of omeprazole and probably other antisecretory drugs. This may hasten relapse and make it difficult to withdraw the drug until gastrin levels return to normal.

Prokinetics

The argument for the use of prokinetics in GERD is that, unlike acid-suppressing drugs, they attack the basic defects (see Chaper 27). They speed stomach emptying, tighten the LES, and perhaps even improve the esophageal housekeeper. The fallacy, however, is that when the drug stops, so do the beneficial effects. Despite some favorable reports, I believe these drugs will prove less helpful than acid-suppressing medication, especially omeprazole. Because of side effects, bethanechol and metoclopromide should not be used for this purpose. Domperidone and cisapride are apparently safer, but only the latter consistently shows benefit in trials of treatment and maintenance therapy.

Cisapride, 20 mg before meals and at bedtime, will heal grade 1 or 2 esophagitis. However, it is a third-string drug for GERD. In company with an H_2 antagonist the drug is more effective, but the combined cost and inconvenience begs the question, "Why not switch to a proton pump inhibitor?"

Omeprazole or lansoprazole, in sufficient doses, will heal most esophagitis. Rarely, a prokinetic such as cisapride must be added, especially in complicated esophagitis. However, recurrence is inevitable once the drug is stopped. As pointed out above, the choice of treatment and maintenance drugs can be designed on the basis of the degree of esophagitis. Vignari *et al.* demonstrate that for a range of severity, omeprazole 20 mg per day is the best maintenance option over 12 months. It is superior to cisapride 10 mg three times per day or ranitidine three times per day in the prevention of heartburn, esophageal pain, and regurgitation. The addition of cisapride to omeprazole is no better than omeprazole alone. The poor performance of cisapride and ranitidine when used alone is improved when they are combined, but is still no better than omeprazole alone. In all five of these drug programs, adverse events are minor.

Combination therapy is expensive, requires several pills each day, and is seldom necessary. It may have a place in special circumstances where regurgitation threatens lung or laryngeal complications. All these considerations are likely also true for the prevention of esophageal complications such as bleeding, stricture, and perhaps even Barrett's esophagus and cancer.

Surgery

Medical failure should be rare. However, there are special circumstances where surgery is advisable (see Chapter 29). Despite acid suppression and cisapride, regurgitation may be so severe that it threatens the lungs or larynx. A young person who has become dependent on omeprazole may seek a permanent, cheaper solution that eliminates any theoretic risk of drug-induced cancer.

The surgeon's objective is to restore LES competence. Repair of a hiatus hernia is inadequate by itself, but it is still a part of the procedure. There are several operations available, all bearing the names of their inventors: Nissen, Hill, and Belsey. They have in common an attempt to reinforce the sphincter with gastric tissue, so that when the stomach contracts, the sphincter closes. These operations require much surgical skill and are described in Chapter 29.

SUMMARY

GERD manifests itself clinically as heartburn or regurgitation, and in a minority of instances, causes esophagitis. Usually, heartburn is recognized by the patient's description of a burning retrosternal pain or discomfort that is worse with straining, bending, and reclining, and improved with antacids. GERD is very common and is usually well managed by the family doctor and the patient through diet and lifestyle measures. Severe or resistant cases require endoscopy to assess the presence and severity of esophagitis. Sometimes a careful barium swallow will help, but uncomplicated GERD needs no other tests. Mild esophagitis and heartburn respond to H_2 antagonists, but recurrence is the rule.

Maintenance requires full doses. Severe esophagitis and disease resistant to other drug treatments necessitate a proton pump inhibitor, often indefinitely, to heal the esophagitis and prevent recurrence or complications. Prokinetics, especially cisapride, are useful when regurgitation and fear of aspiration exist. Antireflux surgery is rarely necessary now.

CHAPTER SEVENTEEN

Complications of Gastroesophageal Reflux

Heartburn and regurgitation are troublesome, but usually harmless. However, they sometimes have serious consequences. Esophagitis may stealthily damage the esophagus and come to medical attention only when bleeding, obstruction, or even cancer, occurs. This chapter discusses the complications of gastroesophageal reflux disease (Table 17-1).

COMPLICATIONS OF HEARTBURN

Misdiagnosis is the most important complication of heartburn. Because of poor communication or a genuine misperception, physicians may mistake heart pain for heartburn and lose an opportunity for life-prolonging therapy. Usually, coronary pain (angina) is a characteristic retrosternal pressure, squeezing, or heaviness that occurs with exertion. Sufferers often know their exact limits and are able to prevent angina by measured exertion. Cold air also causes angina. Heart pain is usually central in the breast, and the discomfort sometimes extends up into the neck and inside the left arm. The lower esophagus lies just behind the heart, so it is not surprising that its pain distribution is similar to angina. When these two conditions occur together, interpretation is doubly difficult.

Vigorous exercise may provoke reflux as well as angina. Nonetheless, most patients recognize the burning, position-related nature of their heartburn. While mistaking angina for heartburn is the more

TABLE 17-1
Complications of Gastroesophageal
Reflux

Complications of heartburn
Misdiagnosis
Confusion with coronary heart disease
Complications of regurgitation
Aspiration pneumonia
Nonallergic asthma
Acid laryngitis
Dental erosions
Complications of esophagitis
Hemorrhage
Stricture
Barrett's esophagus
Cancer of the esophagus
Other complications
Perforation of esophageal ulcer
Unwanted effects of treatment
Impaired quality of life

serious error, mistaking esophageal pain for angina is more common. In cases of doubtful chest pain, coronary heart disease must be ruled out. Noncardiac chest pain is discussed in Chapter 19. An imprecise history can mistaken heartburn for musculoskeletal inflammation, dyspepsia, or biliary colic.

COMPLICATIONS OF REGURGITATION

Aspiration Pneumonia

Debilitated or elderly patients who have reduced pharyngeal sensitivity may aspirate regurgitated material into their lungs. This is a particular danger when such patients undergo endoscopy or other intubation, and it is why the procedure is done while the patient is fasting and with careful monitoring. Patients in the intensive care ward are very prone to aspirate, but this is rare in ambulatory persons.

Asthma

There is an interesting relationship between nonallergic (nonseasonal) asthma and gastroesophageal reflux. Respiratory symptoms such as coughing or wheezing produce reflux by sudden, violent changes in the intra-abdominal and intrathoracic pressures. Reflux also may occur with the deep inspiration taken before forceful expiration by an asthmatic. Conversely, acid reflux irritates the larynx and causes a reflex constriction of the bronchi in experimental animals.

It is difficult to prove that reflux causes asthma. The best proof is improvement of both with effective antireflux therapy. In one study, both antireflux surgery and cimetidine improved asthma. While the surgery-treated patients remained better 5 years later, those given cimetidine relapsed when the drug was withdrawn. Thus, if reflux is suspected as a cause of nonallergic asthma, the sensible course is to intensively treat the reflux. Today, a proton pump inhibitor would be the drug of choice. However, in some cases reflux itself is the villain, making a prokinetic drug a better option.

Acid Laryngitis

Sometimes gastric juice refluxes through the esophagus and upper sphincter and spills into the larynx or voice box. The ensuing inflammation of the posterior larynx causes hoarseness. Probes detect acid reaching the larynx in some reflux episodes, and the damage is visible through a laryngoscope. Diagnosis may be difficult. There may be no heartburn to warn the individual of a reflux episode. Just as in heartburn, the esophagus may look normal, so laryngitis may occur with a normal-appearing larynx.

The symptoms include hoarseness, persistent nonproductive cough, a pressure sensation, and the need to continually clear the throat. Omeprazole improves some cases. More importantly, the individual should undertake the lifestyle changes necessary to minimize reflux. Silent regurgitation may, through stealth, be more dangerous than that accompanied by symptoms.

Dental Erosions

Severe gastroesophageal regurgitation of acid has also been associated with dental erosions. Unlike dental caries, dental erosions occur on the exposed surface of the tooth.

COMPLICATIONS OF ESOPHAGITIS

Hemorrhage

Severe esophagitis includes erosions and ulcers that may bleed. Hemorrhage may be inconsequential or may present with a chronic, unnoticed blood loss and iron-deficiency anemia. Once recognized, the esophagitis can be treated and the iron deficiency corrected by iron therapy. In the elderly, it is not safe to assume that iron deficiency or occult blood loss is caused by esophagitis. Cancer of the colon is also a possibility and should be excluded by colonoscopy or barium enema.

Occasionally, bleeding is acute with melena and the patient vomits blood. The diagnosis is confirmed endoscopically, and management is similar to that for bleeding ulcers described in Chapter 13. Bleeding esophagitis is seldom life-threatening, except in the frail.

Stricture

Gastroesophageal reflux promotes repeated cycles of mucosal damage and repair. Repair includes the production of fibrous tissue or scar, which hardens, shrinks, and narrows the esophagus. Stricture is the most common complication of esophagitis, and the principal symptom is *dysphagia*, or difficulty swallowing (Figures 17-1 and 17-2). This is always an important symptom and should prompt an endoscopy.

Causes of Dysphagia

Sometimes dysphagia results from severe esophagitis and will subside with drug treatment, but usually the cause is a motor or mechanical disorder. Some examples are in order.

Pharyngeal Dysphagia

It is important to distinguish *pharyngeal* from esophageal dysphagia. The problem here is in the throat: an inability to initiate a swallow. In neuromuscular disorders or strokes, pharyngeal dysphagia may cause aspiration of food into the lungs or redirec-

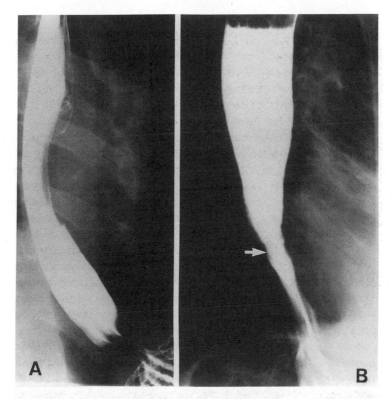

Figure 17-1. (A) Normal X ray of the esophagus after ingesting barium. Note the white barium filling the patent lower esophagus just before it passes through the narrow LES into the stomach (lower right). (B) Stricture of the esophagus caused by GERD. Here the barium passes through a tapered lower esophagus that cannot open further (arrow). Liquids can pass through this stricture, but a hurriedly swallowed piece of meat will lodge there. (Courtesy of Dr. H. Tao, Department of Radiology, Ottawa Civic Hospital, Ottawa, Canada.)

tion of food through the nose. The *globus* sensation, which occurs occasionally in most adults, is the feeling of a lump in the throat. Globus means ball, and the condition was unfairly called *globus hystericus*. Globus is unrelated to or relieved by swallowing and is often precipitated by strong emotion. Its only importance is that it not be confused with true dysphagia.

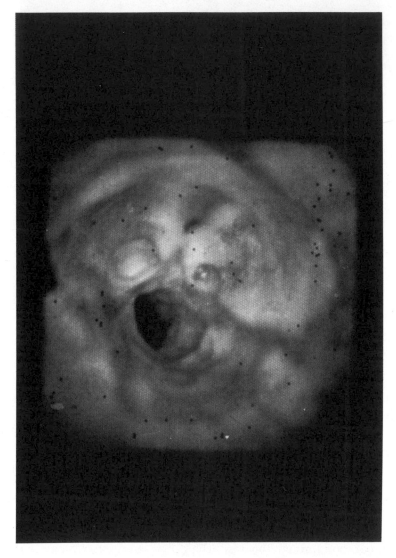

Figure 17-2. Endoscopic view of acutely inflamed lower esophagus with a narrow stricture. This severe narrowing will require guidewire or balloon dilatation.

Motor Dysphagia

The most important motor disorder causing dysphagia is *achalasia* (Figure 17-3). In this condition, the LES fails to relax and permit food and liquids to enter the stomach. This is due to damage to the myenteric plexus in the esophagus. At a late stage the atonic esophagus dilates. Characteristically, the person with achalasia suffers dysphagia for solids and liquids, while someone with mechanical obstruction notices solid dysphagia first. Since air swallowing is the principle source of stomach gas, an upright X ray shows no gastric air bubble. Treatment is surgery or forcible balloon dilatation of the hypertonic LES.

Scleroderma destroys esophageal muscle, so there is no peristalsis or LES function. Occasionally a stricture will develop (see Figure 14-2).

Mechanical Dysphagia

Stricture is the most common cause of mechanical dysphagia. The patient first notices difficulty swallowing solids, especially meat and bread, but can usually force them down with liquids. There may or may not have been heartburn in the past. If neglected, a large piece of meat will impact in the scarred and narrowed lower esophagus. Attempts to wash out the obstruction with fluid are futile, and the liquid overflows into the mouth. Although the obstruction is usually near the LES, the victim often points at the throat to indicate the trouble.

Two other mechanical obstructions of the esophagus deserve attention here. The most common is a Schatzki ring, named for one of the two radiologists who described it in 1953 (Figure 17-4). This is a circumferential, perforated, diaphragm-like structure located at the squamo-cutaneous mucosal junction of esophagus and stomach. The cause is unknown, but there is usually a hiatus hernia. If the aperture is sufficiently narrow, food may impact. The dysphagia is intermittent, often occurring at long intervals when a meal is eaten rapidly with insufficient chewing. Occasionally, esophagitis causes a ring, but it is thicker than a Schatzki ring and there is nearby inflammation. Usually bougies achieve satisfactory dilatation. Recurrences do occur, requiring repeat bougienage. Some-

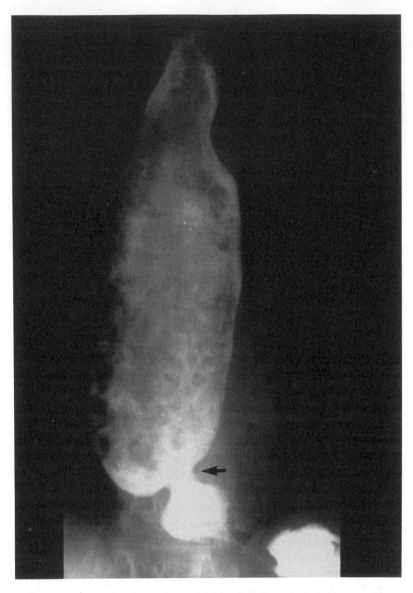

Figure 17-3. Achalasia. Barium fills a grossly dilated esophageal body that narrows at the waistlike LES (arrow) into a small hiatus hernia. Barium from the hernia passes through the diaphragm into the stomach (lower right). The large atonic esophagus is full of food, which accounts for the mottled appearance of the barium column. The LES (arrow) is uncharacteristically open, yet the flaccid esophagus does not empty. (From Thompson, 1989.)

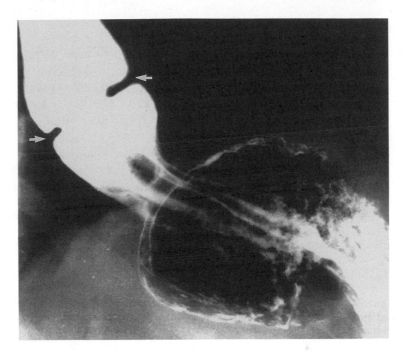

Figure 17-4. Schatzki ring. The thin circumferential diaphragm (arrows) causes intermittent dysphagia. A small hiatus hernia lies below the ring and above the stomach.

times, dilatation is followed by GER, necessitating antireflux measures.

The most important cause of dysphagia is cancer of the esophagus. The cancer originates in the esophageal mucosa and gradually encroaches on the lumen. The result is a steadily progressive dysphagia and profound weight loss. This highly fatal cancer is discussed in Chapter 21.

Odynophagia and Pill Esophagitis

Odynophagia means painful swallowing and is unusual in reflux esophagitis. It is more likely with esophageal infections such as candida, herpes, or cytomegalovirus (CMV). These are best diagnosed by biopsy. Some medications, notably tetracycline, potassium chloride, and quinidine, can lodge in the esophagus and

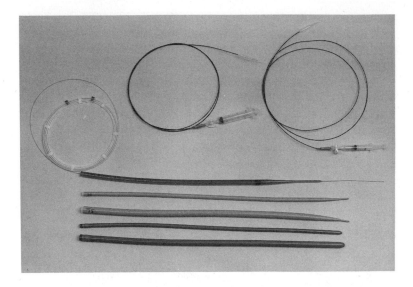

Figure 17-5. Esophageal dilators. From below: Hurst #56F; Hurst 44F; Maloney 56F; Maloney 36F; Savory #45F with guidewire; top left, Regiflex™ 18 mm balloon dilator; top right, Regiflex™10 mm balloon dilator.

damage the mucosa. Potassium is especially dangerous. Even young people are subject to *pill esophagitis* if while recumbent they carelessly swallow medication with insufficient fluid.

Treatment of Stricture

The treatment of a reflux stricture is dilation. One needs to proceed cautiously because there is a risk of perforation. There are three common types of dilators (Figure 17-5):

1. Mercury-filled bougies are very useful for mild to moderate strictures. Tapered (Maloney) bougies fit gradually into the stricture and are usually preferable to the blunt-tipped Hurst bougies.
2. Tighter strictures are dilated over a guidewire. The endoscopist feeds a soft-tipped wire through the biopsy port past the stricture into the distal stomach. After removing the endoscope, he or she pushes a firm, hollow dilator such as the Savory over the guidewire through the stricture. The

passage of bougies or guidewire dilators of increasing size progressively widens the stricture. Usually, only three sizes are passed per session, and sometimes several sessions are required. Relief achieved by this procedure is remarkable. In some cases the gradual worsening of the stricture is so subtle that the patient is scarcely aware of the disability until after dilation it suddenly disappears.

3. Balloon dilation is a recent innovation that is useful for tight strictures. A deflated balloon introduced through the endoscope is inflated in the stricture. This avoids the shearing force of bougie and guidewire dilations, and the process is sometimes complete after one session. The size of the balloon is limited by the diameter of the biopsy port, and sometimes it is difficult to accurately place it in the stricture.

Stricture dilation should accompany vigorous treatment of the esophagitis with omeprazole, usually 40 mg per day. Since the esophagitis and stricture will recur, the drug must be continued indefinitely. Patients appearing for dilations over many years often cease doing so when given omeprazole. Avoidance of the cost and risks of dilatation and improved quality of life justify the expense of long-term drug therapy.

Treatment of a Foreign Body

A piece of meat or other foreign material may lodge in a stricture. In such an emergency, one may try to relax the esophagus with intravenous glucagon or an anticholinergic drug. However, the situation usually calls for urgent endoscopy and disimpaction. Once certain of the nature of the stricture, the endoscopist may be able to push the impacted piece into the stomach with the endoscope. This procedure risks perforation and aspiration and demands care and skill. An alternative is to attempt to break up the morsel so that smaller pieces may pass. This is sometimes difficult, and retrieval is the only recourse. It is wise to place a protective overtube in the pharynx through which the pieces can be pulled by the retreating endoscope. Alternatively, an endotracheal tube placed under a general anesthetic protects the larynx. These procedures carry risks of their own. It is better to avoid such a calamity by acting promptly at the first hint of dysphagia.

Barrett's Esophagus

In 1950, Barrett, a pathologist, described patients whose lower esophagus was lined with columnar, rather than the normal squamus, epithelium (Figure 17-6). He thought this was likely due to a congenitally short esophagus and believed that ulcers occurring in this columnar epithelium were really gastric ulcers. Today the change is believed to be due to prolonged exposure of the lower esophagus to refluxed gastric juice. The process of cell change from flat, layered squamus to tall columnar epithelium is an example of *metaplasia* (Figure 17-7). Columnar cells are perhaps more resistant to acid and pepsin, and metaplasia may be a defense process. The cells themselves are usually of the *specialized columnar* type and include mucus cells, goblet cells, and a tendency to form villi (Figure 17-8). Cells resembling those of colon, small bowel, pyloric body, and cardia epithelium occur in Barrett's esophagus, and one esophagus may contain several types. Rarely, there are functioning parietal cells that compound the problem by producing acid locally.

Diagnosis of Barrett's esophagus is by endoscopy and biopsy of the mucosa. Normally, the red gastric mucosa sharply demarcates the gastroesophageal junction where the paler pink squamus esophageal mucosa begins. In Barrett's, the demarcation is above its normal position. It may appear as tonguelike projections of gastric tissue extending up into the esophagus, islands of gastric mucosa amongst the squamus, or a variable retreat proximally even as high as the upper esophageal sphincter. Normally, the endoscopist easily recognizes the metaplastic tissue, but an overlying esophagitis can obscure it. Peptic ulcers that can be quite large sometimes occur in Barrett's epithelium (Figure 17-9).

The management of newly discovered Barrett's esophagus has two objectives: the treatment of the esophagitis and the early detection of cancer (see below). The aggressive treatment of severe esophagitis with omeprazole is discussed in Chapter 16. Although the metaplastic changes are believed to be due to esophagitis, medical or surgical treatment does not reverse them.

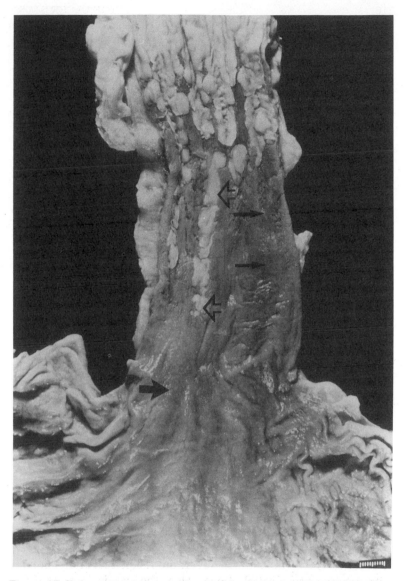

Figure 17-6. A postmortum specimen of the lower esophagus and upper stomach illustrating Barrett's esophagus (thin black arrows). The thick black arrow points to the anatomic gastroesophageal junction, but the columnar cell–squamus cell interface is much higher. Hollow arrows point to islands of squamus mucosa within the Barrett's mucosa. (Courtesy of Dr. Maha Guindi, Division of Anatomical Pathology, Ottawa Civic Hospital, Ottawa, Canada.)

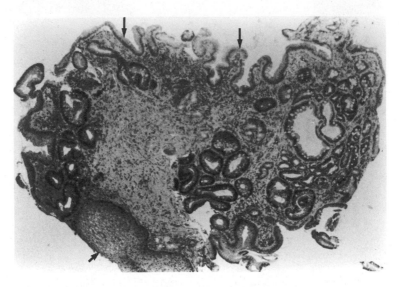

Figure 17-7. Histological specimen of the metaplastic esophageal mucosa of a patient with Barrett's esophagus. The short black arrow points to the normal squamus epithelium that one expects to find in the esophagus. The thinner arrows point to the metaplastic columnar epithelium that is the result of prolonged, severe esophagitis. This tiny biopsy was obtained by pinch forceps through the endoscope, which explains why the epithelium is curved on itself. (Courtesy of Dr. Maha Guindi, Division of Anatomical Pathology, Ottawa Civic Hospital, Ottawa, Canada.)

Esophageal Cancer

The importance of Barrett's esophagus is its quoted thirtyfold to fiftyfold increased risk of esophageal cancer. The exact figure is difficult to obtain because an unbiased estimate of the prevalence of Barrett's is unavailable. However, the risk is real and is greater with tobacco and alcohol abuse. Also, the risk is greatest if the metaplastic epithelium is of the specialized columnar type, and it increases with the extent of metaplasia. As in the cervix, precancerous changes can be detected in those destined to develop cancer. Called *dysplasia*, these changes are an indication for close observation. Indeed, high-grade dysplasia may coexist with an adenocarcinoma. Low-grade dysplasia can result from inflammation and

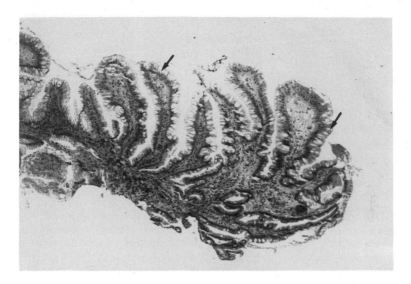

Figure 17-8. Histological specimen of a biopsy taken from a man with extensive Barrett's changes. This is specialized columnar epithelium and has the greatest cancer risk. Note the villus formation that mimics small bowel mucosa and the numerous goblet cells in the epithelium (arrows). (With permission from Thompson and Barr, *Gastroenterology*, 1978.)

subside with treatment of the esophagitis. Failure to do so should prompt close surveillance.

Early detection and prevention of cancer are difficult. One cancer detection program was proposed by an international working team at the 1990 Ninth World Congress of Gastroenterology in Sydney, Australia. For this purpose, Barrett's esophagus is defined as a squamocolumnar mucosal junction 3 or more centimeters above the anatomical gastroesophageal junction or specialized columnar epithelium at any level of the esophagus. Newly detected cases should be biopsied in each quadrant at 2-cm intervals within the metaplastic esophagus. If there is doubt about the interpretation of the biopsies, they should be repeated promptly. Severe dysplasia seen at multiple sites in a young person may be an indication for esophagectomy. Such major surgery is risky in the old and frail, where close observation at 6-month intervals may be safer. If low-grade dysplasia persists after adequate treatment of the esophagitis, it should by checked for worsening every 12

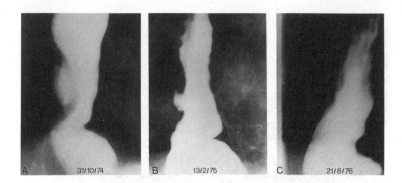

Figure 17-9. Barium-filled esophagus in a series of X rays taken of the patient in Figure 17-7. (A) In October 1974, there was a large ulcer that slowly healed (B) over several months on the newly available cimetidine. (C) By August 1976 the Barrett's esophagus persists, but the ulcer is gone. The patient took cimetidine until his death of other causes a decade later. (With permission from Thompson and Barr, *Gastroenterology*, 1978.)

months. Otherwise, some recommend that all cases should be endoscoped and biopsied every 18–24 months.

Complicated? You bet it is! Not all experts subscribe to such an aggressive and expensive program, nor has it been shown to save lives or improve quality of life. However, few question the ominous implications of high-grade dysplasia. Better databased guidelines are undoubtedly forthcoming.

OTHER COMPLICATIONS

Boerhave's syndrome is a rare spontaneous esophageal perforation that evidently results from gluttony. Spontaneous rupture of an esophageal ulcer is very rare, but it can erode into the aorta with disastrous results. The need to endoscope and biopsy an inflamed esophagus creates a small risk of perforation. While the side effects of drugs are generally mild and reversible, those of antireflux operations are not. Severe GERD and its complications impair quality of life. Happily, with modern treatment and a sensible lifestyle, living with GERD is now usually possible.

SUMMARY

Complications of GERD are due to heartburn, regurgitation, or esophagitis. The principal complication of heartburn is its possible confusion with coronary heart disease. Regurgitation risks aspiration and may trigger nonallergic asthma. Acid laryngitis sometimes occurs without prior heartburn. Esophagitis may progress to bleeding, stricture, or Barrett's esophagus. These complications require vigorous treatment of the esophagitis and long-term drug maintenance. In Barrett's esophagus, concern about cancer should prompt endoscopic biopsies to detect dysplasia, an ominous harbinger of esophageal cancer.

PART FIVE

Topics Related to Ulcers and Heartburn

CHAPTER EIGHTEEN

Functional Dyspepsia

Non-Ulcer Dyspepsia

When the endoscopist sees a peptic ulcer in a patient with dyspepsia, the outlook is excellent. Anti-ulcer drugs promptly relieve the dyspepsia and heal the ulcer over 6 weeks in at least 80% of cases. By ridding the stomach of *H. pylori*, drugs even cure the disease. No such effective drug treatment awaits dyspeptics without ulcers, whose symptoms will likely continue. This chapter begins where Chapter 10 ended, with a discussion of endoscopy-negative functional or non-ulcer dyspepsia.

IMPACT OF DYSPEPSIA

Functional dyspepsia affects at least 6 million Americans and accounts for 1–3% of family doctor visits. It adversely affects quality of life and causes considerable absenteeism. A Swedish survey indicates that patients with non-ulcer dyspepsia require more sick leave than those with peptic ulcer. Several factors other than the dyspepsia contribute to the absenteeism. A study of Mayo clinic patients suggests that those with functional dyspepsia have a poorer quality of life than those with other upper gastrointestinal disorders. These data may be misleading. Dyspeptics who find their way to a tertiary care clinic may be a particularly disturbed subgroup compared to patients with structural disorders. Nevertheless, for some, "Dyspepsia is the ruin of most things! Empires, expeditions and everything else." (De Quincey, 1823).

DIAGNOSIS

Confirm Dyspepsia

Diagnosis is essential to sensible management. Once endoscopy has excluded peptic ulcer, gastric cancer, or other upper gastrointestinal disease, the doctor should again confirm that the symptoms are dyspepsia. If the pain is defecation-related, consider the IBS. If worsened by bending or lying, it is likely GERD. If precipitated by exercise, it may be angina. The pains of pancreatic or biliary disease are characteristic.

Dyspepsia may occur coincidentally with other diseases, and the careful doctor will inquire about ominous features of these such as weight loss, anemia, melena, vomiting, or fever. Physical findings should be absent. Too often the chronic dyspeptic's abdomen has a surgical scar, mute reminder of a futile cholecystectomy: "We see too many scarred abdomens with persistence of symptoms, too many 're-operations' and operations undertaken for pain." (Ryle, 1928).

Subgroups

Frustrated by the lack of a physiological explanation for functional dyspepsia, clinical scientists describe symptom-based subgroups that imply mechanisms. The notions of ulcerlike or motility-like dyspepsia are not new. In his famous textbook a century ago, Osler proposed that some dyspepsia was due to disturbed stomach function. Hutchison described secretory and motor derangements of the stomach in a 1927 monograph called *Lectures* on *Dyspepsia*. This tradition has echoes today.

The latest incarnations are the Rome criteria developed by an international working team (Table 18-1). The term *ulcerlike* dyspepsia is reminiscent of *Moynihan's disease* described by Spiro. He believed that dyspepsia, duodenitis, and duodenal ulcer were a continuum; that is, they are stages of the same disease. A hole in the mucosa is thus incidental to dyspepsia, and the symptoms should be treated the same whether or not an ulcer was present. This implied that neutralization of gastric acid and other contemporary ulcer treatments should be employed in both ulcer and non-ulcer dyspepsia.

However, Spiro wrote in 1972, before the availability of the powerful anti-ulcer drugs. These have turned out to be ineffective in non-ulcer dyspepsia. If functional symptoms were part of the ulcer spectrum, basal and poststimulation gastric acid levels should be intermediate, between those of normals and peptic ulcer patients. They are not. If non-ulcers are destined to become ulcers, the progression should be recordable. It is not (Table 18-2). Finally, *H. pylori* found in most peptic ulcers is no more common in ulcerlike than in other dyspepsias or in normals. Thus, the term ulcerlike dyspepsia makes no clinical or pathological sense. Indeed, it is misleading.

The term *motility-like* dyspepsia has similar limitations. Symptoms like postprandial bloating and fullness, early satiety, and perhaps nausea and eructations tempt one to think of delayed gastric emptying. Indeed this is the case in diabetic gastroparesis that damages the nerves to the stomach. Other rare motility disorders where gastric motor function is faulty are described in centers equipped to measure gastric emptying. However, it is a mistake to extrapolate this information to the large numbers of patients seen in primary and secondary care with common functional dyspepsia.

Originally, the Rome group proposed the subgroup *reflux-like dyspepsia*, but this is heartburn. This designation is omitted from the latest Rome documents. For those dyspeptics who do not fit any subgroup, the designation *unspecified (nonspecific) dyspepsia* ensures completeness.

The subgroups serve no clinical purpose. They do not indicate specific treatments, nor do they yet define mechanisms. Talley found that half of dyspeptics fit more than one subtype, and some fit none of them. He concluded that subtyping was inappropriate. Indeed, the attempt to fit all dyspeptics into the complicated classification in Table 18-1 could give us all dyspepsia!

Nevertheless, careful analysis of symptoms is essential if we are to identify explanatory mechanisms for them. Clinical trials of dyspepsia treatments must include a careful symptom record of the study patients and a means of measuring and recording their

TABLE 18-1
The Rome Criteria for Functional Dyspepsia[a]

Functional dyspepsia
1. Three months or more of pain or discomfort centered in the upper abdomen
2. No clinical, biochemical, endoscopic, or ultrasonographic evidence of known organic disease that is likely to explain the symptoms

Ulcer-like dyspepsia—Three or more of the following are necessary, but *upper abdominal pain must be the predominant complaint:*
1. Pain that is localized in the epigastrium (ie., can be localized to a single area by pointing with one or two fingers)
2. Pain after relieved by food (>25% of the time)
3. Pain often relieved by antacids and/or H_2 blockers
4. Pain often occurring before meals or when hungry
5. Pain that at times wakens the patient from sleep
6. Periodic pain with remissions and relapses (periods of at least 2 weeks with no pain interspersed with periods of weeks or months when there is pain)

Dysmotility-like dyspepsia—Pain that is *not* a dominant symptom. Upper abdominal discomfort should be present in all patients; this discomfort should be chronic and characterized by three or more of the following:
1. Early satiety
2. Postprandial fullness
3. Nausea
4. Retching and/or vomiting that is recurrent
5. Bloating in the upper abdomen *not* accompanied by visible distension
6. Upper abdominal discomfort often aggravated by food

Unspecified (nonspecific) dyspepsia—Dyspeptic patients whose symptoms do not fulfill the criteria for ulcerlike or dysmotility-like dyspepsia

[a]From Drossman *et al.*, 1994.

improvement on treatment. Only in this way will we know if true subgroups exist and in whom a study treatment might be effective.

CAUSE

The cause of functional dyspepsia is unknown. As with any vacuum, theories rush in to fill the void. Characteristic of functional disturbances, there is no pathophysiological marker by which the disease may be universally recognized. In this respect, *ulcer* dyspepsia enjoys an enormous advantage. We only know of the existence of functional dyspepsia through reports of those who have it. No animal model can help us understand symptoms. Any definition of functional dyspepsia thus depends upon the patients' symptoms and the absence of structural disease (see Table 10-1).

TABLE 18-2
Prognosis of Dyspepsia

Investigator	Number of patients	Years of follow-up	Percent still dyspeptic	Percent developing peptic ulcer
Brummer, 1959	102[a]	5–6	66	12
Gregory, 1972	102	6	24	3
Talley, 1987	110	2	70	3
Sloth, 1988	37	5–7	80	0

[a]X-ray diagnosis.

Motility

Many circumstances frustrate our understanding of the pathophysiology of dyspepsia. Subdividing dyspeptics into ulcerlike or dysmotility-like fails to identify those who might share physiological characteristics. Motility studies are invariably carried out in tertiary care centers, where patients are not representative of dyspepsia at large. Reports that up to 50% of patients have delayed gastric emptying or gastroduodenal reflux are meaningless if diabetes and other diseases known to cause these phenomena are included.

The task is to prove that putative abnormalities cause the symptoms. No controlled data confirm that abnormal gut movements cause dyspepsia. Even in tertiary care, most "dyspeptic" patients have normal gastric emptying and transit. The response of such patients to gastrokinetics is not so great that we can accept it as evidence of a motility disorder. There are reports that peptide hormone blood levels (motilin, gastrin) are altered in dyspepsia, but no systematic study. Cholecystokinin causes satiety, and estrogen, progesterone, and prolactin all affect smooth muscle contraction. Their role in functional dyspepsia is speculative.

Helicobacter pylori

If H. pylori caused symptoms, it would be useful to subdivide dyspeptics into those who do or do not have the organism. The former would be treated with antibiotics, and they at least might be cured. However, present data do not confirm the notion that H. pylori causes dyspepsia. While the organism does cause gastritis, older studies indicate that gastritis is asymptomatic. Therefore, antibiotics can cure the gastritis, but not the symptoms. Figures vary considerably, but the prevalence of the organism in those with functional dyspepsia seems similar to that of the background population. In 1995, several European studies found no relationship between the presence of *H. pylori* infection and functional dyspepsia. A Canadian study found that eradication of the organism does not improve symptoms in patients with nonulcer dyspepsia.

Psychosocial Issues

Without a known pathophysiology, stress and psychosocial causes are invoked as causes of IBS. Beaumont, Wolf, and Wolfe and others demonstrated that emotion alters gut motility. However, it is another matter to determine that emotional disturbance causes the chronic and repetitive symptoms of dyspepsia. Dyspeptics who seek healthcare, especially by specialists, are often emotionally distressed. As demonstrated in irritable bowel syndrome (IBS), psychosocial issues may be a hidden agenda, the real reason a dyspeptic seeks care. This does not imply cause and effect.

In IBS, the gut is hypersensitive to distension. The symptom threshold is lowered in the anxious and the stressed. In dyspepsia, there is also a decreased threshold for perception of balloon distension within the stomach. As in IBS and heartburn, data support the notion that psychosocial distress causes gut hypersensitivity.

TREATMENT

The sheer number of treatments proposed for dyspepsia bear witness to their collective fruitlessness. The absence of effective therapy no doubt contributes to Talley's conclusion that quality of life is more impaired in sufferers of functional dyspepsia than in those with peptic ulcer. There are many impediments to objective treatment trials, and those that are published are flawed. The placebo response in controlled studies is 40–60%, so uncontrolled studies must be disregarded. Few trials clearly indicate their entry criteria. Almost none employ tight definitions such as the Rome criteria (Table 18-1). Doubtless, many dyspepsia trials include subjects with IBS, gastric motor diseases, and even peptic ulcer. If heartburn is included, improvement will occur with many drugs, yet will reveal nothing of their benefit to dyspeptics. In 1989, Van Zanten pointed out that only two therapeutic trials in dyspeptic patients (both negative) measured symptoms when determining outcome. The use of a meta-analysis to pool uncontrolled data from polyglot symptoms with no outcome measures is absurd.

With an unproved pathophysiology, it is difficult to generate treatment hypotheses. Extrapolation from the treatment of peptic ulcer or diabetic gastroparesis is untenable. Yet, such is the enthusiasm of the pharmaceutical industry and the size of the dyspepsia market that drug trials of disputable validity are encouraged. Expanded indications are sought for drugs already available, so no regulatory approval is required. A publication bias of unknown magnitude exists. Negative studies are less likely than positive ones to make it into print. Trials that answer several questions increase the likelihood of a chance positive result.

Several authors and working teams criticize the methodology of existing studies. Ironically, after pointing out trial weaknesses and doubts about drug efficacy, these critics often recommend that individual dyspeptic patients should try the drug anyway. This author believes that this is illogical and that no drug should be recommended for most patients with functional dyspepsia. The onus is on industry and clinical research to prove efficacy and identify potential responders. Certainly, the public purse should no more underwrite unproved drugs than quackery, lest they become synonymous.

General Measures

Unproved benefit applies to all dyspepsia treatment, even the general measures that follow. Here logic must give way to common sense. In some cases, the cause of dyspepsia may be obvious. Alcoholic excess can render even the most resilient stomach dyspeptic. Fat delays gastric emptying. This supports anecdotal reports that cream, and fatty and fried foods, leaves one full, bloated, and sated. Many lifestyles cry out for advice: the harassed executive grabbing a sandwich at a greasy spoon; the busy lawyer, no time for lunch, gorging himself late at night; the chemical worker devouring a sandwich in a smelly lab; the bored secretary augmenting her breaks with extra coffee; the dedicated accountant smoking up a storm as he does the weekly payroll; the overachieving salesman clocking a 14-hour day. Many drugs include dyspepsia among their side effects, and almost all of us can attest to the dyspeptic effects of stress. Discovery of such lifestyle failings requires careful interviewing by the doctor and insightful interpretation by the patient. Surely, the patient's responsibility to deal with such issues should not be subverted by the notion of a pharmacological quick fix.

It is always useful to consider the reason a dyspeptic person seeks medical care. Many do not. With IBS, sufferers in the community have a psychosocial profile that is similar to the symptom-free population. However, those studied after referral to tertiary centers have a high prevalence of anxiety, depression, and panic and a variety of personality disorders. It is likely the same with dyspepsia.

Why do some regard this symptom complex as nonmedical, perhaps part of living, while others cannot cope and seek specialist care? We cannot measure severity, but there is often a less obvious agenda. This hidden agenda might be a fear of serious disease. In one series, 71% of dyspeptic patients feared cancer. The freshly endoscoped patient is well positioned to be reassured that he or she has no ulcer or cancer. In the end, such reassurance may be the most powerful therapy available.

In other dyspeptics, the impulse to consult may be more complex. Anxiety, depression, and other psychological and psychiatric syndromes may be very subtle. A stressful event may precipitate the symptoms, or at least prompt the trip to the doctor. Sympathetic assistance with these and other psychosocial issues may not cure the dyspepsia, but it may reestablish it as a nonmedical problem that the patient can self-manage.

Patients who do not respond to advice and reassurance are overrepresented in secondary or tertiary care. In many, the hidden agenda has not been successfully addressed. Such patients should not have repeated tests. By raising false hopes of diagnosis and cure, they undermine confidence in the diagnosis. Psychological treatments, self-help, hypnotism, and stress management may be tried if they are available. Efficacy of such treatments is unknown, but the reassuring, caring attitude they convey is at least a powerful placebo. Continuing care falls to the family doctor, who can best manage to reassure and support the patient through regular, brief visits. Such people are unlikely to be cured of their dyspepsia and the psychosocial burden they carry, so the objective of care must be improved social and vocational functioning.

Drug Therapy

Many dyspeptics improve on drugs, yet no drug is much better than a placebo. The placebo effect is a powerful force, and, when caringly used, it can be of therapeutic benefit (see Chapter 30). Nevertheless, drugs are expensive, and none is completely without side effects. For details on individual drugs, consult Part 6.

So many drugs have been recommended for dyspepsia that a detailed discussion of their collective failure is impractical. Drugs such as anticholinergics, opiate antagonists, and calcium channel blockers delay gastric emptying and are therefore unlikely to be helpful. Anti-ulcer drugs and prokinetics require further discussion.

Anti-Ulcer Drugs

Antacids fail to demonstrate efficacy in clinical trials. Nevertheless, in *small* doses an antacid may serve as a cheap, safe placebo if one is desired. Pirenzepine is an anticholinergic. Misoprostyl and sucralfate compound gut symptoms and may interact with other drugs. There is no basis their use. Indeed, such treatment may do more harm than good.

Because they are so safe and readily available, it is more difficult to dismiss the histamine H2 antagonists. Where they are available over the counter they are not a liability to the public purse. Nevertheless, based on available data, several reviewers conclude that they are ineffective in dyspepsia. Since abnormal acid secretion is not a causative factor, there is no reason why they should be. They *are* costly and bear some unwanted effects. Most importantly, they distract from lifestyle issues that are more important in the long run.

Despite their unproved benefit there is great compulsion to use H2 antagonists in dyspepsia. The placebo effect and the resemblance of dyspeptic symptoms to those of an ulcer lend these drugs a superficial credibility. They are widely used without scientific justification, but so are laxatives, vitamins, and many other proprietary drugs. This should not delude us into believing that they are effective. Even if the patient believes they help, their prolonged, uncritical use should be discouraged.

Prokinetics

Metoclopromide is too toxic for use in a benign complaint such as dyspepsia. Domperidone and cisapride have better safety profiles, but they may alter the absorption of other drugs. Cisapride often causes diarrhea. The proposed role of prokinetics is to speed up gastric emptying and improve antroduodenal coordination, but abnormal gastric motility is not always present in functional dyspepsia. Despite some positive clinical trials, exponents have not convincingly demonstrated that prokinetics are useful. They are expensive prescription drugs that should be reserved for difficult cases where lifestyle changes fail and delayed gastric emptying is suspected.

Antibiotics

Since functional dyspeptics are no more likely than others to have *H. pylori*, there is no rationale for treating them with antibiotics. One study showed that eradication of *H. pylori* failed to relieve dyspepsia immediately, but there was a benefit 1 year later. Veldhuyzen van Zanten and his colleagues recently found that eradication fails to benefit such patients. In view of the expense, side effects, and risk of bacterial resistance attributable to such treatment, we need much better supporting data before we can recommend it.

SUMMARY

Unlike peptic ulcer, functional dyspepsia has no proven treatment. When faced with a non-ulcer dyspeptic the doctor must confirm that dyspepsia is the problem and then emphatically use the negative endoscopy as reassurance. A careful analysis of lifestyle may identify aggravating factors such as alcohol and diet that are within the patient's control. There is no proven pathophysiology and no clinical justification for subgroups such as ulcerlike and dysmotility-like dyspepsia. In secondary and tertiary care, dyspepsia may be accompanied by psychosocial problems that not only impair coping but also require management in their own right. No drugs are proven to be effective in functional dyspepsia, and since the disease is chronic, their long-term use should be avoided.

CHAPTER NINETEEN

Noncardiac Chest Pain
The Irritable Esophagus

Of the half million Americans annually investigated for chest pain, up to 30% have normal coronary arteries and no other evidence of heart disease. A few have diseased microscopic blood vessels in the heart, but most have noncardiac chest pain. For some, a negative investigation is small comfort. The pain continues, and, without an explanation, worry about heart disease may continue as well. Perhaps because of its proximity to the heart, physicians next turn to the esophagus to explain the pain.

Pinning the blame for chest pain on the esophagus is a troublesome and unsatisfactory exercise. Yet, what else is there? Lungs are insensitive. Inflammation of the outer lining of the lungs and heart causes pleurisy or pericarditis. The breathing-linked pain of pleurisy is quite unlike cardiac pain. Tender ribs and chest muscles are aggravated by movement and breathing and are tender to touch. When these are excluded, the esophagus is the handiest scapegoat.

Chest pain due to esophageal spasm must be distinguished from heartburn due to gastroesophageal reflux. While heartburn is very common and usually identified as such by the patient, it may occasionally be impossible for physician and patient to distinguish it from other types of chest pain. Indeed, acid reflux may trigger motility events that cause a pain other than heartburn. It is this connection of noncardiac chest pain to acid that warrants its inclusion in *The Ulcer Story*.

PHYSIOLOGICAL OBSERVATIONS

Motor Abnormalities

Science has been unhelpful in establishing the esophagus as the seat of chest pain. Esophageal peristaltic waves and sphincter function can be recorded by pressure sensors aligned within the esophagus (Figure 19-1). Motility abnormalities were once thought to indicate esophageal spasm, but when they fail to occur in unison with the pain, their significance is doubtful. The *nutcracker esophagus* is the most commonly blamed motor disorder. In this disturbance, peristalsis is intact, but the pressure generated by the esophagus is exaggerated. Some believe that this phenomenon may become diffuse esophageal spasm with repetitive, nonperistaltic contractions. However, such contractions are observed without chest pain, and it is doubtful if they have much to do with one another. Spasm may be triggered by acid, cholinergic drugs, or balloon distension. Here again, unless spasm occurs with the pain, its etiologic significance is questionable. Occasionally a spasm pattern occurs in the early stages of achalasia (see Figure 17-3).

Manometric recordings of decreased peristalsis, abnormal wave forms, simultaneous contractions, or a high-pressure LES were once considered to be evidence of diffuse esophageal spasm, but no longer. Esophageal spasm itself infrequently causes chest pain. Peters *et al.* studied 24 patients with noncardiac chest pain wearing intraesophageal pH and motility recording devices for 24 hours. Of 92 episodes of chest pain, only 20 coincided with reflux and 12% of pains occurred with abnormal motility, and even here the timing was inexact.

The Hypersensitive Esophagus

The transmission of esophageal pain is a mystery. There are probably mechanoreceptors in the esophagus muscle that transmit changes in esophageal tension through the enteric nervous system to the brain (see Figure 1-9). Many years ago, the British physiologist Hurst caused chest pain by inflating a balloon within the

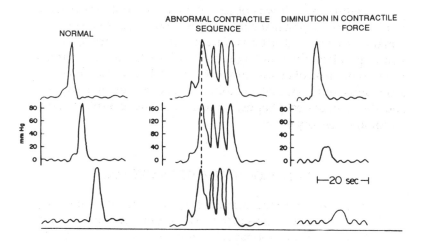

Esophageal Peristalsis

Figure 19-1. Esophageal manometry: recordings from three pressure-sensing devices sited at 5-centimeter intervals within the esophagus. On the left is demonstrated the normal, sequential passage of a peristaltic pressure wave over these sensors from top to bottom. The pressure peak indicated by the scale is 80 millimeters of mercury. In the middle are demonstrated simultaneous, repetitive contractions generating pressures of 160 millimeters of mercury. When such spasm is observed at the same time as the subject experiences his or her pain, the cause may be concluded to be diffuse esophageal spasm. Such a coincidence of pain and esophageal event is uncommon. Recordings on the right show one of the many other motility disturbances whose relationship to chest pain is very obscure.

esophagus. Richter (1986), in North Carolina used calibrated balloon distension to reproduce the noncardiac chest pain of 68% of 30 patients. The pain was often felt at a lower balloon pressure than that required to produce chest pain in normal individuals. Similar observations in the colons of patients with IBS suggest a hypersensitive gut. Patterson *et al.* add further evidence that esophageal chest pain occurs in a hypersensitive esophagus. Repeated intraesophageal balloon distensions are accompanied by increasing pain in those with noncardiac chest pain, but not in controls. These painful sensations occur with no abnormal esophageal contractions. Esophageal chest pain may not be a motor disorder after all.

A century ago, it was observed that cold, hot, or carbonated drinks evoke esophageal contractions. Loud noises cause asymptomatic tertiary contractions. In contrast, a cold drink can transiently paralyze the esophagus so that it distends. Air that is not released because of an inability to belch probably also distends the esophagus. In functional gastrointestinal disorders like dyspepsia and the irritable esophagus, there is a subtle interplay between motor and sensory events.

PSYCHOLOGICAL OBSERVATIONS

Stress causes esophageal irritability. Stressful interviews induce nonpropulsive contractions in the lower esophagus. In a study of 50 patients referred for esophageal manometry, half had one of the following manometric abnormalities: increased amplitude of contraction, increased wave duration, or triple peaked waves. Of the 25 patients with abnormal tracings, 83% had criteria for depression, anxiety, or somatization disorder, compared to 32% of the remaining 25 with normal manometry. While this suggests that emotion causes manometric abnormalities, it is uncertain how these translate into symptoms. In another study, patients with noncardiac chest pain who were deliberately stressed by problem-solving exercises had increased esophageal contractions and anxiety. While the emphasis in the past was on the identification of motor abnormalities that cause pain, newer research attempts to elucidate how mental or physical stress can affect motility or alter esophageal sensation.

CARDIAC OR NONCARDIAC?

Cardiac pain indicates serious disease, and its exclusion is the first step in someone complaining of chest pain. Sometimes a physician cannot decide if a pain is cardiac or noncardiac. Both heart and esophageal pain can be "squeezing," "tight," or "pressurelike." Nitroglycerin may relieve both pains and is not a reliable discriminator. To make matters worse, both pains may occur in the same patient. Pain radiating to the arms and occurring with exertion is most likely to be cardiac. Pain that lasts several hours, repeatedly awakes the patient at night, or occurs with recumbency is more likely esophageal. Esophageal pain may be severe, radiate to the back and occur with heartburn and dysphagia. However, the overlap is so great that if heart pain is a possibility, cardiac investigation is essential.

Usually heartburn is identified by its relationship to meals, relief with antacids, and worsening with bending, reclining, or straining. Pleurisy and pericarditis are brief, usually infectious illnesses that cause a sharp pain that "catches" with breathing or coughing. Injury or inflammation of the chest wall, such as arthritis of the joints between ribs and sternum, are tender to touch and aggravated by cough or movement.

ESTABLISHING AN ESOPHAGEAL CAUSE

A barium swallow will exclude most mechanical causes of esophageal pain such as cancer or stricture (see Figure 19-2). However, recognition of esophagitis requires endoscopy. As can be seen from the forgoing discussion, the results of esophageal manometry are often inconclusive, and the most practical use of this test is to exclude achalasia. If the infusion of acid, a cholinergic drug, or balloon distension simultaneously provokes the pain and a characteristic motor disturbance, the physician may be convinced. However, such concordance is unusual.

Experts sometimes recommend 24-hour observation with intraesophageal apparatus to record changes in pressure and pH. Pressure-sensing instruments and a pH probe are placed one within the LES and two more at 5-cm intervals above in the the esophagus. Over 24 hours, pH and pressure are recorded while the patient pushes a button to indicate pain episodes. For the test period, the subject goes about his or her daily activities. Association of pain episodes with pH or pressure changes in the esophagus is evidence for esophageal chest pain. Ward *et al.* showed that such reassuring evidence improved the outlook for patients. They subsequently have fewer symptoms and were back to work sooner. However, this study predated the introduction of the proton pump inhibitors.

The positive diagnosis of esophageal spasm as a cause of chest pain is elusive, and it is probably less common than formerly thought. However, once cardiac disease is ruled out, patients can be comforted that the chest pain does not represent a fatal disease and will likely improve over time. X ray, endoscopy, and sometimes manometry should satisfy the physician that no other esophageal

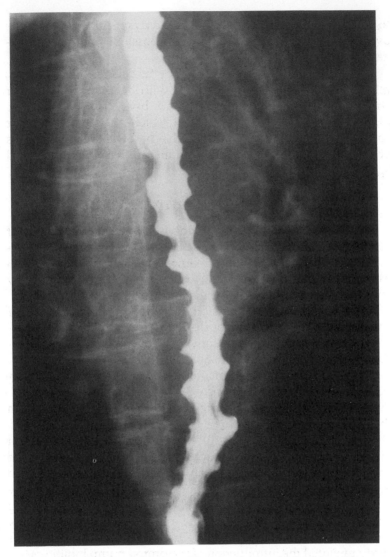

Figure 19-2. An X ray of a barium-filled esophagus. In this case there are muscular indentations indicating forceful and uncoordinated esophageal contractions. When this can be demonstrated to occur at the same time as chest pain or dysphagia, one suspects esophageal spasm as the cause of the pain. In this case the patient was asymptomatic; the X ray was done for other reasons. This illustrates the difficulty of attributing chest pain to abnormal esophageal motility.

disease exists. Chest pain triggered by acid is much more common than that due to spontaneous esophageal spasm, and a patient may not describe it as heartburn. Aggressive antacid therapy should therefore be tried before pH and manometric studies or drugs directed against spasm. Such a policy will leave few patients without a diagnosis.

TREATMENT

Even if endoscopy shows no esophagitis, the pain may be due to acid. Therefore, the first step should be aggressive treatment of gastroesophageal reflux. The antireflux measures discussed in Chapter 16 are sensible, but rendering the stomach achlorhydric is more likely to promptly relieve pain. One double-blind study showed that a single dose of 80 mg omeprazole reduced chest pain in 60% of 20 patients when compared to placebo—as convincing a diagnostic result as can be achieved by 24-hour pH and manometric monitoring. In practice, if a prolonged course of omeprazole improves or prevents the chest pain, one need go no further. Since precise diagnosis is neither easy, nor a virtue in itself, a symptom-free patient is a satisfactory objective.

A few patients will continue to have chest pain, and for them treatment is unsatisfactory. A nitroglycerin tablet placed under the tongue may help some for a while. Those who are depressed may get relief from physical and psychological pain through antidepressants. Nifedipine prevents coronary artery spasm by blocking calcium influx into the smooth muscle cells of the blood vessel wall. It also affects esophageal smooth muscle, and decreases the contractions of the nutcracker esophagus. Nifedipine seems logical in the treatment of esophageal spasm. However, despite anecdotal reports, it is no better than placebo in reducing the duration, severity, or frequency of chest pain. These observations again demonstrate the uncertain relationship between esophageal contractions and chest pain.

Mercury-weighted bougies are sometimes used for esophageal chest pain. A double-blind crossover trial compared therapeutic bougienage (large bougie) and placebo bougienage (small bougie), and both were equally effective. Winters et al. (1984) suggest that the close physician–patient interaction necessitated by bougienage is more important therapy than any effect of the bougie itself. It is also likely that such close attention to the esophagus draws attention away from fear of cardiac disease.

PROGNOSIS

In the aforementioned nifedipine trial the investigators presented evidence that even in the placebo group the pain improved over 1–2 years. In another 22-month study, they followed 119 patients, 63 of whom had manometric evidence for an esophageal cause. Pain continued in them all, but the 63, who could be convinced that the esophagus was the cause, were less disabled and required less physician care. Reassurance is an essential component of treatment.

SUMMARY

Esophageal spasm is blamed in up to one-third of patients with noncardiac chest pain. However, not only is the abnormality in esophageal function difficult to explain, but it is also exceedingly difficult to apprehend a physiological abnormality in the act of causing pain. Both manometric abnormalities and pain are influenced by stress, and often the triggering incident may be gastroesophageal reflux of acid. That an esophagus may be hypersensitive to acid, distension, or emotional distress is undoubted, and it is likely that esophageal chest pain will have both motor and sensory components. There is increasing realization that esophageal chest pain is as much influenced by perception of esophageal events as by the events themselves. Once cardiac disease has been excluded, barium X ray and endoscopy constitute the minimum esophageal investigations to detect esophagitis, strictures, and other esophageal disease. Since no treatment is effective even if a manometric abnormality is found, motility studies are mainly justified for the reassurance that a positive study might engender in someone who is fearful of heart disease. In this context, the uncertainty of a negative result should be weighed before undertaking such tests. Sensibly, any possible effect of acid reflux should be eliminated by aggressive proton pump inhibition before embarking on specialized tests of esophageal function. As with other functional disorders, reassurance, good doctor–patient interaction, attention to physical and mental stressors, and the passage of time are key therapeutic tools.

CHAPTER TWENTY

Burbulence

Functional Abdominal Bloating

I feel as unfit as an unfiddle, and it is the result of a certain turbulence
of the mind and a certain burbulence in the middle
Ogden Nash, "New Year's Day 1964"

Bloating is a common symptom, that is very often found with IBS. If it occurs without IBS or other organic or functional disorder, it is designated *functional abdominal bloating* with the following Rome criteria:

1. Symptoms of gaseous distension, borborygmi, or farting for at least three months
2. Symptoms unrelated to maldigestion or other gastrointestinal disease causing similar symptoms
3. Insufficient criteria for IBS, dyspepsia, or other functional disorder

This definition embraces three unrelated phenomena. Farting is a physiological phenomenon caused by the production of gas by colon bacteria. Excessive belching or burping is associated with aerophagia (air swallowing). This is also partly physiological, but it may become exaggerated through habit. The mechanism of bloating, distension, or epigastric fullness is obscure. Bloating seems to be unrelated to the other two phenomena, yet they often

241

occur together. Here we will discuss all three phenomena, since they often accompany dyspepsia.

GAS, WIND, FLATUS

Composition of Flatus

Like defecation, the passage of flatus is a normal excretory process. Although some nitrogen from swallowed air may reach the colon, most emitted gas originates there. Some carbohydrates, such as cellulose, glycoproteins, and other ingested materials, are not assimilated in the small intestine. They arrive intact in the colon, where resident bacteria digest them to produce hydrogen, carbon dioxide, methane, and trace gases. In intestinal obstruction, or postoperative ileus (paralyzed intestines), gas accumulates and distends the gut to cause discomfort and pain. Nevertheless, the very common sensation of bloating usually occurs with no increase in intestinal gas.

Production of Gas

Passing gas is part of the human condition, and is a welcome sign of recovery after abdominal surgery. Normally, the gut contains 100–200 ml of gas. In 1906, Fries collected gas by rectal tube and determined that an average person on a normal diet emits about 1 liter per day. Someone has recorded that we pass 50–500 ml a mean of 13.6 times per day. There is great variation in amount and frequency from person to person and from time to time. Those prone to produce more than average amounts of gas or who are unduly sensitive may suffer socially.

Nevertheless, flatus is here to stay. Most flatus consists of hydrogen, carbon dioxide, and methane. Hydrogen is exclusively the product of unabsorbed substrates that are fermented by colon bacteria. These substrates include cellulose from coarse vegetables and grains, glycoproteins, and complex saccharides such as stachyose and raffinose found in beans. Intestinal floras differ from person to person. Some bacteria produce hydrogen, while others consume it. In one-third of people, an organism called *Methanobrevibacter smithii* converts hydrogen to methane. The methane-producing trait is familial, but is a result of early environment rather than genes. Spouses do not share the trait with one another. These factors account for the great variation in the composition and volume of flatus.

Carbon dioxide is released when hydrochloric acid reacts with bicarbonate secreted in the intestines, bile ducts, and pancreas. However, most of this gas is quickly absorbed. Carbon dioxide, too, is a product of local fermentation. Nitrogen, hydrogen, carbon dioxide, and methane comprise 99% of colon gas. The remaining 1% are trace gases that compensate for small quantities by strong odors. Hydrogen sulfide accounts for the "rotten egg" smell. Other smelly gases include ammonia, skatol, indole, and volatile fatty acids.

Farting has been the subject of literary mirth and misery since the days of Chaucer. *Borborygmi* is not some Third World tribe, but the name given to the noises generated as air and fluid gurgle through the gut. These phenomena are normal and do not account for bloating. They have little impact on *The Ulcer Story*. So...

Where're ye be, Let ye'r wind gang free.
Robert Burns, 1759–1796

AEROPHAGIA

Mechanism

Air swallowing is also normal, although unlike farting it contributes no discernible benefit. Newborns begin life with gasless intestines until they draw their first breath. Subsequently, air appears progressively down the gut. Loss of innocence marks the onset of burbulence.

During inspiration, the normally negative intraesophageal pressure falls, attracting the ambient air. Forced inspiration against a closed glottis (willfully closed windpipe) draws even more air into the esophagus. The air may be forced out again as intraesophageal pressure increases with expiration. The resulting sounds delight adolescents who love to shock their elders. More practically, those who have lost their larynx because of cancer put this learnable skill to use generating esophageal speech. Commonly, aerophagy is an unwanted habit in those who repeatedly burp in response to a sense of bloating.

About 5 ml of air is ingested with each swallow of saliva, perhaps more with food. Nervous patients undergoing abdominal X rays accumulate more intestinal gas than those who are relaxed. Other mechanisms include thumb sucking, gum chewing, rapid eating, and poor dentures. Stomach gas has the same composition as the atmosphere, and the volume increases about 10% when heated by body temperature. Carbonated drinks and antacids reacting with hydrochloric acid produce carbon dioxide and traces may diffuse from the blood. Air forced into the stomach during endoscopy often appears by rectum in 15 minutes.

Virtually all stomach gas is ingested. In achalasia, where the lower esophageal sphincter cannot relax, the stomach is gasless. Exceptions include bowel obstruction or a gastrocolic fistula where colon gases reach the stomach. Sometimes gastric stasis permits gastric bacteria to grow and produce hydrogen in situ. One man made achlorhydric by previous surgery happened to belch while lighting a cigarette and suffered burns to his nose and hair.

Clinical Manifestations of Aerophagia

To belch is to bring forth wind noisily from the stomach. The word "burp" does not appear in some dictionaries, but it seems to mean to "cause to belch" as one would burp a baby. Colloquially, the terms are interchangeable. A belch after a large meal is a physiological venting of air from the stomach. In some societies it is a gesture of appreciation to the host. It also has comic associations, as with Sir Toby Belch in *Twelfth Night*. It is still a reliable source of mirth in male societies, as in the military or on a fishing trip.

Gaseous distension augmented by a meal stretches nerve endings in the muscle of the accommodating stomach, and distress occurs with little increase in intragastric pressure. A satisfying belch eases the discomfort. The ability to tolerate intragastric pressure varies, and some individuals seem unduly sensitive. If release of gas relieves the distended feeling, even transiently, a cycle of air swallowing and belching may be established. People with gastroenteritis, heartburn, or ulcers swallow more frequently, but the ensuing belch is probably a counterstimulus of no lasting benefit. The swallow–belch cycle may continue long after the original discomfort is forgotten.

Of course, venting gas is important, as those unable to do so will attest. When the lower esophageal sphincter is reinforced by antireflux surgery, belching may be impossible. The patient's position may hinder a belch. Swallowed air is lighter than food and reaches only the esophagus, from whence it is readily returned. Bedridden patients, such as those recovering from surgery, however, may trap air in their stomachs. In the supine position gastric contents seal the gastroesophageal junction so that air cannot escape. Relief is achieved through assumption of the prone position (Figure 20-1). Sometimes sleeping on the left side favors a belch and may reduce gastroesophageal acid reflux (see Chapter 14).

Repetitive belching is not physiological. While the patient insists that his stomach is producing prodigious amounts of gas, in reality, air is drawn into the esophagus and released. A little may even reach the stomach. Some can belch on command, and the inspiration against a closed glottis is demonstrable. Others must examine themselves during an attack to gain insight. Most sufferers are relieved to have their habit pointed out, but some are incredulous. Quitting the habit is often difficult. Repeated and intractable belching is termed *eructio nervosa*.

FUNCTIONAL ABDOMINAL BLOATING

The wind bloweth where it listeth, and we hear the sound thereof, but cannot tell whence it cometh and whither it goeth

John 3:8

Mechanism

Those complaining of bloating and distension are often convinced that it is due to excess intestinal gas. Although the sensation may induce aerophagia, it seldom results from it. Farting may temporarily relieve bloating, but intestinal gas production doesn't cause it. Lasser *et al.* infused the inert gas xenon into the gut to wash out the resident gases. He demonstrated that gas volume and composition in bloaters was no different from nonbloaters. Despite visible distension, X rays and computerized tomography (CT) show no large collections of intestinal gas. The distension disappears with sleep and general anesthesia. It is difficult to interpret

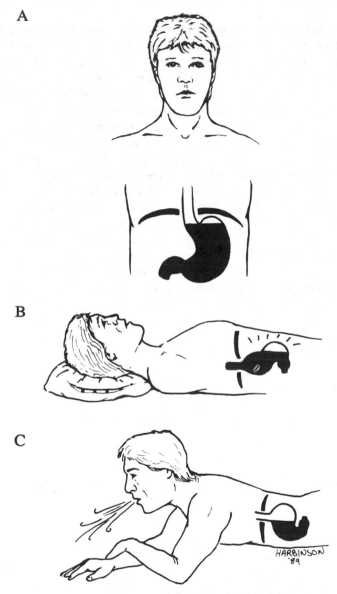

Figure 20-1. Effect of position on the ability to belch. (A) Erect: Air that lies in the fundus above the gastroesophageal junction cannot escape. (B) Supine: Air collects anteriorly and cannot be easily passed distally through the pylorus or retrograde through the esophagus. (C) Prone: Air may now escape through the gastroesophageal junction.

the psychodynamics of this common problem, but horses bloat to avoid the saddle.

Observable bloating has been called *pseudotumor* or *pseudocyesis* (false pregnancy). In 1838, Robert Bright described this condition in neurotic females. One of his patients had surgery for an ovarian tumor, but none was found. Dickens describes bloating in Sam Weller's mother, who "always goes and blows up, downstairs for a couple of hours arter tea." In the 1930s, Walter Alvarez of the Mayo Clinic described *hysterical nongaseous bloating*. Of 150 bloating patients, he collected 92 whose abdomens became clinically distended without increased gas in the gut. He also observed a forward arching of the spine so that when the patient was supine, he could insert a fist between the back and examining table.

As in other functional gastrointestinal disorders, gut hypersensitivity may explain the sensation of abdominal bloating. The hypersensitive gut feels distended at lower than normal filling, and abdominal muscles relax to accommodate the perceived distension. The stomach is and feels distended with normal amounts of air. The idea is not new. In 1927 Hutchison ascribed gastric flatulence to stomach "hyperesthesia."

Maxton and colleagues (1991) studied the abdominal girth of 20 female IBS patients who complained of distension. It increased 3–4 cm over an 8-hour day. CT demonstrated the change in profile despite unchanged gas content or distribution. There were no corresponding changes in 20 control subjects. Lumbar lordosis (arching of the spine) was increased in eight patients, and decreased in seven. When the women deliberately protruded their abdomens, the configuration was different from when they were bloated. Therefore, a conscious mechanism is unlikely. Sullivan (*New Zealand Med J*, 1994) found that 26 of 46 patients with visible abdominal bloating had increased abdominal girth that he blamed on weak abdominal muscles. These data partly confirm Alvarez's observations of one-half a century ago. The reality of the phenomenon is indisputable; the how remains a mystery.

Clinical Features

The symptom of bloating occurs in 30% of adults and is frequent in 10%. Among those with IBS and dyspepsia the figures

are much higher. It is often their most troublesome feature. Typically, the abdomen is flat upon awakening, but distends progressively through the day only to disappear with sleep. Women
complain of the need to let out their clothing and sometimes
volunteer, "It's as if I'm 6 months pregnant." Many report that
bloating can occur quickly, in some cases within 1 minute. It is often
aggravated by eating and relieved by lying. Menstruation and
stress affect a few cases. Usually, it is most obvious in the lower
abdomen, but many report it near the umbilicus or all over the belly.

Upon examination there is usually nothing to see. However, if
the distension is present at the time of the examination (more likely
late in the day), the features described by Alvarez and Maxton may
be observed. There is no abdominal tympany to suggest gaseous
intestines, and sometimes the distended abdomen can be mistaken
for ascites or a tumor, as in Robert Bright's case. Bloating's importance to *The Ulcer Story* is its association with dyspepsia. On its own,
it is not a symptom of peptic ulcer and should prompt no ulcer
investigation or treatment.

Treatment

Functional abdominal bloating, or bloating as part of the IBS
and dyspepsia, is frustrating to treat. The temporary disappearance
of distension during sleep and anesthesia suggests a voluntary
mechanism. Stress or psychological factors likely contribute, but
there are few data. Nevertheless, some claim success with hypnotherapy or dynamic psychotherapy.

Carminatives such as peppermint are volatile oils that relax
the lower esophageal sphincter, permitting a belch. Peppermint in
various forms is popular to help settle meals and is a common
antacid flavoring. Ingestion of activated charcoal may absorb some
gas, but it is too messy to use. Surfactants such as the silicone-con-
taining compound simethicone are directed against gas. Through
their surface activity, air bubbles coalesce in the gut. This improves
the view on gastroscopy or X ray, but the gas must still be there.
Since intestinal gas is not increased in bloating, these treatments
seem beside the point.

SUMMARY

Bloating is a common symptom on its own and is commonly part of IBS and dyspepsia. Although intuitively considered a result of increased intestinal gas production or aerophagia, there is no excess intestinal gas. Distension usually increases throughout the day and is abolished temporarily by sleep, anesthesia, or hypnotherapy. There is no satisfactory explanation of the phenomenon, but patients' abdominal girth increases as they bloat, and on lateral CT one can sometimes demonstrate forward abdominal protrusion. Bloating has no definitive treatment. The discomfort greatly troubles some bloaters, who are able to tolerate only loose-fitting clothing.

CHAPTER TWENTY-ONE

Cancer of the Upper Gut

Cancer has an impact on *The Ulcer Story* in several ways. In its early stages, cancer's physical appearance and symptoms may resemble those of peptic ulcer or esophagitis. *H. pylori* may cause gastric cancers. Severe esophagitis may progress though metaplasia and dysplasia to esophageal cancer.

GASTRIC CANCERS

Carcinoma of the Stomach

Epidemiology

Fifty years ago, carcinoma of the stomach was the most common cancer in the United States. The annual deaths from this cancer were about 23 per 100,000 and are now about 6 per 100,000. There is much variation in prevalence worldwide. Death rates are very high in Costa Rica and Columbia. In Japan the annual mortality is 63 per 100,000. Intense screening for early cancer in Japan may account for a recent decline in mortality there. Japanese who migrated to Hawaii in the 1890s suffered cancer at the Japanese rate, but the next two generations adopted the lower rate of the native Hawaiians. The environmental explanation for this change is unknown.

Gastric cancers are more likely to occur in individuals with blood group A and in the so-called cancer family syndrome (Lynch II). First-degree relatives of cancer patients have a two-to three-fold increase in risk, and it may occur in identical twins. In one set of twins the disease occurred simultaneously.

Cause

There are several pathological classifications of gastric cancer that need not concern us here. The intestinal type of cancer is the most common, and it occurs in people with gastric atrophy and intestinal metaplasia of the mucosa. Dysplasia in this tissue is an ominous precancer sign (see the discussion of Barrett's esophagus in Chapter 17.)

Normally, gastric acid suppresses bacterial growth in the stomach. Sixty percent of patients with gastric cancer are achlorhydric when fasting, and 20% remain so after stimulation of the gastric mucosa by pentagastrin. Bacterial overgrowth in the achlorhydric stomach may change ingested nitrates into nitrosamines and carcinogenic nitrosamides. Thus, lack of gastric acid may help account for the increased risk of cancer in pernicious anemia. Twenty or thirty years after a partial gastrectomy, the relative risk of cancer is three-to five-fold. Cancer in the achlorhydric stomachs caused by widespread use of the proton pump inhibitors has fortunately not occurred.

The most important and exciting causative agent may be *H. pylori*. Carriers of this organism have an estimated sixfold increase in risk of developing gastric cancer. *H. pylori* and gastric cancer are becoming less common in Western countries, but not in the Orient and some parts of Latin America. Over 2 billion people are infected, but most do not develop cancer. Therefore, the organism must interact with other factors for malignant change to occur.

The reduced risk of cancer in expatriate Japanese suggests that the environment is important. Some suspect smoked fish. Those with a high salt intake may be at greater risk. The concordance in identical twins supports a genetic cause. However, it uncertain if the observed family clustering is due to genes or exposure to a carcinogenlike *H. pylori*.

Prevention

Dysplasia of the gastric mucosa has the same sinister implications as it does in the colon or Barrett's esophagus. When found, dysplasia should be treated as a harbinger of cancer. *Early gastric cancer* is a familiar concept in Japan, where the great prevalence of cancer prompts aggressive surveillance. This asymptomatic stage may precede advanced cancer by 8 years. If removed promptly, the outlook is good. Early gastric cancer exists worldwide, but most countries have not undertaken Japanese-style early detection programs. There is debate whether achlorhydric states such as pernicious anemia or gastrectomy are precancerous. The current view is that they are, but the rate is insufficiently high to justify an early detection program.

Eradication of *H. pylori* might reduce the likelihood of cancer. However, the huge human reservoir of infection will not permit its extermination through antibiotic therapy. The cost, side effects, and risk of bacterial resistance with the existing antibiotics are too high. The eradication rate under optimal conditions is only about 80%. In Western countries the problem may be resolving spontaneously. Succeeding generations have less infection and less gastric cancer. It is uncertain if this is due to less crowding and better hygiene or if it is another manifestation of the transitory nature of some human diseases. Better living conditions in the Third World may help, but extermination will only be achieved through the development and worldwide distribution of a vaccine. Such a program is a formidable challenge.

There are genetic markers of stomach cancer. In the future it might be possible to identify carriers of stomach cancer genes and to target for tests and treatment those who also have *H. pylori* infection. However, we must know much more before any prevention program can proceed.

Gastric Cancer and Peptic Ulcer

Cancer of the stomach may ulcerate and initially resemble a benign gastric ulcer both in the presence of dyspepsia and in its endoscopic appearance (see Figure 3-3). Bleeding and obstruction may occur with both lesions, and the endoscopist must distinguish one from the other. Ulcerated cancers look benign in about one-fifth of cases and may appear to heal with anti-ulcer medication. Most gastric ulcers should thus be biopsied. Seven biopsies plus cytology will achieve greater than 95% accuracy. In suspicious gastric ulcers, a repeat endoscopy 6–8 weeks later will ascertain complete healing.

In the past, many worried that a benign gastric ulcer could turn malignant. Rarely, a small patch of cancer occurs in a gastric ulcer. It is more likely that malignant ulcers are cancer from the start. The early diagnosis of gastric cancer is desirable, and prompt gastric surgery is the only hope of cure.

Warning Signs

While a gastric cancer may initially cause dyspepsia, more sinister symptoms soon appear. Early satiety and weight loss are very important. Bleeding may be subtle, and an iron-deficiency anemia should draw attention to the gut. The pain becomes intense and relentless. Vomiting often follows eating. Unlike patients with dyspepsia or ulcer, a cancer victim begins to appear very ill. There may be a mass in the upper abdomen. Often, the diagnosis is made by discovery of a metastasis at a distant site: a lung shadow on a chest X ray, a large liver and jaundice, an ovarian mass (Krukenberg tumor), or a malignant lymph node above the clavicle (Virchow's node). Endoscopy confirms the cancer, and computerized tomography (CT) assesses the extent of spread. While a barium meal may discover a gastric tumor, barium obscures the endoscopist's view. This may delay a biopsy diagnosis.

Gastric Lymphoma

A lymphoma is a cancer of lymph tissue. There are many types of lymphoma, but we are only interested in those that originate in the stomach. Mononuclear cells such as lymphocytes occur in the mucosa and submucosa of the entire gut, and those in the stomach are most prone to become malignant. Gastric lymphoma is much less common than gastric cancer, but their symptoms and endoscopic appearances are similar. Causing dyspepsia at first, it later produces satiety, weight loss, vomiting, and anemia. Here again the diagnosis depends upon biopsy. Lymphomas generally have a better prognosis than carcinomas. Current treatment includes surgery, radiotherapy and chemotherapy in various combinations, and the 5-year survival is about 50%.

Of great interest to *The Ulcer Story* is a slow-growing gastric lymphoma known as a mucosa-associated lymphoid tissue (MALT) lymphoma. This cancer is invariably associated with *H. pylori*. Prospective studies in the United States, United Kingdom, and Japan indicate that killing the organisms with antibiotics achieves a complete remission in the cancer, and there is hope for a lasting cure.

Other Gastric Tumors

Benign gastric polyps are usually discovered incidentally during endoscopy. Metastatic tumors and tissues of the fatty, fibrous, or muscle tissue of the stomach are of little interest here. Muscle tumors that bulge into the stomach lumen, called leiomyomas or leiomyosarcomas, occasionally have a peptic ulcer at their summit.

ESOPHAGEAL CANCER

Carcinoma of the esophagus is one of the most common cancers worldwide. It is especially common in the Orient but is not as common as gastric cancer in the West. Nevertheless, it is one of the deadliest of all malignant tumors, principally because it usually is discovered too late for curative surgery or radiotherapy. Esophageal cancers arise from two different epithelial cell types: squamus cells and the columnar cells that are seen after many years of gastroesophageal reflux called Barrett's epithelium (see Chapter 17). Until recently, adenocarcinoma from columnar cells accounted for as few as 5% of all esophageal cancers, but it now is responsible for about one-third.

Squamus Cell Carcinoma

This lethal cancer is especially common in smokers who are also alcoholics. Its principal symptom is difficulty in swallowing, so it must be differentiated from esophageal stricture. Despite the bad outlook, squamus cancers are radiosensitive, so radiotherapy can achieve limited remissions and rare cures. Since these carcinomas usually occur in the upper esophagus near the great vessels from the heart, surgical treatment, even for palliation, is often impossible.

Adenocarcinoma

Like squamus cancers, adenocarcinomas cause dysphagia and must be distinguished from a stricture due to esophagitis. They tend to occur at the lower end of the esophagus, so that a surgical approach is often possible. This is important since radiation for adenocarcinomas is not an option even for palliation.

The principal importance of these cancers to *The Ulcer Story* is that nearly 90% of them are found in Barrett's epithelium. This permits physicians to discover the lesion early through a screening program aimed at patients with specialized columnar epithelium resulting from chronic esophagitis (see Chapter 17). Finding the cancer at an early stage is the only hope of cure. By the time symptoms occur, the disease is already incurable.

DUODENAL CANCER

Duodenal cancer is so uncommon that endoscopists seldom consider it a possibility when viewing a duodenal ulcer. However, a masslike lesion near the ulcer or failure of the ulcer to heal with conventional therapy should arouse suspicion.

SUMMARY

Gastric and esophageal cancers are important to *The Ulcer Story* because they must be excluded in patients with gastric ulcer or esophageal stricture. Gastric cancers cause dyspepsia, and esophageal cancers cause dysphagia. Both produce weight loss and may present with bleeding or an iron-deficiency anemia. There is great interest in the possible role of *H. pylori* in gastric carcinoma. The rare MALT lymphoma appears to result from this infection, and eradication of the organisms may cure the cancer. Adenocarcinoma appears to develop in the specialized columnar epithelium found in the lower esophagus after many years of gastroesophageal reflux (Barrett's esophagus). Regular screening of such patients for the dysplastic changes that signal malignant development may lead to earlier diagnosis and more cures.

PART SIX

Treatments for Ulcers and Heartburn

CHAPTER TWENTY-TWO

Antacids

You might ask, "With modern anti-ulcer medication, why bother with antacids?" Why indeed! Antacid benefits do not compare with the ulcer-healing properties of H_2 antagonists, the virtual anacidity obtainable with omeprazole, or the ulcer-curing power of antibiotics. Nevertheless, antacids are an important part of the ulcer and heartburn stories because of their long history, low cost, and safety. Their very availability ensures that people will continue to use them for minor dyspeptic or reflux complaints.

Antacids are the oldest effective anti-ulcer medications. Chalk (calcium carbonate) has been chewed for centuries to ease dyspepsia. Indeed, before the arrival of cimetidine in the early 1970s, antacids were the only useful anti-ulcer drugs the physician had to offer. Patients whose disease was uncontrolled by antacids and diet had recourse only to surgery. Now antacids transcend medical practice. They occupy large sections on pharmacists' shelves and are almost obligatory components of the household medicine chest. Antacids are cheap and safe, except in heart or renal failure. Ever popular for heartburn and ulcer symptoms, it is ironic that proof of their efficacy in healing ulcers came only *after* release of the H_2 antagonists.

Since people will likely continue to use antacids for "acid complaints" with or without medical approval, we need to know about them. Also, ulcer healing or reflux control is seldom immediate with any agent, so antacids may relieve symptoms for the short term. Antacids are no better than placebo in treating non-ulcer dyspepsia, but they themselves can be a safe and inexpensive placebo.

WHAT ARE ANTACIDS?

Most commercially available antacids are combinations of aluminum and magnesium hydroxide. Calcium carbonate (Tums™) is chalk. Some effervescent antacids contain sodium bicarbonate, and who has not resorted to good old baking soda for a tummy-ache? Our discussion will concentrate on these four chemicals, but there are others. Antacids are often peppermint-flavored. Many contain the antiflatulent simethicone. For heartburn, an alginate combined with antacid floats on gastric fluids and protects the esophagus from acid exposure.

CLINICAL PHARMACOLOGY

The objective of antacid therapy is to neutralize gastric acid. In chemical terms this implies reducing the free hydrogen ion (H^+) concentration in gastric juice, thereby raising its pH. This not only reduces the corrosive effect of the acid itself, but also, by raising the pH above 4, inactivates the digestive effect of pepsin.

The concept of acid neutralization is simple enough, but consistent elevation of gastric pH is difficult to achieve. This is because the fasting stomach empties within an hour. Doubling or tripling the dose may increase the overall neutralizing power, but it will not raise the stomach pH for more than an hour. This disadvantage may be overcome by constant infusion of antacid through an intragastric tube or by hourly dosing. Both solutions are impractical in ambulatory patients. After a meal, food takes time to be processed and emptied. Therefore, antacids given 1 hour after a meal can raise the intragastric pH for longer. This is the rationale for their postprandial administration (Figure 22-1). Unfortunately, patients who experience heartburn or ulcer pain in the middle of the night benefit little from a bedtime antacid.

Antacids heal peptic ulcers as well as H_2 antagonists do. However, to be effective, the antacid must be taken seven or more times a day. Few will comply with such a regimen, especially if they

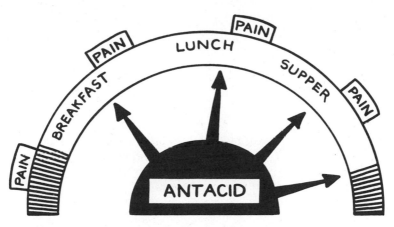

Figure 22-1. Antacid regimen that was frequently recommended for peptic ulcer. Typically, ulcer pain occurs 1 or 2 hours after meals as the stomach empties and acid reduces the pH. It also occurs in the night, when the stomach is empty. Thus, antacids were prescribed for 1 hour after meals and at bedtime to anticipate the fall in pH and onset of pain. Such a predictable pain pattern is unusual today. This plan often failed to relieve night pain, and antacid was required when the patient awakened. With modern drugs for peptic ulcer, such treatment is no longer necessary. However, antacids are useful for mild heartburn and might be given in a pattern not unlike that in the illustration.

can achieve the same benefit with a single daily dose of another drug. Liquid antacid preparations are faster-acting and have greater neutralizing power than the equivalent antacid tablet. This is because the tablet must be chewed and may not interact as well with gastric juice. For most, the convenience of tablets far outweighs these slight disadvantages.

ANTACID COMPONENTS

The basic antacids are reviewed in Table 22-1.

Sodium Bicarbonate [$NaHCO_3$]

$$NaHCO_3 + H^+ \rightarrow Na^+ + H_2O + CO_2$$

TABLE 22-1
The Basic Antacids

Antacid	Formula[a]	Neutralizing power	Side effects
Magnesium hydroxide	$Mg(OH)_2$	high	Diarrhea, magnesium toxicity
Aluminum hydroxide	$Al(OH)_3$	modest	Constipation, drug and phosphate binding
Calcium carbonate	$CaCO_3$	very high	Constipation, acid rebound
Sodium bicarbonate	$NaHCO_3$	low	Sodium, alkalosis

[a]Al, aluminum; Mg, magnesium; Ca, calcium; Na, sodium.

Sodium bicarbonate is the least effective basic antacid. It rapidly empties from the stomach, so the antacid effect is short. While generally a safe household remedy, its high sodium content is a disadvantage. It is unlikely to be recommended by doctors, but "bicarb," or "baking soda," is a common component of several patent medicines. Its effervescent property has commercial appeal, which explains the survival of Alka-Seltzer™ and Bromo-Seltzer™. The interaction of bicarbonate with gastric hydrochloric acid releases carbon dioxide gas (CO_2) that is quickly absorbed. Sometimes the CO_2 elicits a satisfying belch.

Overuse of bicarbonate may result in systemic alkalosis. This is doubly harmful if chloride or potassium are depleted through vomiting or diuretic therapy. Individuals who require sodium restriction for high blood pressure or heart disease should not use sodium bicarbonate.

Magnesium Hydroxide [$Mg(OH)_2$]

$$Mg(OH)_2 + 2H^+ \rightarrow Mg^{++} + 2H_2O$$

Magnesium hydroxide is best known as milk of magnesia. Akin to magnesium citrate or magnesium sulfate, it is a very effective laxative. Therein lies its chief disadvantage as an antacid. Were it not for its tendency to cause diarrhea, magnesium hydroxide would be a cheap and effective choice. To counter the diarrhea effect, most manufacturers add aluminum hydroxide, which is constipating. The combination substantially raises the price, and dilution of the magnesium compound with the less effective aluminum hydroxide reduces the antacid effect.

Magnesium hydroxide is insoluble and is not absorbed by the intestine. However, its interaction with hydrochloric acid results in the formation of soluble magnesium chloride that can be absorbed. Magnesium has many functions in human cells, including the heart, and may cause deleterious effects if blood levels rise. This is not a risk with healthy kidneys, but magnesium is best avoided if there is renal failure.

Aluminum Hydroxide [Al(OH)$_3$]

$$Al(OH)_3 + 3H^+ \rightarrow Al^{+++} + 3H_2O$$

Compared to magnesium hydroxide, aluminum hydroxide is a weak, slow-acting antacid. Because of differing chemical properties among commercial products, the reaction of Al(OH)$_3$ with hydrogen ions varies. At best it raises the intragastric pH to 4.5. Aluminum hydroxide not only inactivates pepsin but also binds the enzyme. In animal experiments, aluminum seems to protect the stomach mucosa from the damaging effects of alcohol and other irritants. This "cytoprotective" effect involves the release of prostaglandins. Aluminum is a smooth muscle relaxant that delays gastric emptying and slows gut transit. The principal reason for its inclusion in commercial antacid preparations is to counteract the diarrhea effect of magnesium.

Aluminum hydroxide binds phosphate in the gut lumen to produce insoluble aluminum phosphate. It is useful in kidney failure when the serum phosphate is elevated. It is also useful for patients who tend to form phosphate kidney stones. A very small amount of aluminum is absorbed, and brain damage (encephalopathy) may occur with its long-term use in kidney failure. Nevertheless, a suspected link with Alzheimer's disease is unproved. Chronic use of aluminum hydroxide may deplete the body of phosphate and risk bone loss (osteoporosis, osteomalacia) and spontaneous fractures. Alcoholics and malnourished people are especially at risk. By delaying gastric emptying and binding drugs such as digoxin or propanalol, aluminum hydroxide may alter their absorption.

Calcium Carbonate ($CaCO_3$)

$$CaCO_3 + 2H^+ \rightarrow Ca^{++} + H_2O + CO_2$$

Calcium carbonate (chalk) is the most potent basic antacid. It can achieve an intragastric pH of 9. However, it is not the best choice for regular use for several reasons. About one-third of the administered calcium is absorbed, and high blood calcium (hypercalcemia) or calcium-containing kidney stones are slight risks. Binding of phosphate by calcium in the gut or bone may deplete the serum phosphorus in patients with kidney failure. A systemic alkalosis rarely produces metabolic consequences. Another disadvantage is the tendency for gastric acid secretion to rebound after calcium is given. Calcium stimulates parietal cells directly and indirectly through the release of gastrin from the antral G cells.

Popular calcium antacid preparations include Tums™ and Titralac™, which are only available in tablet form. The dose should not exceed 3 grams per day if hypercalcemic consequences are to be avoided. Like aluminum hydroxide, calcium carbonate binds phosphate in patients with renal failure. Oral calcium supplements are often needed for pregnancy and lactation, metabolic bone disease (osteomalacia, osteoporosis), and malabsorption states. Another important use of calcium carbonate is to prevent bone loss in postmenopausal women. When these requirements coexist with the need for an antacid, then calcium carbonate is doubly useful.

Flavoring

Peppermint is the most common antacid flavoring. It is a carminative that relaxes smooth muscle, and, without convincing data, it is used to treat the irritable bowel. Peppermint's carminative action encourages the release of a postprandial belch. Hence the popularity of after-dinner mints. However, by relaxing the lower esophageal sphincter to release gas, it may inadvertently encourage reflux. In antacids there are probably insufficient quantities of peppermint to have a clinical effect.

TABLE 22-2
Some Liquid Antacids[a]

Product	Ingredients[b] (mg/5 ml)	Neutralizing capacity (meq/5 ml)	Sodium content (mg/5 ml)	1994[c] price/100 ml ($Cdn)
Mylanta extra-strength™	Al(OH)$_3$ 650 Mg(OH)$_2$ 350 Simethicone	32.4	1.0	1.98
Amphogel™ 500	Al(OH)$_3$ 500 Mg(OH)$_2$ 500	31.92	2.5	1.84
Gelusil extra strength™	Al(OH)$_3$ 650 Mg(OH)$_2$ 350	31.9	0.8	2.09
Maalox TC™	Al(OH)$_3$ 600 Mg(OH)$_2$ 300	27.06	1.0	1.83
Diovol Ex™	Al(OH)$_3$ 600 Mg(OH)$_2$ 300	26.84	2.2	1.66
Amphogel Plus™	Al(OH)$_3$ 300 Mg(OH)$_2$ 300	20.4	6.0	1.37
Phillips' Milk of Magnesia™	Mg(OH)$_2$ 408	13.95	na	1.25
Maalox™	Al(OH)$_3$ 225 Mg(OH)$_2$ 200	13.5	0.9	1.56
Diovol™	Al(OH)$_3$ 200 Mg(OH)$_2$ 200	13.38	2.0	1.32
Diovol Plus™	Al(OH)$_3$ 200 Mg(OH)$_2$ 200 Simethicone	13.20	9.2	1.49
Maalox Plus™	Al(OH)$_3$ 228 Mg(OH)$_2$ 200 Simethicone	12.85	0.9	1.66
Univol™	Al(OH)$_3$ 200 Mg(OH)$_2$ 200	12.75	10.6	0.60
Gelusil™	Al(OH)$_3$ 200 Mg(OH)$_2$ 200	12.49	1.8	1.77
Mylanta Regular™	Al(OH)$_3$ 200 Mg(OH)$_2$ 200	12.42	5.0	1.50
Amphogel™	Al(OH)$_3$ 320	10.17	9.5	1.52

[a]Adapted from Thompson, 1989; updated, 1994.
[b]Al, aluminum; Mg, magnesium; Ca, calcium; Na, sodium.
[c]Ottawa Civic Hospital Pharmacy, 1994.

Antiflatulent

Simethicone is a surfactant that breaks down bubbles within the gut, presumably rendering gas available for absorption. Despite the lack of evidence that it is clinically effective, simethicone is included in some popular antacids (Tables 22-2 and 22-3).

TABLE 22-3
Some Tablet Antacids[a]

Product	Ingredients[b] (mg)	Neutralizing capacity (meq)	Sodium content (mg)	1994[c] price($Cdn)
Maalox™	Al(OH)$_3$ 400 Mg(OH)$_2$ 400	23.3	0.9	1.09
Amphogel™	Al(OH)$_3$ 600	22.2	0.9	1.03
Gelusil ES™	Al(OH)$_3$ 400 Mg(OH)$_2$ 400	19.9	1.8	0.58
Mylanta Double Strength™	Al(OH)$_3$ 400 Mg(OH)$_2$ 400 Simethicone	19.3	1.8	1.39
Amphogel Plus™	Al(OH)$_3$ 300 Mg(CO)$_3$ 300 Mg(OH)$_2$ 300 Simethicone	17.6	5.3	1.10
Maalox Plus™	Al(OH)$_3$ 200 Mg(OH)$_2$ 200 Simethicone	11.7	0.9	1.16
Gelusil™	Al(OH)$_3$ 200 Mg(OH)$_2$ 200	11.4	0.5	1.24
Diovol™	Al(OH)$_3$ 300 Mg(OH)$_2$ 100 Mg(OH)$_2$ 100 Simethicone	11.2	6.4	0.93
Phillips' Milk of Magnesia™	Mg(OH)$_2$ 310	10.8	NA	0.44
Tums™	CaCO$_3$ 500	10.3	3.0	0.27
Digel™	Mg(OH)$_2$ 85 CaCO$_3$ 280 Simethicone	9.9	11.7	0.80
Titralac™	CaCO$_3$ 420	8.8	0.3	1.02
Mylanta™	Al(OH)$_3$ 200 Mg(OH)$_2$ 200 Simethicone	7.5	0.4	1.05

[a]Adapted from Thompson, 1989; updated, 1994.
[b]Al, aluminum; Mg, magnesium; Ca, calcium; Na, sodium.
[c]Ottawa Civic Hospital Pharmacy, 1994.

Alginic Acid

Alginate is not an antacid. Prepared from kelp (seaweed), it acts as a physical barrier to gastroesophageal reflux. When ingested, this tasteless, and apparently harmless, substance floats on gastric fluid to prevent the reflux of acid and pepsin into the esophagus. Preparations such as Gaviscon™ or Algicon™ combine alginate with antacids and are very popular heartburn remedies. There are no satisfactory clinical trials, but these preparations have little neutralizing power and are probably of little benefit in esophagitis.

COMMERCIAL PREPARATIONS

Most commercial antacids contain two or more components. Those commonly employed in Canada and the United States appear in Tables 22-2 and 22-3. There are other antacids that sacrifice efficacy in the interests of taste and acceptability. One such brand is Rolaids™ (dihydroxyaluminum sodium carbonate). Another is Riopan™ which contains magaldrate, an aluminum–magnesium compound.

SUMMARY

As a primary treatment for peptic ulcer, antacids are cumbersome and less convenient than other treatments. Nonetheless, they do provide symptom relief for many and might be considered a harmless placebo in those with burbulence or non-ulcer dyspepsia. The most practical antacid is magnesium hydroxide, but, because of its laxative effect, most commercial preparations combine it with aluminum hydroxide. By raising the intragastric pH above 4, antacids inactivate pepsin, relieve symptoms, and permit an ulcer to heal. Antacids by themselves or combined with alginate are very helpful for the treatment of heartburn, but they are ineffective for esophagitis.

CHAPTER TWENTY-THREE

Histamine H₂ Antagonists

The H_2 antagonists were the first effective drugs for peptic ulcer. In the 1970s and 1980s they were the backbone of treatment for ulcers and esophagitis, and they remain among the world's largest-selling drugs. Now that omeprazole has proven so effective in treating gastroesophageal reflux disease and antibiotics cure non-NSAID ulcers, H_2 antagonists face an uncertain future as prescription drugs. Nonetheless, they are very safe and effective for healing and symptom relief. Because they are available over the counter, they will likely remain widely used.

HISTORY AND RATIONALE

Histamine stimulates the parietal cells in the gastric mucosa to secrete hydrochloric acid. In the days when measuring acid output was thought to be important, physicians stimulated gastric acid secretion with histamine to test secretory function. The total acid produced in a defined period after histamine injection was called the "maximal acid output" (MAO). This reflects the number of parietal cells in the stomach, that is, the parietal cell mass (see Chapter 6). However, histamine has profound effects elsewhere, notably in the nasal mucosa, the bronchi, and the skin (see Figure 6-1). To counter these effects, patients undergoing a histamine stimulation test were pretreated with an antihistamine such as diphenhydramine (Benadryl™). The British pharmacologist Sir

James Black reasoned that, if an antihistamine blocked systemic histamine effects, but not the gastric acid secretory effects, then there must be a second histamine receptor. He and his colleagues described the histamine H_2 receptor in 1972 (see Figure 6-2).

Based on this hypothesis, Black synthesized and tested histamine-like molecules until he found some that inhibited acid secretion, yet had no effect elsewhere. The prototype, metiamide, damaged the bone marrow in two patients, prompting its withdrawal. Subsequently, cimetidine became a great success story. For this pharmacological tour de force and for development of the beta-blocking drugs for heart disease, Black received the 1988 Nobel Prize in Medicine.

THE HISTAMINE H_2 ANTAGONISTS

There are four commercially available H_2 antagonists (Table 23-1). Although they differ in potency (effect per given weight), there are few to choose among them based on efficacy and safety. Cimetidine and ranitidine are by far the most widely used, and we know the most about them. Because cimetidine causes confusion in some older people and may alter the metabolism of certain drugs, ranitidine is probably the best choice in elderly patients who are taking other medications. Young patients will choose according to cost (see Table 16-2). Since the four H_2 blockers are equally effective and compete for the same receptor, switching to another when one fails is likely to be futile. Increasing the dose may help.

ACTION

The H_2 antagonists compete with histamine for H_2 receptors on the gastric parietal cells. They bind but do not permanently inactivate the receptor. Large amounts of histamine will displace the drug. This explains the large doses required in the Zollinger–Ellison (ZE) syndrome, where gastrin excess releases histamine. By displacing histamine, the H_2 blockers reduce both basal and stimulated gastric acid secretion, no matter whether the stimulus is histamine, pentagastrin, or food. Ranitidine depresses acid secretion for at least 5 hours after a 150 mg dose. A reduced volume of gastric juice accounts for decreased pepsin activity.

TABLE 23-1
The H2 Blockers

Drug	Trade name	Dosage form	Dose[a]	Notes
Cimetidine	Tagamet™	300 mg(Can)	300 qid	Alters drug
		600 mg(Can)	600 bid	metabolism,
		200 mg(US, UK)	200 qid	
		400 mg(US, UK)	400 bid	gynaecomastia,
		800 mg(US, UK)	800 hs	confusion
Ranitidine	Zantac™	150 mg	150 bid	
		300 mg	300 hs	
		50 mg IV	500 bid	
Nizatidine	Axid™	150 mg	150 bid	
		300 mg	300 hs	
Famotadine	Pepsid™	20 mg	20 bid	Use with caution
		40 mg	40 hs	in heart failure

[a]qid, four times daily; bid, two times daily; hs, at bedtime.

H2 antagonists inconsistently raise gastrin serum levels. These agents protect the gastric mucosa against experimental aspirin damage, but they do not alter gastric mucus production or pancreatic secretion. Cessation of prolonged ranitidine treatment (300 mg for 60 days) provokes a marked rebound gastric secretion of hydrochloric acid. The BAO and MAO are more than double the pretreatment levels and the effect may last up to 10 days. This may explain the rapid resurgence of heartburn seen clinically when the drug is stopped.

UNWANTED ACTIONS

Central Nervous System

H2 antagonists cross the blood–brain barrier and interact with histamine H2 receptors in the brain. However, central nervous system (CNS) side effects are unusual. They include headache, dizziness, anxiety, somnolence, and depression. Rarely, confusion and delirium occur in the elderly. Side effects are more common when H2 antagonists are taken with other drugs, and attribution is often difficult.

Heart

As with the brain, cardiac side effects are most common in the elderly and the ill, where drug interactions are also more likely.

Reported unwanted effects include hypertension, hypotension, and irregular or slow heartbeat. Famotidine may reduce the force of heart muscle contraction. However, such effects are unlikely to occur in a healthy heart.

Endocrine

Cimetidine is weakly anti-androgenic and may have feminizing effects in men. These include breast development (gynecomastia), impotence, loss of sex drive, and elevation of the pituitary hormone *prolactin*. While disconcerting, these effects are rare and are thankfully reversed when the drug is stopped. They are more likely to occur when large doses are used for a long period, as for the ZE syndrome. Although these attributes are less for the other H_2 blockers, all are capable of causing gynecomastia.

Other Side Effects

During their widespread use, H_2 antagonists have been accused of many incidents. They depress suppresser T cells in the immune system, but any fallout from this is difficult to prove. Pancreatitis and abnormal liver function tests are reported. There is reduced production of intrinsic factor, a gastric protein essential for absorption of vitamin B_{12}. This seems insufficient to result in deficiency of the vitamin, let alone to cause its associated anemia and neuropsychiatric complications. The truth is that the H_2-blocking drugs are very safe. Side effects requiring their cessation occur in 1.5% of cases in clinical trials, compared to 1.2% for the placebo! Even an accidental overdose of cimetidine was without consequence.

DRUG INTERACTIONS

Alcohol

Alcohol dehydrogenase (ADH) is the enzyme principally responsible for the metabolism of alcohol. It is located mainly in the liver, but ADH in the gastric mucosa metabolizes 20% of ingested alcohol. Therefore, alcohol injected through a tube into the duodenum (unlikely to become a social pastime) produces a higher alcohol blood level. A meal slows gastric emptying, so alcohol taken with meals is subject to more gastric metabolism and lower Breathalyzer values. Women have less gastric ADH than men, accounting for their greater susceptibility.

Except for famotidine, the H$_2$ antagonists seem to inhibit gastric ADH. If true, this risks higher-than-expected blood alcohol levels. At least one legal action is based on this. However, the drug is unlikely to serve as an adequate alibi, and some studies cast doubt on this ADH effect. Meanwhile, if you drink, especially while taking an H$_2$ antagonist, you should not drive.

Altered Drug Absorption

When coadministered, antacids or sucralfate bind H$_2$ antagonists in the gut and can reduce their absorption by as much as 30%. This may be critical if a bedtime dose fails to adequately suppress nocturnal acid secretion. Because these drugs raise intragastric pH, they delay absorption of weak bases such as ketoconazole. Also, proton pump inhibitors require an acid medium to convert to their active metabolite. Therefore, an H$_2$ antagonist may delay the effect of omeprazole or lansoprazole. Taking the two types of drugs together is costly nonsense anyway.

Altered Drug Metabolism

Most drugs are lipid soluble and cannot be excreted into bile or urine until they are converted to water-soluble metabolites. This is accomplished by a family of liver enzymes, called cytochrome p450, that catalyze their oxidative biotransformation. Genes determine the mix of cytochrome enzymes that account for individual variations in drug tolerance.

Cimetidine has an imidazole ring that inhibits the cytochrome p450 system and delays the metabolism of some drugs. The other H$_2$ blockers with different ring structures have less effect. Concomitant administration of cimetidine will raise a susceptible drug's blood level and delay its excretion. This is most likely to produce toxic effects of drugs with a narrow therapeutic range such as theophylline, warfarin, or phenytoin. When cimetidine is stopped, a previously satisfactory blood level of a coadministered drug may fall below the therapeutic range.

Cimetidine depresses the metabolism of the anti-asthma drug theophylline by 30%. Warfarin is an anticoagulant that is also slowly metabolized when given with the anti-ulcer drug. After a pulmonary embolism, if cimetidine is withdrawn before warfarin, the latter must be increased to maintain anticoagulation and prevent another pulmonary embolus. Cardiac drugs such as quinidine, lidocaine, nifedipine, verapamil, and propanolol are subject to similar dangers. Patients taking tricyclic antidepressants such as imipramine, amitryptaline, or doxepin should reduce the dose by 50% during cimetidine treatment to avoid toxic effects. Some of the benzodiazepine drugs (e.g., diazepam, midazolam, chlordiazepoxide) are 30% less metabolized when taken with cimetidine. This may be enough to confuse the elderly or, since they depress breathing, decompensate a patient with marginal respiratory function.

Altered Drug Excretion

Cimetidine and ranitidine interfere with excretion of the normal metabolite creatinine. This is of no significance as long as the reduced creatinine clearance is not confused with renal failure. These drugs interfere with excretion of the cardiac drug procainamide and could produce a toxic blood level. In kidney failure, blood levels of the H_2 antagonists themselves may rise. Although of little consequence, the dose should be reduced accordingly.

Comment

Theoretically, many drugs could be affected by their interaction with cimetidine and the other H_2 antagonists. They are, however, very safe, so safe that authorities in some countries permit their sale over the counter. It makes sense to avoid prescribing cimetidine to the elderly or to people taking other medications. The overriding messages are to avoid polytherapy and to not use the H_2 antagonists without an indication. Complacency breeds hubris, wherein lie the seeds of potential disaster.

USE

Indications for the use of the H_2 blockers are listed in table 23-2. For the treatment of acute gastric or duodenal ulcer, the usual doses indicated in Table 23-1 will heal 80–90% in 6–9 weeks. Now that antbiotics cure ulcers, H_2 blockers are needed to speed healing and relieve symptoms. Ranitidine will prevent NSAID-induced gastric erosions and duodenal ulcers. It appears that ranitidine and miso- prostyl are equally effective in preventing NSAID-induced duode- nal ulcers, but misoprostol is superior in preventing gastric ulcers. Once an ulcer is healed, long-term maintenance therapy reduces the likelihood of recurrence. Ranitidine, 150 milligrams per day, reduces the annual ulcer recurrence of 50–80% on placebo to less than 20%. Ulcer prevention is successful for up to 12 years. If the drug is withdrawn after 1 year of maintenance, duodenal ulcers recur at the same rate as if there was no maintenance. However, after many years of continuous H_2 antagonists, the ulcer disease appears to remit, and further maintenance is not required. Smoking greatly increases the chance of ulcer recurrence whether or not an H_2 blocker is used. Nonsmokers without ranitidine do as well as smokers taking the drug.

The H_2 antagonists are effective in most cases of heartburn that do not respond to antireflux and lifestyle measures (see Chapter 16). However, severe esophagitis, especially if complicated by bleeding or stricture, requires a proton pump inhibitor. Fed patients requiring urgent surgery or delivery risk aspiration of acid gastric contents into the lungs. H_2 antagonists reduce the volume and acidity of gastric juice and thereby reduce the danger. Kidney patients undergoing dialysis or renal transplant are liable to peptic ulcer that is prevented by histamine blockade. Gastric acid destroys pancreatic enzymes given for pancreatic insufficiency. Acid sup- pression preserves their activity.

The omeprazole family of drugs have supplanted the H_2 an- tagonists in the treatment of ZE syndrome. Although the H_2 blockers heal ulcers, clinical trials suggest that they have little impact on acute ulcer bleeding. Nevertheless, acid impairs the quality of blood clotting and encourages clot destruction (fibrinolysis). This effect can be prevented by alkalinization, so fast-acting intravenous H_2- blocking drugs make sense. Their use to prevent stress ulcers in

TABLE 23-2
Indications for Histamine H$_2$ Antagonists

Healing peptic ulcers
Healing peptic ulcers while antibiotics eradicate H. pylori
Long-term maintenance of ulcer healing when there is no H. pylori to eradicate or when eradication fails
With NSAIDs to prevent ulcers
Mild esophagitis
Heartburn, without esophagitis, that persists after lifestyle changes
Prevent stress ulcers (controversial)
Prevent ulcers in other high-risk situations such as renal failure
Before emergency surgery or delivery to reduce acid regurgitation
To prevent destruction of therapeutic pancreatic enzymes

seriously ill patients is controversial and may not be cost-effective. The annual U.S. bill for intravenous H$_2$ blockers is $112 million.

H$_2$ antagonists are greatly overused. Many patients take them for dyspepsia, IBS, or other abdominal pains where no effect beyond placebo can be expected. This is an important issue. Should public or collectively funded health plans provide drugs for benign, chronic diseases without proof that they work? It is a lesser problem if the patient pays for the drug himself and is aware of their unlikely benefit. Some European authorities neatly side-step the issue by permitting over-the-counter sales. H$_2$ antagonists are now available over the counter in the United States. The stated indications are heartburn and indigestion for persons over 12 years of age. Note that the tablet strength is one quarter of the usual dose recommended for the treatment of peptic ulcers (e.g. ranitidine 75mg).

DOSE AND ADMINISTRATION

The recommended H$_2$ antagonist dosages appear in Table 23-1. A single bedtime dose achieves results almost as good as divided doses and is cheaper and easier to remember. The elimination of unneeded nocturnal gastric secretion makes sense, since the sleeping stomach is without food or saliva to tame the acid. The H$_2$ antagonist should be given separately from antacids.

SUMMARY

Histamine H2 antagonists competitively inhibit the effect of histamine on gastric parietal cell H2 receptors. By reducing acid and the digestive action of pepsin in the upper gut, these drugs permit 80% of duodenal ulcers to heal in 6–8 weeks. They are less effective in gastric ulcers and are useful in only moderately severe esophagitis. Now that antibiotics cure non-NSAID ulcers and omeprazole controls severe esophagitis, the need for these drugs should decline. Nevertheless, they are remarkably safe and cheap and are still needed to heal acute ulcers while antibiotics kill *H. pylori*. They are also useful in moderate esophagitis and heartburn and in the prevention and treatment of NSAID ulcers. Data do not support their use in functional disorders such as IBS and non-ulcer dyspepsia.

CHAPTER TWENTY-FOUR

Proton Pump Inhibitors

In gastric parietal cells, the proton pump uses the enzyme hydrogen potassium adenosine triphosphatase (H^+, K^+ -ATPase) to produce hydrogen ions. A family of drugs, the benzimidazoles, irreversibly binds to this enzyme, incapacitating the parietal cells. Even in modest doses, these drugs are the most powerful known inhibitors of gastric acid secretion. Omeprazole (Losec™, Prilosec™) was the first commercially available pump blocker in North America. Lansoprazole (Zoton™, Prevacid™) now has been released in Canada, the United States, Europe, and Japan. A third drug, panoprazole (Pantozol™), was introduced in Sweden and Germany in 1994.

ACTION

Omeprazole is a pro-drug. With an inactive weak base, it is concentrated in the acid environment of the parietal cell. Here it acquires a proton and positive charge that prevents its escape through the cell membrane. Safely inside the cell it becomes the active sulphenamide form. The concentration of omeprazole in the parietal cells is so great that its half-life in the blood is only about 1 hour. Perhaps this helps prevent side effects. By blocking histamine and reducing proton pump activity, H_2 antagonists may delay omeprazole uptake in the parietal cells. There is no reason to use these two types of drugs together.

The means by which omeprazole inactivates the proton pump is uncertain. At an acid pH, the drug binds with sulphydryl groups on the H^+, K^+ - ATPase and irreversibly inactivates it. However, acid pumps are continuously synthesized, and about one-third of the stomach's acid secretory capacity is restored 36 hours after taking a 20-mg omeprazole capsule. H_2 antagonists compete with histamine for H_2 receptors on the parietal cell. A stimulus such as a meal may overwhelm this effect, and acid suppression is never complete. In contrast, even modest doses of omeprazole completely block acid production, and the effect of a single dose may linger for 3 or 4 days. Pantoprazole binds the proton pump at a different site than omeprazole and lanzoprazole. Its makers claim greater binding specificity, but so far, this "me too" drug offers little advantage over omeprazole. It bestows the benefits of competition, so more attractive prices ultimately will determine commercial success.

Omeprazole decreases both basal and stimulated acid production, regardless of the stimulation. The effect increases with the dose until there is achlorhydria (pH > 4). The drug also inhibits pepsin production by the chief cells and reduces the volume of gastric juice. Twenty mg of omeprazole daily produces a pH of over 4 for most of a 24-hour period. In most people, 40 mg daily achieves almost complete achlorhydria (anacidity).

Omeprazole so dramatically depresses gastric acid that gastric antrum G cells attempt to compensate by secreting the acid-stimulating hormone gastrin. After 7 or more days of treatment, the serum gastrin levels rise. They return to normal a week or two after the drug is stopped, but rebound hyperacidity may make it difficult to stop. These drugs appear only briefly in the blood and have little effect on other tissues. Extragastrointestinal side effects are unusual.

USE

Omeprazole heals peptic ulcers within 2–4 weeks. Hitherto it has been used for ulcers that fail to respond to H_2 antagonists. However, the discovery that *H. pylori* eradication will permanently cure most non-NSAID-induced ulcers has changed the picture radically. Antibiotics are increasingly used as primary treatment. One popular eradication regimen is to combine omeprazole with an antibiotic such as amoxicillin. Omeprazole has some bacte-

riostatic effect, and the combination achieves about 80% eradication in some trials, but much less in others. Better results are
achieved through the use of omeprazole and 2 antibiotics.This
approach combines a lasting eradication with prompt healing and
relief of symptoms. It is likely that even with triple therapy (e.g.,
bismuth + amoxacillin + metronidazole), physicians will employ
an acid-suppressing drug to control symptoms while the bacteria
are being killed. Recent evidence suggests that short pretreatment
with omeprazole improves the antibiotic kill.

Omeprazole is commonly used to promptly heal bleeding or
NSAID ulcers. However, the most important use for the proton pump
inhibitors is in the management of gastrointestinal reflux disease with
severe (grades 3 and 4) esophagitis where H_2 blockers are less effective
(see Chapters 16 and 17). Omeprazole prevents bleeding and stricture.
Even in milder esophagitis, a proton pump inhibitor may be needed
when H_2 blockade fails. Many elderly patients with esophagitis must
take the drug indefinitely. In one study, omeprazole healed esophagitis after 6 months of treatment in 100% of patients, compared with 53%
of those receiving an H_2 antagonist. Rendering patients dysphagia-
free cost 50% less in those receiving omeprazole since the need for
stricture dilation was diminished.

Omeprazole is the drug of choice for the Zollinger–Ellison (ZE)
syndrome (see Chapter 12). This rare condition is caused by a
gastrin-secreting, slow-growing adenoma, usually in the pancreas.
Before antisecretory drugs were available, only total gastrectomy
could control the aggressive ulcer disease found in this syndrome.
Now omeprazole, often in higher than normal doses, is so effective
against the ulcers that the disease's prognosis now depends upon
the degree of malignancy and rate of tumor growth.

Other than for esophagitis or the ZE syndrome, the long-
term use of a proton pump inhibitor is seldom indicated. Other
cheaper drugs are preferred to prevent gastroduodenal NSAID
damage. Prevention of stress ulceration in an intensive care setting is controversial and probably requires less powerful agents.
There is a risk of lung infections in the achlorhydric and debilitated state. Most other ulcers are curable and should require no
maintenance.

Lansoprazole is claimed after clinical trials to heal ulcers and
esophagitis more quickly than omeprazole, and at a lower price. It

is claimed that replacing omeprazole with this new pump blocker would reduce the annual drug costs of the British National Health Service by £55 million.

UNWANTED EFFECTS

Omeprazole is excreted in the urine in the form of inactive metabolites. The drug is safe in liver and kidney failure, and kidney disease or hemodialysis do not alter its pharmacokinetics. There are few data on toxicity in the very young, the very old, and the pregnant. There are no reports of untoward effects from overdose. Omeprazole seems very safe for short-term therapy.

However, there are theoretical and experimental reasons to be concerned about possible effects of long-term proton pump inhibition. In rats given omeprazole for 2 years, hyperplasia (growth) of the mucosal enterochromaffin-like (ECL) cells occurred, and a few developed gastric carcinoid (neural crest) tumors. This may result from prolonged G-cell stimulation. Such tumors have not occurred in humans over 12 years of clinical use. Nevertheless, serum levels of gastrin rise in those consuming long-term omeprazole, with hyperplasia of gastric ECL cells. Pernicious anemia is another condition associated with achlorhydria and hypergastrinemia. Patients with this disease have gastric atrophy and an increased risk of gastric cancer.

Gastric acid is a natural barrier protecting the intestine from infection. Except for *H. pylori*, most bacteria do not survive in gastric juice and are not normally found in the stomach or duodenum. Bacterial overgrowth occurs in the upper gut when gastric acid is reduced, such as following gastric surgery, or absent, as in pernicious anemia. Bacterial overgrowth also occurs with a 5-week course of omeprazole, even the low 20-mg daily dose. There are several actual and theoretical disadvantages to this.

First, people taking omeprazole are more susceptible to intestinal infections such as salmonella, cholera, and parasites. Those who visit places such as Mexico or North Africa, where turista is prevalent, are more susceptible to traveller's diarrhea. Bacterial overgrowth in the upper gut causes malabsorption of fat by destroying bile acids as bile flows into the duodenum. Small bowel bacteria may consume vitamin B_{12} before it can be absorbed by the ileum. Also, gastric acid separates the vitamin (cobalamin) from protein.

Thus, by more than one mechanism, omeprazole can interfere with vitamin B_{12} absorption and may theoretically lead over several years to a B_{12} deficient anemia and neurological complications.

Possibly more sinister is the production of amines by bacteria surviving in an achlorhydric stomach. These may carcinogenic, that is, they may lead over many years to stomach cancer. This theory is credible considering the cancer risk associated with other anacid states such as pernicious anemia and previous gastric surgery. While of little concern to elderly people receiving omeprazole for esophagitis, young people might be more cautious in using this drug chronically for peptic ulcer, especially now that other treatments are available.

The commonest indication for long-term proton pump inhibitors is severe, or complicated GERD. In those who happen to harbor *H. pylori* in their gastric mucosa, drug-induced achlorhydria may occur. In one study (Kuipers), 30% of *H. pylori*-positive patients taking omeprazole for GERD over 5 years developed atrophic gastritis compared to none in a comparison group treated surgically. The drug treated patients were older and more likely to be male, so more data are needed.

Yet another undesirable consequence of gastric contamination is the reflux of bacteria-rich gastric contents into the esophagus, from whence they might contaminate the respiratory tract. This is a potential problem in debilitated patients in an intensive care unit.

Rare cases of blindness and deafness are reported with omeprazole when the drug is given intravenously. For this reason, intravenous omeprazole was temporarily withdrawn from use in Germany and is unavailable elsewhere. It is now used only in those Germans unable to take oral medication, and there is a warning on the label.

DOSE AND ADMINISTRATION

Omeprazole is available in capsules containing enteric-coated granules that promote absorption in the small bowel. Each capsule contains 20 mg of the drug, and the usual dose is 20–40 mg once daily. The ZE syndrome commonly requires a larger dose. The recommended dose of lansoprazole is 30 mg per day; of pantoprazole, 40 mg per day.

The cost is considerable for patients who require long-term therapy with proton pump inhibitors. To economize and perhaps minimize untoward effects, a variety of strategies are proposed. These include pulse therapy such as 3 consecutive days weekly, drug holidays, and second-day dosing. These are not validated, but they might be tried in individual patients.

SUMMARY

Omeprazole and the related proton pump inhibitors are the most powerful gastric acid suppressants available. In a 40-mg dose, omeprazole causes virtual anacidity and rapidly heals peptic ulcers and esophagitis. However, it is expensive and the anacidity carries several actual and theoretic risks through bacterial proliferation in the stomach and upper small bowel. The intestine becomes liable to enteric infections, pulmonary contamination may occur in the debilitated, and malabsorption of fat and vitamin B_{12} might be anticipated. Long-term achlorhydria may permit hypergastrinemia or gastric contamination with carcinogenic byproducts. These might increase the risk of gastric cancer. Nonetheless, proton pump inhibitors have few proven disadvantages. They have a firm place in the treatment of reflux esophagitis in the elderly and in the acute management of severe or refractory ulcer disease.

CHAPTER TWENTY FIVE
Sucralfate

Sucralfate (Sulcrate™, Antipepsin™, Carafate™) is an aluminum salt of sucrose octasulphate. It was developed in Japan for the treatment of peptic ulcers. Its principal action is to bind to the protein material at the base of the ulcer and thereby prevent further digestive tissue damage. This interesting drug is still used, but others have surpassed it as a first-line treatment for ulcers.

ACTIONS

Sucralfate acts locally; very little is absorbed into the blood. It binds to damaged gastric and duodenal mucosa for about 6 hours and forms a protective barrier at the ulcer site. When exposed to gastric acid, sucralfate becomes a viscous, adhesive paste, yet it retains acid-buffering activity. The drug forms stable complexes with proteins and consequently resists the proteolytic (protein-digesting) action of pepsin. It inactivates pepsin itself and increases gastric bicarbonate secretion. In addition, it stimulates the generation and release of prostaglandins, particularly prostaglandin E_2. Sucralfate also binds bile salts and might prevent the damaging effects of bile refluxed from the duodenum into the stomach or esophagus. While mucosal protection has been the proposed means of healing, we now learn that sucralfate suppresses acid secretion in *H. pylori*-positive duodenal ulcers. It seems that the drug suppresses but does not eradicate *H. pylori*. This reduces gastrin release and basal and stimulated acid secretion by 50%.

USES

Sucralfate is as effective as the H_2 blockers in the treatment of gastric and duodenal ulcers. It may also be of benefit in esophagitis. Some propose it for maintenance of ulcer healing. However, despite its safety, there are several reasons why it has not become the drug of choice for the treatment of peptic ulcer disease.

First, the pills themselves are large and difficult to swallow. Ideally they should be crushed and dispersed in water before use, especially if esophageal lesions are being treated. Second, because the drugs bind to the damaged mucosa for only 6 hours, multiple daily dosing is required. One gram four times a day is the norm, although the results of one study suggest equal clinical benefits with 2 grams twice daily. Third, since the drug may bind to food protein, it is best given well before meals. Why bother with these inconveniences if equal benefits can be achieved with single or twice daily doses of an H_2 blocker? There is little difference in cost. With the prospect of ulcer cure using antibiotics, sucralfate has become almost obsolete.

Sucralfate has been proposed as an alternative to the H_2 antagonists for the prevention of stress ulcers in intensive care patients. Since it does not suppress acid, it might minimize lung infection caused by aspiration of gastric contents. However, in such very ill patients, the medication must be given through a nasogastric tube. Even in slurry or liquid form it may clog the tubing.

ADVERSE EFFECTS

The drug is poorly absorbed, so systemic effects do not occur. However, some aluminum is assimilated, and this may increase blood levels if the drug is administered to patients with kidney failure. Almost half of those receiving this drug become constipated. Binding with phosphate could have consequences for bone metabolism. It may bind other drugs and thereby impair their absorption and depress their therapeutic effect. Warfarin, digoxin, phentoin, and tetracycline are examples of drugs potentially affected in this way. It clearly is not ideal for treating peptic ulcers when antibiotics are given for *H. pylori*.

It is not rare to find these large pills lying intact in the esophagus of patients confined by illness to the recumbent position. One elderly, disabled patient taking opium developed a sucralfate bezoar (ball of retained material) in his stomach.

ADMINISTRATION

The tablets contain 1 g sucralfate. The recommended dose is one tablet four times per day, but good results are claimed with 2 g twice daily. Since binding to an ulcer base is optimal at an acid pH, patients should consume the pills 30–60 minutes before meals. A suspension may be more suitable for esophagitis and 10 milliliters contain 1 gram of sucralfate.

SUMMARY

Sucralfate is an interesting and effective anti-ulcer drug that, if introduced before 1970, might have enjoyed widespread employment for the treatment of peptic ulcers. However, its awkwardness of administration, constipating effect, and intraintestinal drug interactions make it no match for the H_2 blockers. Newer treatments that cure ulcers threaten to eclipse its use altogether.

CHAPTER TWENTY-SIX
Prostaglandins

Prostaglandins are naturally occurring fatty acids that are produced to some degree by virtually every human cell. Among many other things, they support the inflammatory process and protect the gastric and duodenal mucosa against insults such as the digestive effects of acid and pepsin. By inhibiting the production of prostaglandins, nonsteroidal anti-inflammatory drugs (NSAIDs) reduce the inflammation of arthritis and permit mucosal damage in the upper gut. NSAIDs and their effect on prostaglandins are discussed in Chapter 7.

BIOCHEMISTRY

In 1936, Euler described a substance with vasodilating and smooth muscle-stimulating effects from the accessory genital glands in men and animals. That is why prostaglandins came to be named after the prostate gland. Many prostaglandins with many and assorted actions that have little to do with the prostate are now known. They are produced from a fatty acid called *arachadonic acid* through the actions of the enzyme *cyclo-oxygenase.*

Prostaglandins are a family of 30-carbon fatty acids designated PGA, PGB, PGC, PGD, PGE, and PGF. Our interest centers on the PGE series. A subscript number indicates the number of double bonds, as in PGE_2. Vane reported in 1971 that aspirin and other NSAIDs inhibit cyclo-oxygenase. Subsequently it became known that prostaglandins could reduce the injury to gastric mucosa by alcohol, NSAIDs, and even boiling water. This phenomenon was christened *cytoprotection*, a notion that inspires controversy. It is the centerpiece activity to those who promote prostaglandins for the treatment and prevention of NSAID gastropathy.

ACTIONS

The actions of the various prostaglandins are diverse and often conflicting. Some increase blood flow through vasodilation (PGE_2), while others decrease it through vasoconstriction (PGE_2). Many, including these two, stimulate smooth muscle contraction. They also stimulate mucosal bicarbonate secretion and inhibit gastric acid secretion through parietal cell receptors. In sufficient doses, prostaglandins suppress acid secretion as effectively as the H_2 antagonists.

The idea of cytoprotection invites controversy. Although the phenomenon may be demonstrated experimentally and the mucosal damage inflicted by NSAIDs appears to be due to prostaglandin inhibition, the mechanism of cytoprotection is obscure. It has been attributed to many factors: increased mucosal mucus and bicarbonate secretion; increased mucosal blood flow, increased epithelial integrity, inhibition of the release of free radicals and enzymes from polymorphonuclear leucocytes (granulocytes); stabilization of mast cells and lysosomal membranes, and relaxation of smooth muscle. None of these is of proven importance, and it is possible that several of them are operating. Cytoprotection is an important theoretical and practical consideration. If the benefits of prostaglandins depended solely upon their ability to suppress acid secretion, then untoward effects would make them less attractive alternatives to the H_2 antagonists.

Unwanted effects of the prostaglandins used in ulcer treatment are mainly caused by their effects on the smooth muscle of uterus and gut. Authorities in some countries take advantage of this effect by employing them as abortifacients. They cannot safely be used in pregnant women. Ten to twenty percent of those taking misoprostyl report significant diarrhea. This is also used to good effect for the treatment of obstinate constipation.

PROSTAGLANDINS IN ULCER DISEASE

In peptic ulcer disease, prostaglandins are effective only in doses that inhibit gastric acid secretion. They therefore offer no advantages over other anti-ulcer drugs. However, they are effective in the treatment and prevention of NSAID-induced gastropathy and ulcers, and that has become their market niche. Misoprostol (Cytotec™) is a synthetic PGE_1 prostaglandin that has been developed for this purpose. When taken with NSAIDs in doses of 100 or 200 µg four times a day, misoprostyl will prevent or heal more gastric and duodenal ulcers due to NSAIDs than will a placebo. However, Feldman has pointed out that this success may not apply to symptoms or complications.

The diarrheagenic effects of the drug, its inapplicability in pregnant women, and its cost are daunting disadvantages. In 1990 it was estimated that for all NSAID users, each life-year saved through the prevention of ulcer bleeding by misoprostol cost $664,400. For those over 60, the cost was $186,700 per life-year saved, and for those with rheumatoid arthritis the cost was $95,600. Primary prevention against ulcer bleeding for all NSAID users is thus too expensive to contemplate. Secondary prevention may be more practical. When used in those with a recent history of gastro-intestinal bleeding, the cost per life-year saved fell to $40,000.

Treatment of NSAID Ulcers

If an ulcer develops while a person is taking NSAIDs, the drug should be stopped. It will then heal rapidly with a proton pump inhibitor or an H_2 antagonist. Continued use of the NSAID delays healing. If the drug is indispensable, the patient should take a double dose of an anti-ulcer drug, possibly twice a day. When the NSAID is continued, misoprostol is probably no more effective than H_2 antagonists or omeprazole.

Prevention of NSAID Ulcers

Raskin and colleagues have shown that misoprostol and rani-tidine will prevent duodenal ulcers equally, but that the former drug is superior in preventing gastric ulcers. However, prevention of NSAID-induced endoscopic ulcers is of secondary importance. The serious complications, perforation, obstruction, or bleeding, are of more consequence. Silverstein *et al.* have shown that misoprostol given concurrently with non-aspirin NSAIDs reduces by 40% the serious NSAID-induced ulcer complications in elderly patients with rheumatoid arthritis.

It seems practical to use misoprostol only in those at greatest risk of developing NSAID-induced complicated peptic ulcers. These would include those with rheumatoid arthritis who need their NSAID and who possess the risk factors outlined in Table 7-1. Of course, the risk is even greater if they have had a previous ulcer or NSAID damage. The dose and type of NSAID may also alter the risk (see Table 7-2).

Administration

Misoprostol is usually prescribed in a dose of 200 µg four times per day. While effective in preventing NSAID injury, its benefit to those taking aspirin is unknown. It is also uncertain if it prevents small intestinal injury. It should not be given in women who are at risk of becoming pregnant, and diarrhea may force discontinuance of the drug.

New combinations of NSAID and prostaglandin are cheaper and should encourage compliance. One such drug combination contains 200 µg misoprostol and 50 mg diclofenac (Arthrotec™). Another, is 200 µg misoprostol and 500 mg naproxen (Napratec™). Prostaglandins also reduce the mucosal injury caused by alcohol, but we know of no plans to add misoprostol to whiskey.

SIDE EFFECTS

Other than diarrhea and risk of abortion, prostaglandins occasionally cause headache, fatigue, cramps, and vomiting.

SUMMARY

Prostaglandins are varied and ubiquitous biological substances. Their principal interest in *The Ulcer Story* lies in their gastric cytoprotective effect. As acid-suppressing drugs, they are less attractive than the H_2 antagonists because of their diarrheagenic and abortifacient effects and their cost. However, there is evidence for a cytoprotective effect that justifies their use to prevent NSAID ulcer complications.

CHAPTER TWENTY-SEVEN

Bismuth and Antibiotics

Treatment of *H. pylori*

> Be not the first by whom the new are tried,
> Nor yet the last to lay the old aside.
> Alexander Pope, *An Essay on Criticism*, 1688–1744

A decade ago, a chapter on antibiotics in a book about peptic ulcers would have been distinctly out of place. Such has been the revolution in our understanding of this disease that eradication of *H. pylori*, the cause of most peptic ulcers, has become central to its management. Unlike most other bacteria, this most ubiquitous of all pathogens is only weakly susceptible to a single antibiotic, so several drugs must be employed. The ideal combination, however, is not yet discovered. Even very aggressive triple or quadruple therapy seldom cures more than 90% of infections, and such therapy generates significant cost and side effects. *H. pylori* is a clever organism, with many strains and a canny capacity to adapt or become resistant to antibiotics. This chapter discusses the drugs used in the treatment of *H. pylori*, some therapeutic problems, and a brief discussion of currently used regimens.

ANTI-*H. pylori* DRUGS

The following are the most-used drugs in the treatment of *H. pylori* infection. There will be many more. Some terms need explanation. *Anaerobic* bacteria grow in the absence of air. A *gram stain* is applied to a bacteriological specimen that crudely divides bacteria into two groups: *gram-positive* (black) or *gram-negative* (red). Penicillin-sensitive organisms are generally gram positive. Drugs such as tetracycline attack members of both groups and are called *broad spectrum* antibiotics. Bacterial *resistance* is the ability of bacteria, normally sensitive to an antibiotic, to develop tolerance to it. *Bactericidal* drugs kill organisms, while *bacteriostatic* ones merely interfere with their already dull sex life.

Bismuth

General Description

Two bismuth salts are commonly used to treat peptic ulcer. For many years, tripotassium dicitratobismuthate (TDB) (De Nol™) was widely used in Europe. Bismuth subsalycylate is sold as a patent medicine in most Western countries and is called Pepto Bismol™. This product is taken for many digestive disorders, including dyspepsia and diarrhea, and binds the *Eschericia coli* toxin responsible for traveller's diarrhea. While Pepto Bismol is used in some *H. pylori* treatment regimens, especially in the United States, most studies have tested TDB.

Clinical Data

In Britain and Europe, TDB was used to treat peptic ulcer even before *H. pylori* was known to play a role in the disease. It is as effective in healing gastric and duodenal ulcers as the H_2 antagonists, but it requires several doses a day. Its beneficial effect was thought to be due to the binding of the bismuth salt to proteins and glycoproteins in the ulcer crater. In an acid medium TDB coats the ulcer to prevent further attack by acid and pepsin. Bismuth also inhibits pepsin and increases mucosal mucus. These activities seem to be forgotten as science's attention focuses on the drug's antibiotic effect.

The first indication that TDB was more than an ulcer-healing drug was an almost ignored report that ulcers healed with De Nol™ were less likely to recur than those healed by an H_2-blocking drug. Bismuth is able to eradicate the organisms in only a small number of cases. Nevertheless, it is ironic that *H. pylori* was being treated before we even knew about it.

Bismuth is bactericidal and rapidly destroys the organism's outer cell wall. It suppresses, but seldom eradicates, *H. pylori*. However, bismuth enhances the efficacy of several antibiotics. For example, the addition of bismuth to an omeprazole–clarithromycin combination increases the kill from 50% to 80%. Bismuth salts may form complexes with antibiotics and concentrate them at sites colonized by *H. pylori*.

Precautions, Adverse Effects

Bismuth is poorly absorbed from the gut, so systemic effects are unusual during short-term use. However, the drug can accumulate over long periods. Since the principal route of excretion is in the urine, the risk is greater in patients with kidney failure. Bismuth neurotoxicity occurs with other bismuth salts but not with suggested doses of TDB. Since it appears in the placenta it is wise not to use TDB in pregnancy.

TDB works best in an acid medium, so it makes little sense to use it with an acid-suppressing drug for its anti-ulcer (not antibacterial) effect. Bismuth salts bind with antacids and tetracycline in the gut lumen, so they should be taken remotely from these drugs.

Bismuth darkens the stool. This may alarm the patient and can be mistaken for melena (blood pigment in the stool). Moreover, if the drug is used in a controlled trial, black stools may uncover who is receiving bismuth rather than the placebo.

Administration

De Nol™ is available in Europe as a 120-mg tablet or as a liquid in which 5 ml contains 120 mg. In the United States it is available only as a liquid called Ulcaron™. Pepto Bismol™ is available over the counter in tablets containing 151 mg of bismuth subsalicylate. It also is sold in a pink suspension.

Amoxacillin (Amoxyl™, Almoden™)

Amoxacillin is a member of the penicillin family. Like penicillin, it is effective in the treatment of gram positive infections such as *Pneumococcus pneumonae* and *Streptococcus pyogenes*, which commonly cause pneumonia and ear infections. Unlike penicillin, it has a benzyl side chain that extends its effectiveness to many gram-negative bacteria. It is useful in surgical, urinary, and enteric infections, such as those due to *Salmonella*. Penicillins kill bacteria by damaging their cell walls so that they swell and burst. Like penicillin, amoxacillin has a beta-lactam ring that may be destroyed by a bacterial toxin produced by resistant *staphylococci* called *penicillinase*. Resistance also occurs in some gram-negative infections such as those due to *Hemophylus influenzae*, *Proteus mirabilis*, and *Salmonella*.

Clinical Data

Amoxacillin by itself is poorly effective against *H. pylori*. Combined with other agents, such as metronidazole and bismuth, it becomes quite useful. Amoxacillin achieves very good results with omeprazole in some trials, but it is disappointing in others. When it does work, the two-drug regimen has many practical advantages.

Precautions and Adverse Effects

Because it is a penicillin, amoxacillin may cause a hypersensitivity reaction. It should be avoided in those who have had a penicillin rash. Skin lesions include urticaria (hives) or, more commonly, a maculopapular eruption. Anaphylactic shock is rare. This drug is a leading cause of antibiotic-associated diarrhea which, in its extreme form, can be a life-threatening colitis. The drug suppresses the normal gut bacterial flora permitting the overgrowth of another bacteria called *Clostridium difficile*. Although cured by metronidazole, antibiotic colitis can be troublesome and recurrent. It may occur even several weeks after amoxacillin is stopped.

While unwanted effects are uncommon, they cannot be taken lightly. Patients receiving the drug for an unconfirmed infection or an ulcer that is not present will not be amused to discover that *H. pylori* has been exchanged for *C. difficile*.

Administration

The drug is available in 250-mg and 500-mg capsules, 500-mg tablets, or a syrup. The usual dose in treatment programs for *H. pylori* is 500-mg three or four times daily.

Ampicillin (Penbritin™ and Others)

General Description

Ampicillin is a penicillin with many of the properties of amoxacillin. A side chain adds gram-negative bacteria to its spectrum of antibacterial activity and permits its use in a range of infections similar to amoxacillin. It too kills by destroying the bacterial cell wall and is susceptible to penicillinase.

Clinical Data

Ampicillin's effect on *H. pylori* is modest. Its principle advantage is ready and cheap availability, but it is now less commonly included in triple therapy regimens.

Precautions, Adverse Effects

Like amoxacillin, ampicillin causes skin eruptions and, rarely, anaphylaxis. Because so many use the drug, it is one of the most common causes of antibiotic-associated diarrhea. The diarrhea may interfere with the absorption of birth control pills and permit breakthrough bleeding or unwanted pregnancy.

Administration

Ampicillin comes in 250-mg and 500-mg capsules. For ulcer treatment, 500 mg are normally taken four times per day. Because the drug's intestinal absorption is impaired by food, it should be taken 30 minutes before meals. The dose should be reduced in kidney failure.

Azithromycin (Zithromax™)

General Description

Azithromycin is a macrolide antibiotic related to erythromycin. Macrolides interfere with bacterial intracellular ribosomes to impair protein synthesis. It is bacteriostatic for most organisms; that is, it stops reproduction but does not kill. However, it is bactericidal for *Streptococcus pyogenes, Staphylococcus, Pneumococcus,* and *Hemophylus influenzae.* This drug also is effective against gram-positive and gram-negative bacteria that are responsible for pneumonia, skin sepsis, and sexually transmitted diseases. Some bacteria are clever enough to develop a resistance to azithromycin that carries over to other macrolides.

Clinical Data

Azithromycin is a new anti-*H pylori* drug. It has several advantages that may prove important. It is acid-stable and quickly achieves high concentrations in gastric tissue where it has a prolonged effect. Early trials where the drug has been combined with omeprazole or as a substitute for metronidazole in triple therapy have been small. However, two Italian trials indicate success when a single 500 mg dose of azithromycin is given for the first three days of a 14-day course of double therapy. If validated, this simpler- to comply-with regimen may become more widely used.

Precautions and Adverse Effects

Like the other macrolides, azithromycin rarely causes hypersensitivity, but is responsible for a variety of gut complaints, such as nausea, cramps, and diarrhea. Indeed, macrolides are prokinetic (see Chapter 28). Nausea, sore mouth, bad taste, and facial swelling have been blamed on it. There are alternatives, so it is uncertain that azithromycin will become a first-line treatment for peptic ulcer.

Administration

Azithromycin comes in 250-mg tablets, and early results suggest that it should be given three times a day as part of *H. pylori* triple therapy. It binds with food and antacid and should be given separately. The newer regimens described above employed 500 mg administered two hours after a light breakfast for three days. Drug interactions occur with ergot, digoxin, and cyclosporin. Since the drug is excreted in bile, it is best avoided in patients with liver disease.

Clarithromycin (Clathromycin™, Biaxin™, Klaricid™, Klacid™)

General Description

Clarithromycin is another macrolide, like erythromycin. It inhibits bacterial protein synthesis and is effective in several gram-positive and gram-negative infections and in atypical pneumonia caused by mycoplasma.

Clinical Data

Clarithromycin is used in place of amoxacillin with omeprazole or in place of metronidazole in triple therapy because of penicillin hypersensitivity in the former case and metronidazole resistance in the latter. Expense is a drawback. Nevertheless, clarithromycin is one of the most effective anti-*H. pylori* drugs. It achieves very high concentrations in the gastric mucosa, especially in the mucus layer where the organisms live. This concentration is enhanced by omeprazole. In one trial, clarithromycin alone achieved 50% eradication.

Precautions and Adverse Effects

As with azithromycin, hypersensitivity and gut reactions are risks. Sore tongue, sore mouth, and taste abnormalities occur. Drug interactions occur with theophylline, warfarin, digoxin, and other cardiac drugs. Another choice is prudent if the patient is taking other medicines. There is one report of acute liver failure due to clarithromycin. While such a catastrophe is rare, it should serve to remind us to avoid indiscriminant use of these drugs.

Administration

Clarithromycin is available in 250-mg tablets, or 500-mg tablets in the United States. The ulcer treatment dose is between 250 mg twice daily and 500 mg three times daily. The drug seems unaffected by food ingestion.

Metronidazole (Flagyl™)

General Description

Metronidazole has many antimicrobial uses. It is effective against several protozoan infections, such as *trichomonas* in the vagina, *giardia* in the small intestine, and *ameba* in the colon. The drug is also effective against many bacteria resident in the colon, especially the predominant anaerobes. This accounts for its use as a bowel preparation before intestinal surgery, and for infections generated by fecal organisms. Another important indication for the drug is antibiotic-associated (pseudomembranous) colitis, in which the offending organism is the toxin-producing *C. difficile*.

Clinical Data

Metronidazole is one of the first antibiotics to be employed for the eradication of *H. pylori*, and it is still a frequent component of triple and quadruple therapy regimens. Its principal disadvantage is the agility with which organisms develop antibiotic resistance to it. While said to be low in the Netherlands, resistance in London is 37%; among Asian immigrants in London it is 93%, and in Zaire it is 80%.

Precautions and Adverse Effects

The most serious adverse effects of this drug are neurological. Seizures and sensory peripheral nerve deficits are rare at the low doses and short treatment courses employed for ulcer disease. It interferes with the metabolism of alcohol in a manner similar to that of antibuse, a drug sometimes used to decondition alcoholics. Metronidazole thus imposes abstinence, not in itself a bad thing! A prolonged, high dose may depress white blood cells. Skin rashes are rare. The most common reactions are nausea, vomiting, abdominal pain, loss of appetite, and metallic taste. Fungal vaginal infections occur through suppression of the local bacteria.

Administration

There are many tablet strengths of metronidazole; 250, 400, and 500 mg. A common regimen is 500 mg, two or three times per day. The urine may become dark reddish brown, so the patient should be forewarned.

Tetracycline (Achromycin™, Panmycin™, Tetracyn™, and Others)

General Description

Tetracycline is bacteriostatic against a wide range of bacteria, mycoplasma, and rickettsiae. It is therefore used for urinary tract infections, atypical pneumonia, acne, sexually transmitted diseases, and other conditions. Since it kills gram-positive organisms, it is a useful back-up in case of penicillin sensitivity. Tetracycline inhibits protein synthesis, but many gram-negative organisms are able to develop resistance to it.

Clinical Data

Tetracycline is sometimes used in triple and quadruple therapy for peptic ulcer cure. It is less effective than amoxacillin or clarithromycin.

Precautions and Adverse Effects

Tetracycline hypersensitivity occurs. Photosensitivity is common in fair-skinned persons, and the drug should not be given to sunbathers or those with lupus erythematosis. Tetracycline can stain the teeth of the developing fetus, so it must be avoided in small children and pregnant women. It causes protein breakdown and is excreted with its metabolites in the urine. Therefore, tetracycline should be used cautiously for patients with kidney disease. This broad-spectrum antibiotic often permits overgrowth of organisms resistant to the drug that cause intestinal, mouth, or vaginal infections.

Administration

Tetracycline is available in 250- and 500-mg tablets. The usual dose for *H. pylori* is 500 mg four times a day. Calcium and magnesium bind the drug. Therefore, it is best taken 1 hour before or 2 hours after eating, especially milk or antacids.

Tinitizole (Fasigyn™)

General Description

Tinitizole is a nitroimidazole relative of metronidazole. This drug accumulates within the target bacteria or protozoa to damage the helical structure of its DNA. It is used in protozoal infections such as *Giardiasis* and *Amebiasis* in the gut and *Trichomonas vaginalis*. Tinitizole also treats or prevents anaerobic infections associated with abdominal or pelvic surgery.

Clinical Data

Tinitizole appears to be a worthy substitute in cases of metronidazole resistance or hypersensitivity.

Precautions and Adverse Effects

Severe hypersensitivity reactions, including anaphylaxis, are uncommon. Because there is experimental evidence of possible birth defects, this drug should not be deployed in pregnant women. Like metronidazole, it causes a metallic taste and produces a violent reaction when taken with alcohol. Headache, nausea, and vomiting are nuisance side effects.

Administration

Tinidizole tablets contain 500 mg of the drug and are given four times a day in ulcer patients. Alcohol should be avoided.

THERAPEUTIC PROBLEMS

As of April 1995, there were more than 500 publications on the antibacterial treatment of *H. pylori*. Most of these describe small trials of poor quality and were often published as abstracts, where they are safe from critical analysis. Too few trials compare one therapeutic program to another. There are several multiple drug regimens extant, and those that are cost effective are slow to emerge. None is ideal. Short, simple, and effective therapy is badly needed, ideally in a single drug. The search is vigorous, and, by the time you read this, new and better treatments may be available. As we pass through this rapidly changing era, we must remember the risks and problems that may be encountered while endeavoring to rid stomachs of the most common chronic infection of man.

Indications

Herein lies the greatest difficulty. The United States National Institutes of Health (NIH) published a "consensus" recommendation that all gastric and duodenal ulcers should be treated with an anti-ulcer drug. Those infected with *H. pylori* should also be treated with double or triple therapy. However, this view is not unanimous. Many would go beyond this and treat any infected person with functional dyspepsia. Others feel that, wherever found, the organism should be killed.

At the other extreme, skeptics still challenge the view that *H. pylori* causes or permits non-NSAID ulcers. Graham points out that two of the four postulates of Robert Koch are not yet fulfilled, and therefore peptic ulcer cannot be attributed to the infection. The data, he continues, could equally indicate that *H. pylori* is an opportunist that infects damaged gastric mucosa. He states that no one has yet shown that antibiotics without bismuth or other anti-ulcer drug will heal ulcers better than placebos. These observations oblige us to keep our minds open to new developments.

Nevertheless, the NIH recommendation is the right one for now. The program cures peptic ulcers and kills *H. pylori*. If no ulcer is present we should leave the bugs alone. The evidence that they cause functional dyspepsia is not there, and more harm than good will come of treating them with antibiotics. Moreover, attempts to stamp out *H. pylori* to prevent cancer are doomed to failure. Half the world's population is infected. It is beyond the capability of antibiotics to cure them all, and there is no precedent for such a global antibiotic success. The cost would be unthinkable, and the inevitable spread of bacterial resistance could incapacitate the drugs for those who need them.

Side Effects and Compliance

Hypersensitivity and other unwanted drug effects are discussed with the individual drugs. Gut effects, particularly cramps and diarrhea, are nuisances that may provoke withdrawal from therapy. With more drugs, higher doses, and longer treatment, there will be more unwanted effects. A typical triple therapy regimen requires 11 tablets daily in staggered doses over 2 weeks (see Table 27-1). Even highly motivated individuals have difficulty with such a schedule, and most will be occasionally delinquent.

Bacterial Resistance to Antibiotics

So far, *H. pylori* resistance to amoxacillin and clarithromycin is unusual, but either agent alone is weakly effective. That is because organisms live cozily beneath a blanket of gastric mucus, relatively safe from the reach of antibiotics. Larger numbers of bacteria, as estimated by urea breath test, increase the difficulty in eradication.

Resistance to metronidazole is a major problem. In parts of the Third World, 80% of infections are from organisms resistant to this antibiotic. Indiscriminate use will surely increase the resistance in Western populations as well. Beyond careful attention to the indications for treatment, combination therapy offers the best guarantee of continued efficacy.

Role of Anti-Ulcer Drugs

The ostensible objective of the NIH recommendation is that ulcers be treated with anti-ulcer medication to relieve symptoms and prevent complications while the antibiotics do their work. However, other issues arise. Omeprazole itself has some antibacterial effect. In the past, omeprazole and amoxacillin are more effective in killing *H. pylori* than either alone. However, if omeprazole is started before the antibiotic, the combination is less effective than if the two are given simultaneously. It seems that the organism, shorn of its acid surroundings by the action of omeprazole, assumes a "coccoid" form (the bacterial equivalent of the fetal position) and becomes less susceptible to the antibiotic. For this reason, it has been recommended that the two drugs be started together.

We are no sooner used to this idea when we are forced to think again by a well-conducted Dutch study (de Boer *et al.* 1995) showing improved results when patients are pretreated with omeprazole. Seven-day therapy with bismuth, tetracycline, and metronidazole was compared with the same combination plus omeprazole, 20 mg twice daily started three days before. The object was to quickly induce an achlorhydria inhospitable to *H. pylori* before exposing the organisms to the antibiotics. Quadruple therapy eradicated the weakened bacteria in 98% of cases, compared to 83% without omeprazole. The former had fewer side effects, perhaps because of the antacid properties of omeprazole. In an accompanying *Lancet* editorial, quadruple therapy was described as "hitting *H. pylori* for four." For those with a dim understanding of cricket, I believe that this is something like a "home run"!

At least in the laboratory, omeprazole enhances the efficacy of amoxacillin and clarithromycin. The raised gastric pH ensures greater antibiotic stability, and bacterial overgrowth further hinders *H. pylori*. The reduced volume of gastric juice concentrates the drug. Moreover, administration with omeprazole concentrates clarithromycin in the gastric mucosa. It remains to be seen if H_2 antagonists can achieve similar goals at lower costs. Surely this aggressive and expensive therapy should be reserved for those with proven *H. pylori*-positive peptic ulcers. It may prove wisest to treat with a simpler regimen and save quadruple therapy for the failures or complicated cases.

TABLE 27-1
Some Treatments for *Helicobacter pylori*

Drugs	Dose/time[a]	Quoted success
Dual therapy		
Omeprazole	20 mg bid/14 days	50–80%
Amoxacillin	500 mg tid/14 days	
Omeprazole	20 mg tid/14 days	78%
Clarithromycin	500 mg tid/14 days	
Triple therapy		
Bismuth (TDB)[b]	120 mg qid/14 days	80%
Tetracycline/amoxacillin	500 mg tid/14 days	
Metronidazole	400 mg tid/14 days	
Low-dose 1-week triple therapy		
Omeprazole	20 mg qd/7 days	90–95%
Clarithromycin	250 mg bid/7 days	
Tinitizole or metronidazole	500 mg bid/7 days	
Quadruple therapy		
Omeprazole	20 mg bid/10 days	98%
Bismuth (TDB)	120 mg qid/days 4–10	
Tetracycline	500 mg qid/days 4–10	
Metronidazole	500 mg tid/days 4–10	

[a]qd, daily; bid, twice daily; tid, thrice daily; qid, four times daily.
[b]Bismuth subsalicylate appears to be as effective as TDB.

What Drugs?, How Many?, What Dose, For How Long?

Some commonly employed drug combinations appear in Table 27-1. It is impossible to catalog them all, and the situation is rapidly evolving. When an ulcer is active, a regimen that includes an H_2 antagonist or proton pump blocker is advantageous. Otherwise, one must be added to triple therapy. The attractions of double therapy are simplicity, cost, and safety, but these are in exchange for reduced efficacy. Low-dose and one-week regimens have obvious advantages, and early studies indicate that efficacy is maintained. These modifications are the subject of ongoing clinical trials.

SUMMARY

We are still learning how best to kill *H. pylori*. Bismuth and several antibiotics are employed, but amoxacillin, tetracycline, clarithromycin, and metronidazole have attracted the most attention. For now the only indication for therapy is peptic ulcer in the presence of infection. If the ulcer is active, an H_2 antagonist or proton pump inhibitor accelerates healing. Omeprazole has some antimicrobial activity and may enhance antibiotics. No drug works well on its own, and bacterial resistance is likely, particularly with metronidazole. Double, triple, and now even quadruple therapeutic programs overcome this difficulty. The more drugs, the better the kill. However, a price is paid in cost, side effects, and inconvenience. Recent studies indicate good results with smaller doses for shorter periods. Good, large, comparative trials are needed to determine the best of the current approaches. Meanwhile, we badly need better drugs and simpler, safer, cheaper regimens.

CHAPTER TWENTY-EIGHT

The Prokinetics

Gastrokinetics

Prokinetics, or gastrokinetics as they are sometimes called, are a diverse group of drugs that enhance stomach emptying of solids and fluids. Prokinetic proponents reason that, if slow gastric emptying causes bloating and postprandial fullness, such drugs may be therapeutic. This notion is difficult to validate. Prokinetics are interesting from a pharmacological viewpoint, but they are over-rated as treatments for upper gut disease. They may help those with early gastric paralysis due to diabetes or quickly empty the stomach before emergency surgery, but they are ineffective in dyspepsia. They are second-line treatments for GERD. The available prokinetics are reviewed in Table 28-1.

PROKINETICS IN GENERAL USE

Domperidone (Motillium™)

Domperidone is a peripheral dopamine antagonist that promotes antroduodenal coordination. Unlike metoclopramide, this drug is not cholinergic and does not enter the CNS. Its antinausea and antivomiting effects are mediated through the so-called chemoreceptor trigger zone at the base of the brain, outside the blood–brain barrier. With these properties the drug avoids serious neurological side effects.

TABLE 28-1
Prokinetics

Drug[a]	Mechanism of action	Side effects
Cisapride, 5–20 mg qid	Indirect cholinergic nerve stimulation	Diarrhea
Domperidone 10–20 mg qid	Dopamine antagonist	Rare prolactin effects
Metoclopramide, 10 mg qid	Enhances acetylcholine release from local motor neurons	Neurologic: tremors, dystonia, confusion, etc.; prolactin: lactorrhea, gynecomastia
Erythromycin (macrolide), 250 mg tid	Motillin receptors	Nausea, vomiting, cramps, diarrhea
Bethanechol, 10–25 mg tid, ½ hour before meals	Cholinergic	Hypersalivation, acid secretion Cramps, diarrhea, blurred vision

[a]tid, three times per day; qid, four times per day.

Dopamine is a neurotransmitter that delays gastric emptying through its action on the ENS. By antagonizing dopamine, domperidone speeds up gastric emptying. In gastric paralysis due to diabetes (diabetic gastroparesis), it improves the emptying of fluids and solids. The benefit is greatest early in the disease, because the neurotransmission defect becomes irreversible as the myenteric nerves are destroyed. Also, the effects of the drug itself become exhausted over time (tachyphylaxis).

Like some other gastrokinetics, domperidone increases LES tone. The effect is greater when the dose is doubled from 10 to 20 mg per day. Therefore, some recommend domperidone for the treatment of GERD. However, its benefit is less than that of the acid inhibiting drugs or that of prokinetics that have cholinergic effects. It may help prevent reflux in those at risk of aspiration. This drug also helps prevent and treat nausea and vomiting caused by drugs employed in the treatment of cancer and Parkinson's disease.

Domperidone is used in rare gut motility disorders, including chronic intestinal pseudo-obstruction. Like other prokinetics, some published trials indicate benefit in functional dyspepsia. However, these studies are flawed. When compared with placebo, the effect is marginal at best, and it seems that few dyspeptics will become truly better on this drug.

Although domperidone avoids most of the neurological side effects of metaclopromide, it occasionally causes painful breasts in men and lactation in women. These are due to elevated levels of the pituitary hormone *prolactin*. Domperidone is not available in the United States.

Cisapride (Prepulsid™)

Cisapride is a substituted benzamide related structurally to the cardiac anti-arrhythmic drug procainamide. Unlike domperidone and metoclopramide, it does not affect the dopamine system. It does facilitate release of acetylcholine in the gut myenteric plexus. Acetylcholine is a neurotransmitter substance that increases motor activity at all levels of the gut. Cisapride makes the stomach empty by increasing antral contractions and improving gastroduodenal coordination. It also increases LES pressure and promotes small bowel and colon motility.

Despite its different action, the therapeutic profile of cisapride is similar to that of domperidone. Like domperidone, it is a second-line drug for GERD treatment. It is worth trying in patients with symptomatic gastroparesis due to diabetes or surgery, but its efficacy in dyspepsia and other functional disorders is likely to be nonexistent. Diarrhea is an important side effect, and cisapride is proposed for constipation. However, there are cheaper and more effective alternatives, such as dietary fiber or osmotic laxatives. The drug has no breast or neurological side effects.

WHAT'S NEW

Macrolides

The antibiotic erythromycin causes cramps and diarrhea, which are brought on by faster gastric emptying and shorter gastrointestinal transit. This gastrokinetic effect is mediated through the gut hormone motillin. Migrating motor complexes that are quiescent during the fed state become active during fasting, apparently to keep the small intestine swept clean. Macrolides activate these motor complexes. Erythromycin has been tried in gastroparesis, but there are obvious disadvantages of using an antibiotic in this way. The pharmaceutical industry is examining new macrolides that stimulate gut motility.

WHAT'S OLD

Metoclopramide (Reglan™, Maxeran™)

Metoclopramide, the original dopamine antagonist, has been available in Europe for 25 years and in North America for almost as long. It is less desirable for general use because of its CNS activity. However, sedating, antinausea, and antivomiting effects make it useful for cancer patients made ill by chemotherapy. It also reverses the impairment of gut motility caused by narcotics.

Metoclopramide is a substituted benzamide and forerunner of cisapride. Unlike other prokinetics, it crosses the blood–brain barrier, where dopaminergic activity causes neurological side effects. Atropine, but not vagotomy, inhibits the gastrokinetic effect. Unlike bethanechol, metoclopromide does not stimulate gastric acid secretion. Therefore, it must act through the release of acetylcholine from cholinergic motor neurons in the gut wall.

Metoclopramide improves gastric emptying and, in double doses, increases LES pressure. For dyspepsia and GERD the benefits seldom justify its hazards. These include anxiety, drowsiness, hallucinations, confusion, an odd posturing called dystonia, and a hand tremor that resembles Parkinson's disease. They are reversible, but a condition called tardive dyskinesia may not be. This unusual complication may paradoxically worsen when the drug is stopped. Diarrhea and breast complications also occur.

Bethanechol

Bethanechol is a cholinergic drug with an ability to increase LES pressure and the amplitude of gastric and esophageal contraction, which led to its employment in GERD. However, it has little coordinated effect and does not accelerate gastric emptying or small bowel transit. Therefore, it is arguably not a true prokinetic. Side effects include salivation, increased gastric acid production, cramping, blurred vision, and frequency of urination. These side effects inhibit its use for gastrointestinal disease. The drug may precipitate esophageal spasm and is sometimes given to test for spasm during esophageal manometry.

THERAPEUTIC USES

In some ways, prokinetics are drugs in search of an indication. That they increase gastric emptying in a normal stomach is undeniable; that they significantly improve dyspepsia or heartburn is arguable. The largest potential market for these drugs is for non-ulcer dyspepsia, and researchers have tried to identify a "motility-like dyspepsia" (see Chapters 10 and 18). However, it has proven difficult to relate dyspeptic symptoms to delayed gastric emptying.

It is even more difficult to convincingly establish that the actions of a prokinetic improve dyspepsia. Although some trials seem to show a benefit in functional dyspepsia, it is prudent to be skeptical. In most study patients the hypothetical motility disorder is not identifiable. The entry criteria are not clearly defined, and outcomes are inadequately measured. In severe cases, a prokinetic might be worth a short-term trial, but its long-term use is unjustified.

Sometimes, as in diabetes or the postoperative state, gastroparesis causes symptoms. The stomach will not empty, and in extreme cases a concretion of food called a bezoar may form. Although some of these patients are helped by prokinetics, those who most need help are often refractory.

Rapid stomach emptying and increased LES tension should minimize reflux of gastric contents into the esophagus. Cisapride, in doses of 10 or 20 mg before meals, is the best choice. In some therapeutic trials it seems as effective as ranitidine in healing esophagitis, but the three daily doses are inconvenient. Prokinetics cannot match omeprazole's rapid heartburn relief and esophagitis healing. Domperadone and cisapride are expensive second-line drugs in the treatment of GERD. They are most helpful as adjunctive therapy, especially if the patient is threatened with aspiration of refluxed gastric contents.

Prokinetics are useful to empty the stomach for a diagnostic procedure such as emergency gastroscopy if there is upper gut bleeding. They may be given intravenously before delivery or emergency surgery where a full stomach is an anesthetic risk. These drugs also work postoperatively when the gut is reflexly paralyzed. Cisapride is proposed for the treatment of constipation, but it is likely no better than bran. It is certainly more expensive.

UNWANTED SIDE EFFECTS

An unwanted side effect shared by all gastrokinetics is their potential to alter the absorption characteristics of other drugs by rapidly emptying them into the small intestine. They may then appear suddenly in increased concentrations in the blood. If a drug has a narrow interval between effective and toxic blood levels, such an altered absorption profile may be critical. On the other hand, if aspirin is given with metoclopromide for migraine, there is a faster and higher blood salicylate level than if aspirin is given alone.

Neurological effects of metoclopramide and diarrheagenic effects of cisapride have been mentioned. While safe for most people, cisapride has been reported to cause breathing difficulties in asthmatics and has also been blamed for serious disturbances in heart rhythm. The manufacturer recommends that it not be administered with ketoconazole, an anti-fungal drug. Macrolides cause cramping. Metoclopramide, and to a lesser extent domperidone, may cause lactation in women and breast enlargement in men. These downsides should give one pause before using a prokinetic it for unproved indications.

SUMMARY

Prokinetics speed up gastric emptying and whole gut transit. Their therapeutic benefits are probably greatest in gastroparesis caused by diabetes or surgery. Rapid gastric emptying and increased LES tone are theoretically beneficial in gastroesophageal reflux, but gastrokinetics are secondary drugs in the treatment of GERD. They are without proven benefit in dyspepsia, where they are overemployed. Domperidone and cisapride are the most acceptable gastrokinetics in current use. Metoclopramide has potentially serious neurological effects, but because of its central actions it counters the unwanted effects of cancer chemotherapy. Bethanechol is now seldom employed for upper gut disease. Macrolide prokinetics related to erythromycin are being developed.

CHAPTER TWENTY-NINE

Ulcer and Antireflux Surgery
Postsurgical Problems

> Diseases desperate grown
> By desperate appliance are relieved,
> or not at all.
> W. Shakespeare, *Hamlet* Act IV, Scene ii

The age of surgery for acid peptic disease is past. Modern pharmacotherapy is now the primary treatment used to relieve symptoms and to heal ulcers and esophagitis. Nevertheless, surgery remains important to the ulcer story for two reasons. It is still sometimes required to operate for ulcer complications, and those who have had surgery are subject to the consequences of the operation itself. This chapter will discuss the objectives, nature, results, and adverse effects of ulcer and antireflux surgery.

ULCER (GASTRIC) SURGERY

Gastric anti-ulcer surgery began in Germany and was made possible by the developments of ether anesthesia in 1846 and antiseptic surgery in 1885. In 1881 Billroth successfully removed part of a stomach for gastric cancer and joined the remnant to the duodenum. That year, Wolfler performed the first gastroenterostomy for an obstructing, incurable cancer. Von Rydygier performed

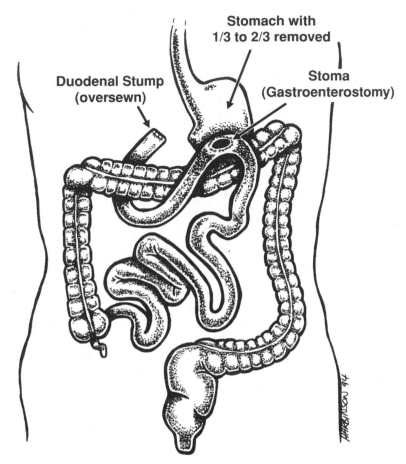

Figure 29-1. Gastroenterostomy and partial gastrectomy. Gastroenterostomy alone was the premier surgical treatment for peptic ulcer for half a century. Much later it was commonly used with a partial gastrectomy. This is the Billroth II operation.

a gastroenterostomy on a 20-year-old man with obstruction from a duodenal ulcer with excellent results. Both operations were quickly adopted for the treatment of peptic ulcer disease. At first, the usual procedure was a gastroenterostomy because of its simplicity and because of the high mortality rate of gastric resection. The Billroth II operation included a partial gastrectomy and gastroenterostomy so that the gastric remnant need not stretch to reach the duodenum (Figure 29-1).

These operations underwent many modifications over the years. Gastroenterostomy was slow to disappear and lingered into the 1930s. It was not until the introduction of vagotomy in 1943 that peptic ulcer surgery acquired a sound physiological basis. Motivations for change were the high recurrence rates after gastroenterostomy and the many complications of partial gastrectomy. Advances in physiology permitted operations directed against the stimulus of acid secretion rather than resection or bypass of the ulcer or removal of parietal cells.

Types of Ulcer Surgery

Gastroenterostomy

Why was this procedure so popular? The stomach is simply drained into the jejunum. In Von Rydygier's case, a duodenum obstructed by a duodenal ulcer was bypassed, but obstruction is an uncommon ulcer complication. The procedure prevents gastric acid from bathing the duodenum, permitting a duodenal ulcer to heal while diverting acid to the jejunum. However, one case in three develops a jejunal ulcer that invariably requires another operation. Despite this, gastroenterostomy was the operation chosen by many famous surgeons for over half a century. Its technical simplicity appealed in the face of the higher mortality of a partial gastrectomy. Improved techniques could have ended it sooner. Most of the other postgastrectomy syndromes were first noticed after this operation. By 1924, gastroenterostomy was called a disease, and some surgeons strove to have it abandoned. Uncommon after 1945, it enjoyed a brief revival as a drainage procedure with vagotomy. Gastroenterostomy drains the stomach in the Billroth II procedure (Figure 29-1).

Partial Gastrectomy

The first gastric resection for gastric ulcer was performed in 1882, but high mortality rates prevented its acceptance as standard anti-ulcer surgery. In the first decade of this century, duodenal ulcer became common, and a new understanding of gastric acid secretion led to its employment for duodenal ulcer. Subtotal gastrectomy came to be used for cancer, while the lesser partial gastrectomy was employed for peptic ulcer.

Partial gastrectomy (Figures 29-1, 29-2) underwent many modifications since 1881. The Billroth II operation permitted larger gastric resections than the original procedure. In 1903, Kocher moved the duodenum closer to the gastric remnant so that larger Billroth I resections became feasible. Controversy over the relative merits of the two types of partial gastrectomy raged long after. Comparisons of peristaltic or antiperistaltic gastroenterostomy or anastomoses before or behind the colon need not concern us here. Suffice it to say that there are many variations on the theme, each eponymously bearing the name of its advocate. In the 1930s, larger resections were done to achieve fewer recurrent ulcers. The trade-off was more postgastrectomy complications. Clearly a better operation was needed.

Vagotomy

After 1911, several surgeons attempted vagotomy based on Pavlov's work (Figure 29-3). However, it did not catch on until Dragstedt adapted it for duodenal ulcer in 1943. Earlier vagotomies were done for several reasons, including the abdominal pain of tertiary syphilis. Vagotomy reduced sensation, motility, and acid secretion. Dragstedt emphasized the latter and improved the completeness of the vagotomy by dividing the nerves above the diaphragm. Early vagotomies required a chest incision.

Vagotomy and Pyloroplasty

In about a third of patients, vagotomy caused gastric paralysis and food retention. Gastroenterostomy was added to facilitate gastric emptying. Later, pyloroplasty became the drainage procedure of choice (Figure 29-4). A commonly used pyloroplasty is that of Heineke and Mickulicz, described in the 1880s. In this operation the pylorus is cut longitudinally and sewn transversely The procedure was originally performed for pyloric obstruction, but reobstruction was common.

Vagotomy and Antrectomy

In the 1950s it became obvious that recurrent ulcers were more common with vagotomy and drainage procedures. Therefore, a

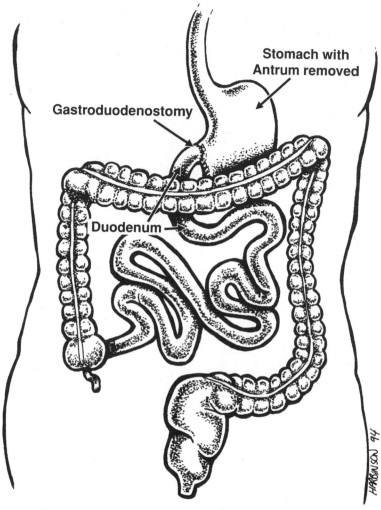

Figure 29-2. Partial gastrectomy with gastroduodenostomy. The original Billroth gastrectomy, it was employed for almost 100 years for peptic ulcer treatment. It became popular as surgical mortality improved in the 1920s and declined with the development of vagotomy.

partial gastrectomy was combined with vagotomy. The removal of the antral and vagal stimuli to gastric acid secretion cured almost 100% of ulcer patients (Figure 29-5). Now surgeons could control both the cephalic (vagus) and gastric (gastrin) phases of acid secre-

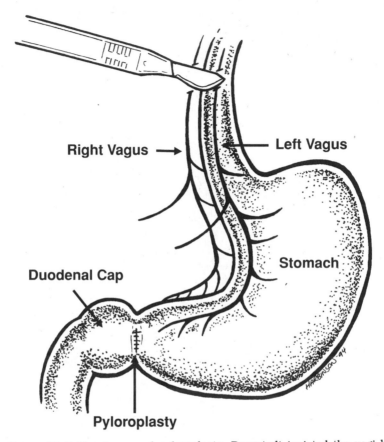

Figure 29-3. Vagotomy and pyloroplasty. Dragstedt insisted the vagi be divided above the diaphragm to ensure completeness. Pyloroplasty was added later to ensure gastric emptying.

tion. Unhappily, this aggressive surgery produced more postgastrectomy syndromes.

Selective and Highly Selective Vagotomy

By preserving the vagal branches to the gall bladder, pancreas, and intestines, surgeons hoped to lessen the disadvantages of dividing the main trunks of the vagus nerves. However, postvagotomy diarrhea and gastric stasis still occurred after selective vag-

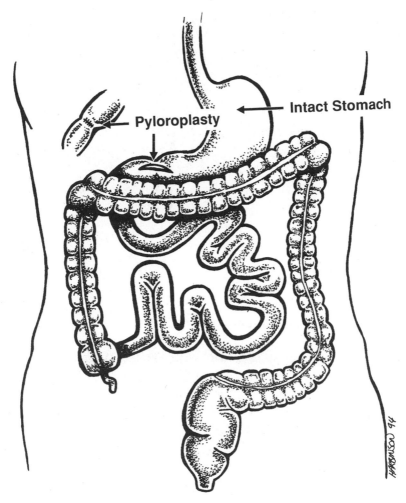

Figure 29-4. Heineke–Mikulicz pyloroplasty. The pylorus is cut longitudinally and sewn transversely.

otomy, and it was soon eclipsed by a highly selective vagotomy (Figure 29-6).

   In 1957 Griffith and Hawkins demonstrated the vagal fibers that enervated the parietal cells. This inspired surgeons to sever them and preserve the fibers supplying motor functions of the upper gut. By 1970, this operation was done without a drainage

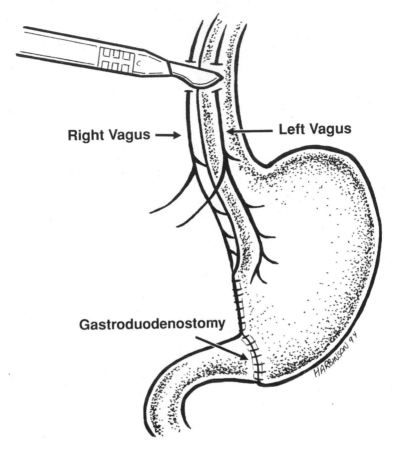

Figure 29-5. Vagotomy and antrectomy. This operation sacrificed less stomach than the partial gastrectomy. By interrupting the cephalic and gastrin stimulation of acid secretion an almost 100% ulcer cure is achieved.

procedure. While recurrent ulcers are more common with this highly selective, or parietal cell, vagotomy, the rarity of postgastrectomy complications established it as the most favored surgery for peptic ulcer. This view was buttressed by the knowledge that modern drugs can easily treat recurrent ulcers. It is ironic that this "ideal" operation should appear on the eve of the great pharmacological and bacteriologic discoveries that have rendered elective ulcer surgery virtually obsolete.

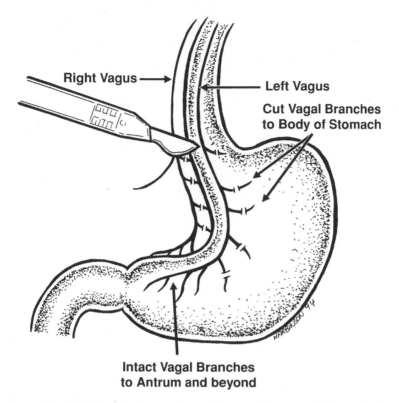

Figure 29-6. Highly selective vagotomy. The vagal branches that supply the parietal cells are divided. Thus, vagal control of upper gut motility is maintained.

Complications of Gastric Surgery

The 100-year search for a satisfactory surgical treatment for peptic ulcer was motivated by the need to prevent recurrent ulcers and minimize postgastrectomy complications. Surgical fashion thus progressed from conservative gastroenterostomy to radical gastrectomy to conservative vagotomy and drainage to radical vagotomy and antrectomy and, finally, to the ultraconservative highly selective vagotomy. While learned controversies over the merits of the various procedures fade into history, contemporary surgeons must select the operation most suitable for the complications of peptic ulcer. Meanwhile, physicians continue to care for that residual, but shrinking, number of patients who had their ulcers treated during the age of gastric surgery. As surgeons and physicians retire, expertise in the prevention and treatment of postgastrectomy syndromes should become a lost art.

Recurrent Ulcer

The lesser the operation, the greater the risk of recurrent ulcer. Hence, ulcers seldom recur after vagotomy and antrectomy, while a highly selective vagotomy risks recurrence in 10–15% of patients. In the highly selective vagotomy, surgical technique is critical, as all parietal cell fibers must be carefully dissected and severed. Recurrent ulcers should suggest the possibility of an incomplete vagotomy or one of the rare syndromes associated with increased gastrin secretion (see Chapter 12).

Highly selective vagotomy may be added to emergency repair of a perforated or bleeding ulcer without significantly increasing the morbidity of the surgery. Some surgeons, unfamiliar with the highly selective technique, will opt for vagotomy and drainage. A vagotomy may be inappropriate for pyloric stenosis and already impaired stomach emptying. These decisions are easier now that most recurrent ulcers are medically treatable. Prompt deployment of anti-ulcer medication may forestall future complications. Management is more difficult when complications occur without warning. Once *H. pylori* is more reliably eradicated, surgery will need only treat complications, and anti-ulcer procedures will be redundant.

Postgastrectomy Syndrome(s)

From the earliest days of gastric surgery, numerous complications were attributed to the operation. The term *postgastrectomy syndrome* is a misnomer because symptoms occur after operations that do not include gastrectomy, and there are several postgastrectomy syndromes. Detailed descriptions of these increasingly uncommon complications are not relevant here. Suffice it to say that at least 50 variations of gastroenterostomy with or without resection have failed to prevent these troublesome surgical sequelae. Only effective medical treatment of ulcers and avoidance of surgery have made them less common. Meanwhile, many a gastric cripple has paid dearly for a surgical ulcer cure. Brief descriptions of the principal syndromes follow. Many patients have several complications, and, in some, precise classification is impossible.

Bilious Vomiting

Bilious vomiting was first caused by food entering the afferent (upstream) loop of a gastroenterostomy. German surgical pioneers described the filling of the duodenum and subsequent discharge of food and bile back into the stomach, from which it is promptly vomited. Modified surgical techniques have made this rare, but a similar phenomenon called the *afferent loop syndrome* survives. Here, the afferent loop becomes kinked or blocked by the arrival of a meal in the stomach. The obstructed loop is distended and painful. As the food passes, kink, obstruction, and pain all disappear and bile is suddenly released into the stomach from where it is vomited. The Roux-en-Y is the preferred surgical remedy. The afferent loop is attached to the jejunum to bypass the kink and prevent bile reflux. This operation generates its own problems, such as malabsorption and gastric stasis.

Delayed Gastric Emptying

Immediately after surgery, the stomach, like the rest of the gut, is atonic. This may last for days or weeks because of technical or metabolic problems. Occasionally, the stomach refuses to empty indefinitely. Some believe that a vagotomy makes this more likely, but Billroth reported the phenomenon long before vagotomy was invented. Rarely, there is an unrecognized motility disorder. Prolonged pyloric obstruction causes a dilated stomach that may fail to regain its contractility with relief of the obstruction.

Whatever the cause, patients experience abdominal discomfort as food accumulates throughout the day and are only relieved by vomiting. Unlike the afferent loop syndrome, the vomitus is not bile stained, and, unlike dumping, the symptoms seem unrelated to meals. Weight loss and nutritional defects are important symptoms. Small, low-fat meals are best for treatment. Gastrokinetic drugs such as metoclopromide or cisapride may help. Reoperation can be contemplated only if there is a mechanical obstruction. Rarely, such patients must be sustained by intravenous feeding.

Dumping Syndrome(s)

The incidence of dumping is greatest after subtotal gastrectomy and least with a highly selective vagotomy. Symptoms result from the dumping of food directly into the jejunum rather than by measured spurts through an intact pylorus. It may also complicate pyloroplasty. There are two types of dumping: early and late. Both result from the sudden arrival in the small intestine of hypertonic, carbohydrate-rich food.

In *early* or *vasomotor dumping*, the hypertonic chyme sets off a number of events. By osmosis, fluid is drawn into the jejunum, distending the gut and transiently reducing the blood volume. Blood flow to the gut increases, and enteric hormones, notably serotonin and bradykinin, are released. The latter probably causes many of the cardiovascular manifestations of early dumping.

Almost immediately after a meal, the early dumper experiences dizziness, weakness, heart palpitations, and sweating. There may also be cramps, vomiting, and explosive diarrhea. He or she learns to avoid sugar and eat small meals. Small, low-carbohydrate meals eaten without fluids are also helpful. Most achieve satisfactory relief with such dietary measures. Recumbency after a meal slows gastric emptying. Dietary fiber, especially pectin, also slows dumping. A somatostatin analogue inhibits the release of many gut hormones, but it is expensive and requires injection. If surgery is necessary, conversion of a gastroenterostomy to a Roux-en-Y may be successful.

Late or *hypoglycemic dumping* is less common than the early variety. A sudden carbohydrate load raises the blood sugar. The consequent release of insulin and enteroglucagon (another gut hormone) sharply lowers the blood sugar again. Symptoms coincide with the hypoglycemia (low blood sugar) that occurs 1–3 hours after a meal. Many of the measures recommended for early dumping also help the late dumper. The patient should limit carbohydrate intake to 50 g daily spread over several meals. A corresponding increase in fat ingestion may slow gastric emptying. During a hypoglycemic attack, a sugar solution will relieve symptoms.

Postvagotomy Diarrhea

After truncal vagotomy, about 20% of people experience diarrhea regardless of the drainage procedure. One or two percent have chronic, frequent, debilitating, watery, often nocturnal diarrhea. Putative causes are obscure and plentiful. Small gut transit is rapid, and there is probably an inappropriate release of cathartic bile salts by the gall bladder into the gut.

Small, spaced, high-fiber meals help some. Few improve on the bile salt-binding resin cholestyramine. Somatostatin use is a current trend in managing obscure diarrheas. However, even if it works, which is doubtful, its cost and need to be injected are prohibitive. Desperate cases are subject to several surgical maneuvers, which usually involves reversal of a segment of intestine. This complication should disappear as the need for gastric surgery declines, and the highly selective procedure replaces truncal vagotomy.

Alkaline Reflux Gastritis and Esophagitis

Removal of a functioning pylorus permits reflux of intestinal contents into the stomach. Since these contents include bile salts, pancreatic digestive enzymes, and even bacteria, gastric mucosal damage can be anticipated. Bile salts and pancreatic enzymes impair gastric mucosal integrity and permit influx of gastric acid into mucosal cells. Damage ranges from severe inflammation to mucosal destruction with little inflammation. The mucosa appears fiery red to the gastroscopist. Tests to quantify bile reflux are unreliable.

Much that is written on this subject must be revised. Most of those undergoing ulcer surgery must have harbored *H. pylori,* which could account for the gastritis. The lack of correlation between gastritis and dyspepsia makes it doubtful that alkaline gastritis causes symptoms. It is believed among surgeons that postgastrectomy syndromes are more likely in those who had no clear indication for the original surgery. Probably some postoperative dyspepsia was there preoperatively. Other causes of abdominal discomfort should be excluded, especially recurrent ulcer, afferent loop syndrome, and dumping.

If the relationship of symptoms to bile reflux gastritis is obscure, the treatment is even moreso. Gastrokinetic drugs and cholestyramine achieve limited success, and anti-ulcer medication is ineffective. The Roux-en-Y operation diverts bile and pancreatic juice from the stomach, but there are no proper trials and many patients fail to improve.

After gastrectomy, bile salts and acidic gastric contents may reflux into the esophagus, causing a severe esophagitis. With slower cell turnover, squamus esophageal epithelium is more susceptible to damage than is gastric epithelium. Symptoms do not improve on antacids, and the efficacy of omeprazole is uncertain. Gastrokinetics and cholestyramine are logical but of little benefit. Antireflux or bile diversion operations may be necessary last resorts.

Nutritional Complications of Gastric Surgery

Gastric surgery causes malnutrition in several ways. Postoperative dyspepsia, vomiting, and the new small stomach are powerful deterrents to eating, causing weight loss and folic acid-deficiency anemia. Anatomical alterations may impair absorption of food. If too much gut is bypassed or transit is hurried, there will be insufficient mucosal contact. A large afferent loop after gastroenterostomy may delay the union of a meal with pancreatic digestive enzymes. Such a loop or any other cause of upper gut stasis may permit bacterial overgrowth, which has two important consequences. The first is inactivation of bile salts, which impair their ability to assist the absorption of fat and fat-soluble vitamins A, D, and K. Second, the interloping bacteria consume ingested vitamin B_{12} and may cause a vitamin B_{12}-deficient anemia. Some iron may be lost from a bleeding marginal ulcer. Gastric acid is important to iron absorption. If surgery reduces acid secretion, iron deficiency may follow. These are powerful arguments for less extensive surgery, such as highly selective vagotomy.

Bacterial overgrowth may be corrected surgically or treated with antibiotics. Vitamin deficiencies are corrected with supplements or injections. If indicated, pancreatic enzymes may be given with meals. Calorie malnutrition is more difficult to overcome, and in severe cases intravenous feeding (total parenteral nutrition) may be the only recourse.

It is important to remember primary maldigestive states such as celiac disease or pancreatic insufficiency. Preoperatively, the presence of a malabsorbtion state may be obscured by ulcer symptoms.

Postoperatively, the added physiologic impairment imposed by the surgery may add to the nutritional consequences of malabsorption.

Gastric Remnant Cancer

It is ironic that duodenal ulcer patients who are normally less prone to cancer should become at risk after curative surgery. The role of *H. pylori* in both of these diseases makes it more understandable. There is probably an increased risk of cancer in the remaining stomach 20–30 years after a partial gastrectomy. However, statistics over such a long period of observation are notoriously unreliable. Bile reflux is suspect, but other candidates include overgrowth of carcinogen-producing bacteria and the evolution of gastritis through intestinal metaplasia, dysplasia, and cancer in situ (see Chapter 21).

Possible gastric remnant cancer is probably an insufficient indication for an endoscopic program aimed at early detection. Nonetheless, dyspeptic symptoms in a vulnerable patient should prompt an examination.

Postgastrectomy Gallstones

Gallstones are more likely after gastric surgery, especially after truncal vagotomy. Again the causes are obscure, but interference with gall bladder emptying and alterations in bile salt metabolism are likely. Bile salts keep cholesterol in solution in bile so that cholesterol stones do not form. Gallstones are very common in unoperated persons, so it is difficult to blame the surgery in individual cases.

ANTIREFLUX SURGERY

Surgical Objective

Antireflux surgery is designed to repair, tighten, or augment the LES to prevent reflux of gastric contents into the esophagus. Such procedures should minimally interfere with swallowing, belching, or vomiting. Many years ago, when heartburn and esophagitis were blamed on a hiatus hernia, it seemed logical to repair the hernia, tighten the diaphragmatic crura, and secure the stomach below the diaphragm. This was usually insufficient, and modern surgery, while repairing the hernia if present, aims to augment the LES. Additional procedures to reduce gastric acid secretion are not helpful. Vagotomy, by slowing gastric emptying, could make matters worse.

Types of Repair

The results of antireflux surgery are variable, and some have claimed that the benefit lasts only 5 or 6 years. However, surgical units that specialize in such operations report 85–95% long-term success. Such success rests on several factors. The indications must be sound. There must be esophagitis, and the symptoms should be convincingly a result of reflux, confirmed by 24-hour intraesophageal pH monitoring. Adequate management must have failed to the extent that the symptoms impair quality of life or continue in a young person where long-term medication is an undesirable option. Surgery also may be necessary when nocturnal reflux risks pulmonary complications.

One must exclude a primary motility disorder through manometric studies of the esophagus. Antireflux surgery in a person with scleroderma will almost certainly cause dysphagia. An esophagus with full-thickness damage due to long-standing reflux may also respond to the procedure poorly. The operation should be one of the standard Belsey, Hill, or Nissen repairs and should be performed by an experienced antireflux surgeon.

Belsey Repair

This English innovation was the first modern antireflux surgery, in which Belsey approached the lower esophagus through the chest (thoracotomy). This technique provides the surgeon with the best view of the lower esophagus, but the need to retract the ribs causes more pain than would an abdominal incision. Sutures placed through stomach and esophagus muscles anchor them to the diaphragm. The LES is strengthened by a 270-degree plication, or pleating, of the cardia. There are several modifications of this operation; the current version is called the Belsey Mark IV. Aside from postoperative chest pain, transient dysphagia, bloating, and inability to belch sometimes occur.

Hill Antireflux Operation

This operation was developed in the United States. Sutures anchor the cardia to its natural attachments in the diaphragm and other supporting structures. This excentuates the flap valve effect of the angle where the esophagus meets the stomach (see Figure 1-3). A plication is also done. This procedure calls for an abdominal incision and is the most difficult to learn and perform. Obesity or other anatomical consideration may make the Hill procedure impossible. Postoperative dysphagia is common and may persist if the operation is incorrectly performed. One surgeon reports that 15% of cases require postoperative dilatations. Some dysphagia is due to edema and inflammation at the operative site that will subside in time.

Nissen Fundoplication

Reported from Europe in the 1950s, the Nissen repair has become the most widely used antireflux procedure, and hence we know more about its good and bad effects. Technically, it is the easiest to perform. The esophagus and stomach are freed up so that the fundus can be wrapped around the lower esophagus and achieve a 360-degree fundoplication. This reinforces the LES and strengthens the antireflux barrier. However, some postoperative problems are formidable, especially if the procedure is inexpertly done. Up to 50% of patients exhibit difficulty swallowing, gas bloat, or inability to belch or vomit. About 10% may have long-term difficulties. If the wraparound is insufficiently tethered, it may slip, causing dysphagia or reflux. Ulcers occur if the wrap is too tight, and fistulas to skin, aorta, and bronchus rarely develop.

Other Approaches

Now that gall bladder and other abdominal operations can be performed through a laparoscope, it is tempting to use a such an instrument for antireflux surgery. A laparoscope is an endoscope that can be inserted through a small abdominal incision into the stomach. Surgery can be performed without a large incision. It is premature to promote this technique for reflux surgery, but its day will undoubtedly come.

Such a day has come and gone for the insertion of an Angel-chick prosthesis. This is a silicone device placed around the LES to prevent reflux. By all accounts it is a failure; by 5 years, many require reoperation. Dysphagia, perforation, and migration of the device into the chest or abdomen are common. The device causes scarring, which makes further repair difficult.

Complications of Antireflux Surgery

It is not always worth the discomforts of major surgery to get minor recovery.

Richard Asher, *A Sense of Asher*, 1983, p.85

The most common complication of antireflux surgery is an inadequate repair with immediate or delayed return of reflux, often more severe than before. Certain preoperative circumstances favor this eventuality. Those who reflux while upright are less likely to enjoy a successful repair than those who have symptoms only when recumbent. If there is a severe stricture or a shortened esophagus, scar tissue poses technical difficulties. After surgery, a persistent or recurrent hiatus hernia is often demonstrable, even before discharge from hospital. If there are no symptoms it is probably best to ignore it. Sometimes after repair, the newly symptomless patient gains weight, which paradoxically causes reflux.

Reoperation should be approached with at least as much caution as the original surgery. Intense medical therapy should be tried first, and all concerned must be convinced that the symptoms are due to reflux. Difficulty swallowing is the complaint most likely to require treatment in the 6 months after surgery. Although more likely with the Nissen repair, it can occur with any antireflux procedure. It may be due to transitory edema and reduced motility from the surgical trauma. Liquid diets, frequent small meals, and time are usually successful, but some patients require dilatation. If the dysphagia persists beyond 6 months, reoperation must be contemplated. A primary motility disorder must again be excluded, and the surgery should be planned by an experienced operator.

Other complications include gas bloat, diarrhea, and inability to belch or vomit. These are more common after Nissen repair and have several explanations. The repair may be so successful that the

LES not only prevents reflux, but also blocks belching or vomiting. There may also be inadvertent vagal damage that impairs esophageal and gastric emptying. Aerophagy often accompanies upper gastrointestinal symptoms such as bloating and dysphagia. The symptoms usually improve with time, but, rarely, the gastric bloat must be decompressed by repeat surgery or a gastrostomy.

SUMMARY

Now that peptic ulcers can be healed and their recurrence prevented with anti-ulcer drugs and antibiotics, elective gastric surgery should become a thing of the past. No longer are ulcers "by desperate appliance to be relieved or not at all." The formidable array of postgastrectomy complications should inspire caution when contemplating an additional anti-ulcer operation in those undergoing life-saving surgery for perforation, bleeding, or obstruction, especially now that recurrence is preventable. Gastrectomy should be rare, and provided that the necessary skills do not become lost, a highly selective vagotomy is the choice anti-ulcer procedure.

A generation of individuals with postgastrectomy syndromes remain in the community as unhappy reminders of the age of gastric surgery and how *The Ulcer Story* has evolved. Recurrent ulcers, dumping, bilious vomiting, postvagotomy diarrhea, afferent loop and surgically induced cancer should gradually fade from the medical vocabulary in the 21st century.

Gastroesophageal reflux disease is not yet curable, even though it can be controlled by aggressive drug therapy. Antireflux surgery will likely retain a small place in treatment of this disease in the foreseeable future. Precision in diagnosis and an experienced surgeon are prerequisites if failed operations and dysphagia are to be avoided.

PART SEVEN

Testing Treatments and Patients

CHAPTER THIRTY

Testing Treatments
Clinical Trials and Placebos

Sometimes new treatments produce such a dramatic change from the inevitable mortality that preceded them that they require no clinical trial. Such was the case with insulin for diabetes or penicillin for pneumococcal pneumonia. The advantages of lancing a boil or setting a fracture are self-evident. However, most therapeutic advances are minimal at best, and, despite the enthusiasm of protagonists, they are difficult to prove effective. The therapeutic experience of one patient or one doctor is insufficient to convince a skeptical profession that it is generally useful. We need to know from collective experience whether a treatment will benefit most patients with similar characteristics most of the time.

At first glance, a clinical trial comparing two treatments conducted by blind observers seems simple enough. It is deceptively complicated. Table 30-1 lists some disciplines with an interest in the conduct of clinical trials and use of placebos. Each brings its expertise and bias to the subject, and no human can master them all. However, physicians must take responsibility for treatment validation. Informed doctors and patients must be able to interpret sound evidence when choosing therapy. Society will then have to decide what it can afford. Here we discuss the pitfalls and principles of clinical trials and the obscure, even mystical, effects of placebos.

TABLE 30-1
Some Disciplines
Concerned with Clinical
Trials and Placebos

Clinical medicine
Consumer
Statistics
Epidemiology
Ethics
Health economics
Pharmacology
Pharmaceutics
Marketing
Politics
Law
Philosophy

CLINICAL TRIALS

It takes less moral courage to administer a pill than it does to swallow it.
Mark Twain

Justification of treatments is very important in *The Ulcer Story*.
Patients with peptic ulcers, gastroesophageal reflux, dyspepsia,
and heartburn have relapses and remissions. Most with symptoms
improve on treatment, but how can we be sure that improvement
would not occur without treatment? Indeed, might patients be
better off with nothing? Patients deserve reassurance that treatments are effective and safe. Health authorities demand proof that
they are cost-effective. Clinical trials attempt to answer these
questions scientifically.

The First Clinical Trial

A British naval surgeon, James Lind, undertook the first clinical trial on board the H.M.S. Salisbury in 1747. During long sea
voyages contemporary sailors suffered from, and died of, scurvy.
We now know that this was due to the dietary lack of vitamin
C-containing fruits and vegetables. As for dyspepsia today, many
nostrums were employed to treat this disease without scientific
validation, and certainly without success. To discredit these treat-

ments and convince naval authorities of the value of fruit, Lind entered 12 shipboard sailors "in the scurvy" into a trial where each of six pairs received a test treatment. Diet and surroundings were similar for all. He gave one group two oranges and one lemon daily, while he treated the others with fashionable but nonsensical substances such as sea water, vinegar, and elixir vitriol. Recovery occurred only in those receiving the fruit.

Lind's work led to the eradication of scurvy at sea. British sailors became known as "limeys" because of their daily ration of citrus fruit. It is important to note that the trial patients had similar disease, surroundings, and diet, so only the treatment varied among the six pairs. With several refinements, such controlled clinical trials are now commonplace in all fields of medicine. It is sobering that future generations will regard many of today's treatments with the same amazement with which we look upon sea water and vinegar. Even now, some 1960s peptic ulcer treatments seem archaic.

Need for Clinical Trials

Many treatments are self-evident, intuitive, and common-sense. No sophisticated trial is necessary to demonstrate that prompt surgical repair of a perforated ulcer is life-saving. However, proof that it is superior to gastric suction and antibiotics would require a controlled trial. A prolonged study would be necessary to prove the need to add an anti-ulcer operation. Gastroenterostomy was brilliant therapy for an obstruction due to a duodenal ulcer, but extrapolation to the treatment of routine duodenal ulcers was an enduring mistake. Elevation of the head of the bed to prevent gastroesophageal reflux is often discovered by the patient himself. In this case a clinical trial confirms common sense.

Cardiac surgeons commonly ligated the internal mammary artery to improve blood flow to a diseased heart. In a controlled trial, this procedure proved to be no better than a sham chest incision, and it was quickly abandoned. During the age of gastric surgery, no trials compared the long-term outcome of ulcer operation versus no operation in such an objective, blinded way. However, there are trials comparing one operation to another that permit us to judge between vagotomy and gastrectomy.

Lack of critical evaluation permitted prolonged employment of useless or inferior treatments such as the Sippy diet and anticholinergics for duodenal ulcer. Some treatments are motivated by desperation and frustration, as in functional dyspepsia, or peptic ulcer before 1970. They owe more to emotion than science. In contrast, properly controlled trials have confirmed the usefulness of new drugs such as ranitidine and omeprazole in the treatment of peptic ulcer and gastroesophageal reflux disease.

Difficulties and Pitfalls

> Over twenty years, we conducted a randomized, double blind trial that included 20,000 patients. Unfortunately, nobody can remember why!
> Anonymous

It is difficult to design a clinical trial that can provide a clear answer. Success is more likely if the endpoint is obvious, such as death, or easily measurable, as is high blood pressure. The disappearance of an ulcer or esophagitis provides such an endpoint. Conclusions are more difficult when the measurement of symptoms is subjective and the normal course of the disease is unpredictable. Such is the case with dyspepsia and heartburn.

Peptic ulcer treatment trials contrast with those of dyspepsia (Table 30-2). Although the symptoms are similar, only the former has an objective finding—the ulcer itself. In trials, investigators can follow the progress of the ulcer by endoscope, comparing the rates of healing on different therapies. In a typical duodenal ulcer trial, the ulcer heals by 6 weeks in 85% of patients on H_2 antagonists compared to 40% of those on placebo. In functional dyspepsia, there is no such endpoint, and trial results depend entirely upon patients' interpretation of their symptoms. There is even disagreement on the definition of dyspepsia (see Chapter 10), so patients entered in trials are often dissimilar. If dyspepsia includes heartburn (and it should *not*), any improvement on an antacid drug would not prove the usefulness of the drug in dyspepsia.

Peptic ulcer is a disease with serious complications, but functional dyspepsia is not. This leads to lack of care and critical evaluation in the conduct of dyspepsia trials. Unlike ulcer, dyspepsia treatments have no therapeutic hypothesis and no clear endpoint. Not only are entry criteria and subgroups seldom defined,

TABLE 30-2
Clinical Treatment Trials in Peptic Ulcer and Dyspepsia

Criteria	Peptic ulcer	Functional dyspepsia
Disease importance	Great	Modest
Endpoint	Objective, single	Subjective, multiple
Outcome	Precise	Imprecise
Entry homogeneity	Precise	Imprecise
Side effects	Small tolerance	"0" tolerance
Placebo effect	Important	Important
Comparison trials	Permissible	Placebo arm essential
Publication bias	Small	Great
Subgroups	Known	Suspected
Conclusions	Solid	Weak, usually indeterminate

but negative trials are also less likely to be published. Some trials compare one drug with another when neither have been shown to be superior to placebo. H_2 antagonists may be a "gold standard" for the treatment of peptic ulcer, but not for non-ulcer dyspepsia.

Another fallacy is to demonstrate a drug effect on stomach physiology and assume that it will improve symptoms. Some propose the term "motility-like" dyspepsia to describe fullness and belching after meals. Delayed gastric emptying might be the cause. However, nobody has proved this, nor has anyone proved that faster emptying improves dyspeptic symptoms. Nevertheless, there are claims that prokinetic drugs are effective for functional dyspepsia. Whether or not there is any physiological change, dyspeptic symptoms must be properly measured and improvement demonstrated if a treatment is to be credible. Investigators measured changes in symptoms in only two of the many functional dyspepsia trials, and there was no benefit in either.

Clinical Significance

How should data from a clinical trial apply to practice? Is the patient similar to those studied? Most clinical trials occur in university hospitals, but most clinical encounters are elsewhere. While specialists make, or think they make, precise diagnoses, family doctors must deal with patients who often have no firm diagnosis. Are conclusions arrived at in one environment appropriate in the other? Is a statistically significant improvement of a treatment *clinically* significant? In a young person with a chronic, benign disease such as dyspepsia, would a marginally beneficial medication be worth the cost, unwanted effects, and drug-taking culture that it inspires?

Bias

A great problem with therapeutic trials is bias. Experience influences us all, and we all want a treatment to work. Forty percent of duodenal ulcers heal on a placebo, a substance with no specific effect on the stomach. This so-called "placebo response" also occurs in functional dyspepsia or heartburn. Should we use a medicine that is no better than an inert pill? The answer to this complex question compels an understanding of placebos.

PLACEBOS

The efficient physician is the man who successfully amuses his patients while Nature effects a cure.
Voltaire, 1694–1778

Words are, of course, the most powerful drug used by mankind.
Kipling, 1923

Derived from Latin, *placebo* means "I shall please." Sugar pills and other harmless remedies have been employed for millennia. The word *placebo* cannot be defined logically, yet it plays a role in almost every therapeutic encounter. Up to half of those receiving inert material during experimental therapy seems to benefit. The need to take something is deeply ingrained in us. Therefore, if placebos work, why not use them? Some have ethical concerns about the implied deception and paternalism, but placebos have some measurable effects that require no deception.

Placebos are much more complex than was originally thought. When patients take them for pain, the tissues release narcotic-like substances called endorphins with analgesic qualities. Naloxone, a narcotic antagonist, inhibits placebo-induced pain relief. Some patients, warned of side effects caused by the active drug in a clinical trial, experience them on the placebo. In several Crohn's disease treatment trials, 6–8% of subjects receiving the inert medication experienced effects that forced them to withdraw. Some people even develop placebo addiction. Thus, an inert medication can also be a *nocebo*, meaning "I will harm."

Doctor–patient interaction is important to the placebo response. The effect depends upon the manner in which the placebo is given. In clinical trials, inert medication prescribed by a physician is more effective than that given by a nurse, and both are superior to a placebo sent in the mail. Any medicine performs better when given by a caring physician. Even removal of a normal organ by a confident and enthusiastic surgeon may have a happy result. Could psychotherapy also be an elaborate placebo? When treating ulcers and non-ulcers or interpreting clinical trials, we must keep placebo and nocebo effects clearly in focus.

Implications of the Placebo Response

...but for Medicine as a whole the placebo is a great deceiver, misrepresenter, and creator of illusions...

...someone in the group found that by showing concern to a sick person and giving a token to symbolize this concern, the sick person could be made to feel better.

Thomas, KB, 1994

The placebo response in treatment trials of functional dyspepsia ranges from 20% to 60%. Lest this tempts us to believe that dyspepsia symptoms are imaginary, we should remember that a similar response occurs in trials of peptic ulcer healing (Table 30-3). This phenomenon is typical of clinical trials in other gastrointestinal disorders such as IBS and inflammatory bowel disease. There are, therefore, important lessons. *First*, no costly or potentially harmful diet or drug is acceptable for the treatment of patients with ulcers, dyspepsia, heartburn, or GERD without proof of efficacy through placebo-controlled, double-blind clinical trials. Scientific underpinning is essential for family practitioners who must daily interpret ill-defined and unstable situations. Some risk of side effects is permissible with ulcer or esophagitis if there are marginal or doubtful benefits. However, undesired effects and cost permit

TABLE 30-3
The Placebo Response: Some Responses to Placebo in Clinical
Trials of Dyspepsia and Duodenal Ulcer

Trial	Drugs tested	Percentage of those receiving placebo who responded
Dyspepsia	Cimetidine, pirenzipine	62
	Cimetidine	54
	Cisapride	28
	Antacid, cimetidine	25
Duodenal ulcer	Antacid	55
	Cimetidine	38
	Prostaglandin	44
	Omeprazole	27

no such indulgence with benign disorders such as functional dyspepsia or heartburn.

Second, placebos are sometimes useful. If a placebo is to work, the patient should believe that there is a favorable pharmacological effect. This may not be entirely true. Clinical trials require informed consent to the possible use of placebo, yet those receiving placebos may still improve. In one trial, a small number of neurotic patients improved even when they knew their pills were inert. The symbolic giving of pills is therapeutic. The use of "logical" placebos, which have a plausible rationale yet do no harm, may be useful in certain circumstances. Such logical placebos might include low-dose antacids or a bland diet for functional dyspepsia.

To achieve a maximum placebo benefit, a positive approach is more effective than a more truthful admission of ignorance. Attempts to encourage analytical thinking about a treatment reduce its placebo value. The benefit is greatest in, but not at all confined to, those who are anxious, dependent, and noncritical. An enthusiastic and respected physician or surgeon will achieve the best result. In their quest to purify the profession, the media and health authorities risk impairing physicians' healing powers. Consider the use of placebos paternalistic or Machiavellian if you wish, but also consider what benefits are at risk.

Placebos are as old as human nature. Suggestion influences the benefits and even side effects of a drug. Large capsules are better than small ones. Yellow and red capsules stimulate, white ones are analgesic, and blue ones depress. Consciously or unconsciously a placebo effect is a mystic, yet scientifically validated, component of every therapeutic interaction.

The *third* and probably most important implication of the placebo response is that it illustrates the benefit of a successful physician–patient encounter. "A clinical approach that makes the illness experience more understandable to the patient, that instills a sense of care and social support, and that will increase the feeling of mastery and control over the course of the illness, will be most likely to create a positive placebo response and to improve symptoms" (Brody). Such a positive doctor–patient interaction is indispensable to the management of dyspepsia and other gut symptoms. Whether or not drugs are employed, careful consideration of the patient's complaints, explanation, and reassurance must be integral parts of any management plan.

PRINCIPLES OF A CLINICAL TRIAL

The most common clinical trials are those carried out daily in a doctor's office. The doctor prescribes a drug or diet to alleviate the patient's symptoms based upon his experience and knowledge. If the symptoms improve with no harmful side effects, all is well. Often the doctor cannot prove from published literature that the treatment is generally effective for that symptom. If the treatment satisfies most patients with similar symptoms, the doctor gains confidence and uses it again. This process, however pragmatic and sensible, is quite unscientific and subject to bias. How else might one explain why blood-letting, megavitamins, anticholinergics, and environmental treatments became so fashionable in their times? After all, most illnesses tend to improve.

The next level of clinical trial is the series. Here someone records the result of treatments given to several patients with the same disease. While a useful means of recording untoward effects and comparing results from one clinical center to another, this technique fails to tell us what might have happened without treatment. The series is an insignificant improvement upon individual experience, and it retains great opportunity for bias.

In a clinical trial, improvement or lack of it should be recognizable by someone other than the doctor and the patient, whose biases cloud their judgment. In dyspepsia there are no objective tests or signs, and symptom changes are subjective and subtle. It may take weeks or months before improvement is measurable. The dyspeptic is seldom cured, so benefit is subject to interpretation, attitude, hope, and the placebo response. To circumvent these biases, doctors conduct controlled clinical trials. Like Lind, they must have controls in place. Patients and their symptoms must be homogeneous. The surroundings, circumstances, and mode of treatment should be comparable. Modern trials require even further controls.

Treatments are usually blinded; that is, the patient cannot know which treatment he is receiving and subconsciously bias the results. Blinding is usually achieved with placebo treatment that is outwardly identical to the treatment under study. The research physician is also biased, and his or her enthusiasm for a new treatment must be controlled. Studies are thus double-blinded; only a third party knows what each subject receives, and the assessment of improvement should be free of bias. Treatments must be administered to subjects randomly so that no external factor can influence the results. Finally, the data must undergo rigorous statistical analysis.

The randomized, double-blind, placebo-controlled clinical trial is an indispensable instrument to judge the efficacy of treatments new and old. This enterprise requires partnerships between patients, physicians, health authorities, and industry. The results are essential to therapeutic progress and sensible public policy. Therefore, participation by all partners is an important community service.

META-ANALYSIS

Meta-analysis is a relatively new fashion. It is useful if there are conflicting results or if individual trials have insufficient data to generate a significant conclusion. Meta-analysis validated the use of prednisone in the prevention of premature birth and the intracoronory injection of streptokinase in acute myocardial infarction. While meta-analyses are very useful, they are subject to the same errors, biases, and the other pitfalls that threaten individual trials. The process makes sense when testing one drug for one disease in comparable people, such as ranitidine for duodenal ulcers in young men. However, functional dyspepsia studies include dissimilar entry criteria, drug regimens, and populations. Outcome measures are difficult to define and may vary from study to study. Some results may not even be published. Meta-analysis is no panacea for faulty data.

SUMMARY

Clinical trials confirm the usefulness of many new drugs in the treatment of peptic ulcer and esophagitis. In dyspepsia, trials thus far have been less useful. The inherent difficulties in their conduct and the economic imperative to sell drugs for this common complaint produce substandard research and a publication bias. Even given that, most suggested treatments show no benefit, and those that do seem hardly of clinical significance. The new frontier for clinical trials is the search for a cost-effective treatment for *H. pylori* and cure of non-NSAID peptic ulcers. We should learn from past mistakes, put our enthusiasm on hold, and ensure the proper conduct and complete disclosure of all clinical trials. We must be mindful of the lessons of the placebo response. It teaches a healthy skepticism of accepted treatments and makes us wary of the claims of enthusiasts. Above all, it illustrates the value of good physician–patient interaction and compels us to strive to understand its mysteries.

CHAPTER THIRTY-ONE

Investigations

Testing Upper Gut Symptoms

Present fears
Are less than horrible misgivings
Macbeth, Act I, Scene iii

Patients with a suspected peptic ulcer or esophagitis usually must undergo some tests. The indications vary from case to case. Tests are expensive, and sometimes uncomfortable. They are necessary to determine the presence or absence of disease or its complications. However, tests should be performed only when the results will influence treatment. An understanding of the principles and methods of these investigations should make them less awesome.

ENDOSCOPY

Modern endoscopy was made possible by fiberoptic technology. If you look at a water fountain, you may notice that light from the base of the fountain follows a stream of water through its arc. A glass fiber has the same property; that is, light that enters it at one end follows the fiber through bends and loops to exit at the other. By bundling many fine glass fibers so that their relationship to one another at each end is identical, the bundle can transmit an image. Thus, a gastroscope transmits light through its length into the duodenum by one fiber bundle. Another transmits an image of the duodenum back around the many twists and turns of the upper gut to the examiner's eye. The technology of endoscopy is still evolving. Through microchips it is now possible for physicians, assistants, and even patients to view the endoscopic image on a television monitor. Videotapes are possible. This technology reduces dependence on delicate fiberoptic bundles, which are now used only to transmit light into the gut.

Endoscopes are equipped with cables attached to dials on the handle of the instrument. These dials move the tip of the scope to the required attitude. At least one tube within the instrument permits intestinal juices to be suctioned or biopsy forceps, cautery, and other devices to be deployed. Not only are these instruments useful in diagnosis, but operations may also be done through the endoscope. These include biopsy, polyp removal, foreign body retrieval, and cautery or injection of a bleeding site.

Esophagogastroduodenoscopy (EGD)

Figure 31-1 shows a video gastroscope. It attaches to a device that contains an external light source and provides suction and air pressure. The shaft is little more than 1 meter in length and has a diameter similar to that of a crayon. It is flexible and light.

A patient undergoing endoscopy must fast for at least 8 hours. Most otherwise healthy patients require no sedation, but policies vary from center to center. In our unit, 90% of outpatients undergoing this test receive no medication other than a local anesthetic throat spray (Xylocaine™). This avoids the risks of drug use, allows full comprehension of the findings by the patient, and permits him or her to return to work soon afterward. Anxious patients are treated with intravenous diazepam (Valium™), intravenous medazolam (Versed™), or sublingual oxazepam (Serax™). There is no justification for the risks of a general anesthetic.

In a series of over 200,000 gastroscopies, perforation, bleeding, infection, or cardiac events occurred in 0.13%. These included patients who were very ill, and such data were collected several years ago when instruments and techniques were more crude. When carried out in an otherwise healthy patient by a trained endoscopist

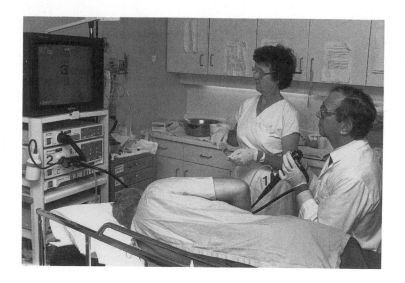

Figure 31-1. Upper gastrointestinal endoscopy (EGD). The endoscope (1) attaches to a device (2) that generates a source of illumination. It also facilitates suction, air to inflate the stomach, and in some cases electrocautery. The monitor (3) displays the image generated by instrument. Control knobs on the handle direct the tip of the scope, and a mouthpiece between the teeth protects the instrument. The endoscopist is introducing the gastroscope with the patient correctly positioned. Note the endoscopy nurse prepared to inject saline to clear the suction port.

with an experienced nurse-assistant, the risk of complications from gastroscopy is very small.

The examination takes place with the subject lying on the left side with the chin against the chest (Figure 31-1). After applying local anesthetic spray, the physician gently places his fingers in the throat to test that the anesthetic has suppressed gagging. This familiarizes the patient with the sensation of something foreign in the anaesthetized throat. Saliva drains into a provided towel. The nurse assistant urges the patient to breathe normally throughout, since this helps to suppress the gag reflex. The examiner places the instrument in the throat and asks the subject to swallow. Although swallowing is difficult under these circumstances, the attempt usually relaxes the upper esophageal sphincter, allowing the gastroscope to pass. A mouthpiece placed between the teeth protects the delicate instrument. An inadvertent bite can be very expensive!

Once the tube is in place the test lasts approximately 5 minutes. It is not comfortable, but there is usually no pain. The physician must inject air into the stomach, inflating it for better visibility. He or she will remove the air before withdrawing the instrument. Sometimes it is necessary to take a biopsy of the stomach or duodenum using forceps delivered through the instrument's biopsy port. This is painless but slightly prolongs the procedure. If no sedation is given, after the test the doctor can explain his findings and discuss how to manage the symptoms.

Other Endoscopic Procedures

Through a side-viewing endoscope placed in the duodenum a cannula can be threaded into the bile or pancreatic ducts. X ray shows the injected contrast material in the duct system. This is called *endoscopic retrograde cholangiopancreatography (ERCP)*. It requires sedation and considerable skill. Serious complications such as pancreatitis or cholangitis may result. The principal indication for ERCP is suspected bile duct or pancreatic disease.

Enteroscopy (endoscopic examination of the small bowel) employs a longer endoscope. For technical reasons it is difficult to maneuver the instrument beyond the duodenum. The test is too lengthy for practical use. The standard gastroscope may transverse most of the duodenum, and a good small bowel X ray usually detects any disease in the jejunum or ileum.

BARIUM CONTRAST X RAYS

X rays blacken photographic film. They pass through a human body and cast light gray shadows of bones or other dense structures onto the film. The gut ordinarily has no shadow, but air in the lumen appears as dark (radiolucent) areas. Feces project a mottled appearance. A plain or "flat film" of the abdomen shows bony structures and gas and feces in the colon. To better outline the gut, a radiopaque substance called barium is swallowed or injected through tubes into the duodenum or rectum. X-ray pictures taken from various angles detect any abnormal configuration of the barium within the gut.

Upper Gastrointestinal X Ray (Esophagus, Stomach, Duodenum)

After a fast, the patient swallows white liquid barium that fills the esophagus, stomach, and duodenum and projects their shadow on the X ray film (Figure 31-2). Sequential films record movement of the barium through the gut. Tumors appear as "filling defects" and an ulcer as a collection of barium in the crater (see Figure 11-3). Properly done, such X rays detect most ulcers or tumors, but superficial lesions such as esophagitis or gastritis are difficult to see. Inexperienced radiologists also tend to "overcall" barium rests in the duodenum (see Figure 10-4). This is not the first choice in the investigation of dyspepsia or heartburn, but it will suffice where endoscopy is unavailable or too expensive.

Small Bowel X Ray

It is sometimes necessary to examine the small bowel in patients in whom Crohn's or small bowel ulcers are suspected. A *small bowel follow-through* is an upper gastrointestinal barium examination in which radiographs are taken as barium travels through the small bowel. Since barium becomes diluted by digestive juices as it makes it way down the gut, radiologists prefer to insert a tube through the nose into the duodenum. They next inject barium to opacify the entire small bowel. The tube is uncomfortable, but quickly removed. This test is quicker than a barium swallow, and the results are superior. It is called *enteroclysis*, or *small bowel enema* (Figure 31-3). The evening before the test, the subject takes a laxative such as two Dulcolax tablets.

ULTRASOUND OF THE ABDOMEN

Like X rays, high-frequency sound waves penetrate the body, casting shadows of body structures on a sensitized film or video. Unlike X rays, ultrasound does not damage tissue. Therefore, ultrasound is a safe and important means to examine the abdomen. This painless procedure can show thickened loops of bowel or abscesses. Ultrasound is also useful in examining abdominal masses or detecting gallstones in patients with episodic right upper quadrant abdominal pain. It may also help identify pancreatitis or tumors. To undergo the test, the subject must be fasting. A techni-

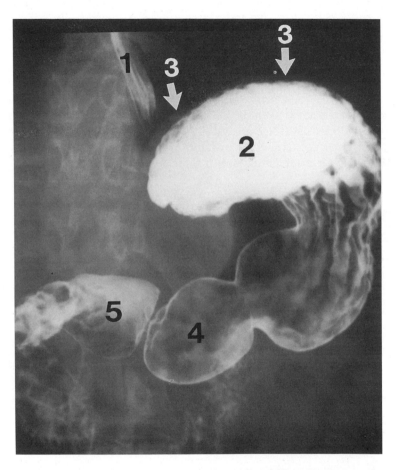

Figure 31-2. Upper gastrointestinal X ray. Swallowed barium fills the upper gut and outlines the esophagus (1), stomach, and duodenum (5) on the X-ray film. Also shown are cardia (2), diaphragm (3), and antrum (4). (Courtesy of Dr. H. Tao, Department of Radiology, Ottawa Civic Hospital, Ottawa, Canada.)

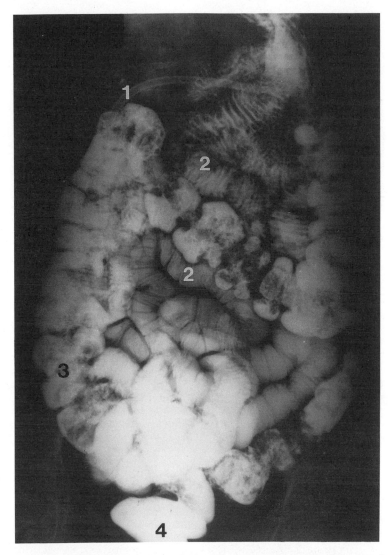

Figure 31-3. Small bowel enema (enteroclysis). A nasogastric tube may be seen passing through stomach into the duodenum (1). Barium injected through the tube quickly opacifies the small bowel (2) to the cecum. Barium has passed into the ascending colon (3) and around to the rectum (4). Note the feathery appearance of the normal small bowel. (Courtesy of Dr. H. Tao, Department of Radiology, Ottawa Civic Hospital, Ottawa, Canada.)

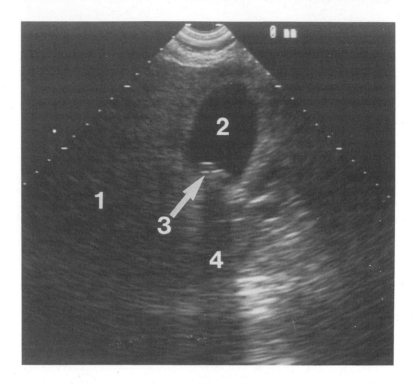

Figure 31-4. Ultrasound of liver (1) and gallbladder (2). The image shows the fluid-filled gallbladder. A gallstone (3) within the gallbladder blocks the sound waves and thus casts an acoustic shadow (4). This technique is 95–100% accurate in detecting gallstones in the gallbladder. (Courtesy of Dr. H. Tao, Department of Radiology, Ottawa Civic Hospital, Ottawa, Canada.)

cian moves a lubricated probe about the abdomen to secure images such as that in Figure 31-4.

COMPUTERIZED TOMOGRAPHY (CT)

This remarkable technologic advance permits cross-sectional views of the body. A CT of the abdomen helps detect complications of peptic ulcer such as perforation or tumors of the upper gut or liver. CT is different from magnetic resonance imaging (MRI). The latter technique detects various elements in tissues and provides a similar image to that of CT. However, the gut is always moving, and MRI requires a stationary subject.

BLOOD TESTS

A complete blood count (CBC) includes a hemoglobin concentration, a white blood cell count (WBC), and sometimes an erythrocyte sedimentation rate (ESR). The hemoglobin concentration is an estimate of the blood's red cell supply. If it is below normal, a person is anemic. Anemia is caused by bleeding, nutritional deficiency, hemolysis (red cell destruction), or chronic inflammation. In the case of peptic ulcers or esophagitis, it indicates chronic bleeding. With chronic blood loss, the body's iron supply becomes depleted. Since iron is a constituent of the blood pigment hemoglobin, the red cells appear pale and small under the microscope; that is, there is a hypochromic, microcytic anemia. A raised WBC or ESR suggests inflammation.

The physician may order blood biochemical tests as well. Serum albumin, for example, may be low because of chronic malnutrition or protein loss. Serum iron and ferritin levels are low in iron deficiency. Calcium, folic acid, and vitamin B_{12} levels are included if anemia or malabsorption is suspected.

Vitamin B_{12} deficiency also causes anemia. This results from a lack of gastric "intrinsic factor" caused by chronic gastritis (pernicious anemia) or total gastrectomy. This factor is necessary for the absorption of vitamin B_{12} in the small bowel. Over a few years, deficiency of vitamin B_{12} results in anemia and, occasionally, neurological consequences. Serum B_{12} levels may be obtained. A Schillings test assesses B_{12} absorptive capacity beginning with a B_{12} injection to saturate liver stores. The subject ingests a B_{12} pill containing a radioactive tracer and collects urine for 24 hours to determine how much B_{12} he or she absorbs and passes in the urine. Repeating the test with and without intrinsic factor distinguishes pernicious anemia from intestinal malabsorption of B_{12} (see also Chapter 6).

TESTS FOR GASTROESOPHAGEAL REFLUX OR DYSMOTILITY

It is difficult to prove that chest pain is caused by the esophagus. Special studies are sometimes helpful. *Esophageal motility* or *manometry* measures pressure waves and the integrity of the LES. The apparatus consists of a series of three electronic pressure sensors arranged along a narrow tube, usually at 5-cm intervals. The tube is placed in the esophagus, where the sensors relay local pressures to a bedside recording device. If the lowest sensor is in the LES, the apparatus produces tracings similar to those in Figure 19-2. Other maneuvers include a "pull-through" of the device through the sphincter and the use of cholinergic drugs to precipitate a contraction. While useful to detect achalasia and early scleroderma, this test is disappointing in the diagnosis of obscure chest pain.

To better associate intraesophageal events with pain, pressure and pH sensors are placed in the lower esophagus. A portable device records lower esophageal pH and pressures while the subject goes about his or her daily activities. The subject indicates pain by pushing a button. As discussed in Chapter 19, the correlation of pain with intraesophageal events is poor. Nevertheless, we can blame the esophagus when reflux of acid or esophageal contractions consistently occur with pain.

We can also study esophageal function when the patient swallows a meal containing a gamma-emitting isotope. Esophageal *scintography* uses a gamma camera to show reflux and abnormal esophageal emptying. As with the two procedures described above, careful interpretation of the results is essential. These are not routine tests.

SUMMARY

A few tests help physicians diagnose acid-peptic disease and its complications. Upper endoscopy is helpful when one suspects esophagitis or peptic ulcer. It is indicated when dyspepsia or heartburn fails to respond to lifestyle and dietary modification, forcing consideration of expensive medication. A barium contrast X ray may be substituted, but it is less accurate and will not detect tiny mucosal lesions. Further tests such as ultrasound, CT, or ERCP are reserved for specific suspicions. Blood tests are necessary if bleeding or inflammation are suspected. While there are tests of esophageal motility, decisions regarding noncardiac chest pain and gastroesophageal reflux often must be made with endoscopy and clinical judgment.

Epilogue

This is not the end. It is not even the beginning of the end. But it is,
perhaps, the end of the beginning.
Winston Churchill, 1942

The Ulcer Story is far from complete. Many unresolved issues promise steady employment for research physicians well into the new millennium. Nevertheless, ulcer disease—particularly duodenal ulcer disease—seems to have passed through this century like a wave cresting at the midpoint and receding at the end. It leaves in its wake many victims and many unsolved dilemmas. Young people today are unaware of the misery with which this scourge threatened their parents and grandparents in their youths. Before leaving *The Ulcer Story*, it is worth looking back at what we have learned and looking forward to challenges that remain.

WHAT HAVE WE LEARNED FROM THE ULCER STORY?

The Evanescence of Disease

Diseases come and go. They attack mankind, sometimes plaguing whole populations and threatening civilizations, only to fade from the scene as mysteriously as they appeared. We like to think we have controlled ulcer disease with hygiene and drugs, but much of the story seems guided by forces beyond our conscious control. It is tempting to attribute the decline of peptic ulcer to improved living standards hostile to the spread of *H. pylori*, belatedly aided by effective treatment. However, this leaves unexplained the apparently sudden increase in peptic ulcers a century ago. Equally perplexing is the variable presence of ulcers in individuals and populations infected with the organism.

As ulcer disease associated with *H. pylori* declines, others take its place. The widespread use of NSAIDs has produced a sharp increase in ulcers in elderly women. The prevalence of complicated ulcers appears, after all, unchanged. Gastroesophageal reflux disease (GERD) is also an increasing problem, masked—but not cured—by antisecretory drugs.

The Frailty of Dogma

If *The Ulcer Story* has taught us anything, surely it is the importance of a skeptical, yet open, mind. Our stumbling, serendipitous search for an explanation and cure for peptic ulcer has left many intellectual casualties. Looking back, it seems facile to attribute ulcers to a faulty diet, or even to propose diet therapy. Gastroenterostomy was an illogical evolution of an operation for obstruction to one for unobstructed ulcer disease. While all diseases are undeniably affected by the psyche, a psychotherapeutic approach must have harmed those with no psychopathology. Throughout the century, observers of ulcer disease were fascinated by the intricacies of acid secretion. While this focus eventually paid off with remarkable pharmacological discoveries, the obsession with acid secretion probably delayed discovery of the truth. Such theories were difficult to dislodge, and they left us totally unprepared for the momentous discovery by Warren and Marshall that ulcers could be an infectious disease. We have been slow to grasp the implications of this development, but previous false starts justify a slow and methodical approach. Undoubtedly, much that we now believe about *H. pylori* will be proven untrue.

We should keep these observations in mind when we contemplate unexplained problems. For example, many patients have symptoms of an ulcer, yet have no ulcer. It is an easy extrapolation to treat this enigmatic syndrome with anti-ulcer medication, just as early gastric surgeons employed gastroenterostomy, but so far, data indicate that this practice is futile, even counterproductive. On the other hand, the lack of objective findings in functional dyspepsia tempts some to regard it as a psychosomatic disease. Unless sensibly and critically applied, this approach may do dyspeptics a disservice. Until the truth is revealed, attractive dogmas must not be permitted to mask our ignorance.

The Burden of Proof

We must increase our efforts to establish the efficacy or noneficacy of treatments. It was problematic enough when physicians persuaded ulcer patients to undergo gastroenterostomy, the Sippy diet, or psychotherapy when the patients had to pay; it will be more difficult to recommend unproved treatment now that costs are increasingly a public responsibility. Not only should the requisite trials be done, but we must also abide by the result. It makes no sense to find no ulcer at endoscopy yet continue with anti-ulcer drugs regardless.

Common Sense and Placebos

Nevertheless, there is therapeutic benefit in a good patient–doctor encounter. Most of us are helped by such an experience. Commonsense advice about diet, drugs, alcohol, tobacco, and other lifestyle issues helps many, but the greatest benefit appears to come from the placebo effect. No matter what the complaint, physicians, patients, and managers must never forget that.

The Indispensability of Clinical Science

None of the triumphs of *The Ulcer Story* could have occurred were it not for skeptical, questioning, yet innovative clinical scientists. While nonclinicians such as Pavlov, Black, and Warren are credited with outstanding scientific discoveries in ulcer disease, clinical scientists were also indispensable to the process. Clinicians describe and classify disease and thus present the questions for science. Only doctors can put scientific hypotheses to the test. Our success with peptic ulcer disease would be nil were it not for the clinical skills of Dragstedt, Marshall, and countless other practicing doctors.

WHAT CHALLENGES REMAIN?

Optimal Treatment for *H. pylori?*

Current triple and double antibiotic regimens achieve less than 100% cure, and the more effective the regimen, the greater the risk of untoward effects. Graham suggests that we insist upon a program that promises a 90% cure and reminds us that the confidence limits of existing trials are small. Comparative trials are rare. The data may not apply to some populations, such as those where metronidazole-resistant organisms are prevalent. The last word will not appear before the next century. We badly need a single, inexpensive, safe drug that is effective after a short course and does not provoke resistance.

Who Should Be Treated?

Consensus is growing that all *H. pylori*-positive ulcers should be treated. Enthusiasts go further, insisting that the organism is evil—a cause of dyspepsia, cancer, maybe even coronary artery disease. They advocate search and destroy. The impracticality of such a policy is obvious. More than 2 billion people are infected, most in places inaccessible to medical care. Antibiotics are unlikely to achieve such global success, and all those cured may not escape carcinogenesis. Closer to home, the urge to treat *H. pylori*-positive dyspeptics seems irresistible, and many poor studies can be cited. But we must resist the urge to treat lest we squander valuable antibiotics and funds on a fool's mission. Such treatments should not take place outside of clinical trials, as we risk repeating past mistakes.

Addressing the larger issue of cancer will involve more data and a different approach. Better hygiene and less crowding will slowly help, but benefits seem generations away. Vaccination of the globe's infants offers the best chance to stamp out the organism worldwide. It is far from certain that such a costly venture is justified or even possible.

How Should We Manage Dyspepsia?

If peptic ulcer treatment has arrived at an age of enlightenment, that of functional dyspepsia idles in a dark age. We need a better definition of the problem, or problems, before we begin to understand its pathogenesis. Without more knowledge, we are unlikely to discover effective treatments. Meanwhile, dyspepsia demands a precise diagnosis—ulcer or non-ulcer—and it is of great public concern that we eschew treatments for the latter that carry risk or significant cost. Surely this excludes currently available drugs. As with those with ulcers before the 1970s, dyspeptics can be helped by firm reassurance, lifestyle advice, and the powerful benefits of the doctor–patient relationship. We should aim to maximize functioning without costly medical care.

How Best to Prevent NSAID Ulcers?

Longer life and potent anti-arthritic medications conspire to cause a growing proportion of peptic ulcers. Each new NSAID is introduced with claims that it is less ulcerogenic than its predecessors. Experience suggests the contrary—or suggests that the price is diminished efficacy. The best solution would be an anti-arthritic drug without ulcerogenic effects, perhaps an NSAID that permits normal gastric prostaglandin synthesis. Until such a drug is available, we should use NSAIDs only where specifically indicated and should remain vigilant with those at high risk: the elderly, steroid users, and the chronically ill. We need better data to determine the best drug to prevent NSAID ulcer complications as well as who should receive it.

What About GERD?

We have several powerful drugs to treat gastroesophageal reflux disease, but we can ill-afford to be complacent. A third of Western adults, probably more, has symptoms of GERD, and, as the population ages, more severe and complicated disease is inevitable. Richer foods, obesity, and sedentary lifestyle confound reflux control, and the drugs fail to reverse it. Long-term drug-induced achlorhydria is expensive and probably harmful, and prokinetics demonstrate tachyphylaxis and cause diarrhea.

We would be remiss to abandon the lifestyle and positional advice designed to minimize reflux, and leave it all to drugs. We need to discover a means to prevent reflux before we are entitled to claim a victory here that is as significant as the discovery of *H. pylori.*

CONCLUSION

We have learned much about peptic ulcers. We have also learned much about diseases generally: their transience, their complexity, their interactions with human circumstances, and their subjugation to forces beyond our understanding. If *H. pylori*-induced peptic ulcer passes from the scene, other diseases will take its place. We must be alert to new understandings of dyspepsia, NSAIDs, and reflux, but must also be sufficiently skeptical to insist upon proof. A knowledgeable and understanding public and open-minded, innovative, yet skeptical clinical scientists are the keys to the successful denouement of *The Ulcer Story.*

Bibliography

CHAPTER ONE

Costa M, Brookes SJH. The enteric nervous system. *Am J Gastroenterol* 1994;89S:129–135.

Hunter J. *Principles of Surgery*. England, 1770.

McGuigan JE, Ament ME. Anatomy and developmental anomolies. In Sleisenger ME, Fordtran JS, eds. *Gastrointestinal Disease: Pathophysiology/Diagnosis/Management* (fifth edition). Philadelphia: W.B. Saunders, 1993;459–469.

CHAPTER TWO

Chesterton CK. *The Man Who Was Thursday*. New York: Modern Penguin Classics, Penguin Books Inc., 1908;14.

Costa M, Brookes SJH. The enteric nervous system. *Am J Gastroenterol* 1994;89S:129–135.

Malagalada JR, Azpiroz F, Mcarin F, Gastroduodenal motor function in health and disease. In Sleisenger MH, Fordtran JS, eds. *Gastrointestinal Disease: Pathophysiology/Diagnosis/Management* (fifth edition). Philadelphia: W.B. Saunders, 1993;486–508.

Meyer JH. Chronic morbidity after gastric surgery. In Sleisenger MH, Fordtran JS, eds. *Gastrointestinal Disease: Pathophysiology/Diagnosis/Management*. (fifth edition). Philadelphia: W.B. Saunders, 1993;731–758.

CHAPTER THREE

Drossman DA, Richter JE, Talley NJ, Thompson WG, Corazziari E, Whitehead WE. *Functional Gastrointestinal Disorders*. Boston: Little, Brown, 1994.

Talley NJ, Colin-Jones D, Koch KL, Koch M, Nyren O, Stanghellini V. Functional dyspepsia: A classification with guidelines for diagnosis and management. *Gastroenterol Int* 1991;4:145–160.

Talley NJ, Nyren O, Drossman DA, Heaton KW, Veldhuyzen van Zanten SJO, Koch MM, Ransohoff DF. The irritable bowel syndrome: Toward optimal design of controlled treatment trials. *Gastroenterol Int* 1994;6:189–211.

Thompson WG. Dyspepsia: Is a trial of therapy appropriate? *Can Med Assoc J* 1995;153:293–299.

Thompson WG, Creed F, Drossman DA, Heaton KW, Mazzacca G. Functional bowel disorders and functional abdominal pain. *Gastroenterol Int* 1992;5:75–91.

CHAPTER FOUR

Abercrombie J. *Pathological and Practical Research on Diseases of the Stomach*. Edinburgh, 1830.

Allbutt TC. The Gulstonion lectures on neuroses of the viscera. *Br Med J* 1884;1:495–499.

Alvarez WC. *Nervousness, Indigestion, and Pain*. New York: Popular Edition, P.F. Collier Inc., 1962.

Allen RN. Dylan PW, Keighley RB, eds. History, epidemiology and mortality. In *Gastrointestinal Haemorrhage*. Bristol: Wright, 1981.

Alexander F. The influence of psychologic factors upon gastrointestinal disturbance. *Symposium Psychoanal Quart* 1934;3:501–539.

Allison PR. Peptic ulcer of the esophagus. *J. Thoracic Surgery* 1946;15:308–317.

Baron JH. History of the gastric ferment. *Gastroent International* 1991;4:143.

Baron JH. The discovery of gastric acid. *Gastroent* 1979;76:1056–1064.

Barrett NR. Chronic peptic ulcer of the esophagus and "esophagitis." *Br J Surg* 1950;37:175–182.

Beaumont W. *Experiments and Observations on the Gastric Juice and the Physiology of Digestion*. Plattsburg: F.P. Allen, 1883.

Black J. Reflections on the analytical pharmacology of histamine H_2 receptor antagonists. *Gastroenterology* 1993;105:963–968.

Clark A. Cases of duodenal perforation. *Brit Med J* 1867; 1:671–684.

Crampton J, Travers B. Rupture of the stomach and escape of its contents. *Med-Chi Trans* 1817;8:228–235.

Cruveilhier J. *Maladies de 1'Estomac de l'Antomie Pathologique du Corps Human*. Vol. 1. Paris;Bailliere, 1835.

Curling TB. Acute ulceration of the duodenum in cases of burn. *Med-Chi Trans* 1842;35:260–281.

Davenport HW. Gastric mucosal injury by fatty and acetylsalicylic acid. *Gastroenterology* 1964;46:245–253.

Davenport HW. *A History of Gastric Secretion and Digestion*. New York: Oxford University Press; 1992.

Doenges JL. Spirochetes in the gastric glands of Macacus Rhesus and of Man without related disease. *Arch Path* 1939;27:469–477.

Doll R. Dietetic treatment of peptic ulcer. *Lancet* 1956:i:5–9.

Doll R, Hill ID, Hutten C, Underwood DJ. Clinical trial of a triterpenoid liquorice compound in gastric and duodenal ulcer. *Lancet* 1962;2:793–796.

Dragstedt LR, Fournier HJ, Woodward ER, Touee ET, Harper PV, Jr. Transabdominal gastric vagotomy. *Surg Gynecol Obstet* 1947;85:461–466.

Dragstedt LR, Owens FM. Supra-diaphragmatic sections of the vagus nerves in the treatment of duodenal ulcer. *Proc Nutr Soc* 1943;53:152–154.

Earlam R, Cunha-Melo JR. Benign oesophageal strictures: Historical and technical aspects of dilatation. *Br J Surg* 1981;68:829–834.

Edkins JS. The chemical mechanism of gastric secretion. *J Physiol Lond* 1906;34:133–144.

Engel GL. "Psychogenic" pain and pain-prone patient. *Am J Med* 1959;26:899–918.

Fenwick WS. *Dyspepsia: Its Varieties and Treatment*. Philadelphia: W.B. Saunders, 1924.

Fry J. Peptic ulcer: A profile. *Brit Med J* 1964;2:809–812.

Fye WB. The history of medicine: An annotated list of key reference works. *Ann Intern Med* 1993;118:59–62.

Ganzer Al and Forte JG. K-stimulated ATPase in purified microsomes of bullfrog oxyntic cells. *Biochim Biophys Acta* 1973;307:169–180.

Gregory RA, Tracy HJ. The constitution and properties of two gastrins extracted from hog antral mucosa. *Gut* 1964;5:103–114.

Gunsberg F. Zur Kritik des magensgeschwurs, inbesonders des perforischenden. *Arch Physiol Heilk* 1852;11:516–527.

Hirschowitz BI. Development and application of endoscopy. *Gastroenterology* 1993;104:337–342.

Hoetzel F. Quoted In: *Samson Wright's Applied Physiology*, 9th ed. Maizels M, Jepson JP (eds.), London: Oxford University Press, 1928: 787.

Jackson C. The diaphragmatic pinch-cock in so-called "cardiospasm." *Laryngoscope* 1922;32:139–141.

Hopkins HH, Kapany NS. A flexible fibrescope, using static scanning. *Nature* 1954;173:39–41.

Kussmaul A. Uber die behandlung der magengenereweiterung durch eine neue methode mittelst der magenpumpe. *Deutsch Arch f.Klin M.* 1869;6:455–460.

Lennard–Jones JE, Barbouris N. Effect of certain foods on the acidity of the gastric contents. *Gut* 1965;6:113–117.

Long J. Post-mortem appearances found after burns. *Lond Med Gaz* 1840;NSi:743–750.

Marshall BJ. Pyloric campylobacter infection and gastroduodenal disease. *Med J Aust* 1985;142:436–444.

Marshall BJ, Warren JR. Unidentified curved bacilli in the stomach of patients with gastritis and peptic ulceration. *Lancet* 1984;i:1311–1314.

Mayo Robson A. The surgery of the stomach. *Lancet* 1900;1:671–684.

Mayo WJ. A discussion on the surgical treatment of duodenal ulcer. *Brit Med J* 1906; ii:1299–1302.

Moynihan BGA. *Duodenal Ulcer* (second edition). Philadelphia: W.B. Saunders, 1912.

Moynihan BGA. Hunterian Lecture: Some problems of gastric and duodenal ulcer *Brit Med J* 1923;1:221–226

Osler W. Principles and Practice of Medicine (first edition). Edinburgh: Pentland, 1892.

Palmer ED. *Functional Gastrointestinal Disease*. Baltimore: Williams and Wilkins, 1967.

Pavlov I., Thompson WH, eds. in *The Work of the Digestive Glands*. London: C. Griffen and Company, 1910.

Phsysick PS. Account of a new mode of extracting poisonous substances from the stomach. *Eclectic Repertory and Analytical Rev* 1813;3:111.

Prout W. On the nature of the acid and saline matters usually existing in the stomachs of animals. *Phil Trans Roy Soc* 1824;1:45–49.

Rawlinson C. Philosophical transactions of the Royal Society 1727;XXXV:361–362.

Rehfuss ME. *Indigestion: Its Diagnosis and Management*. Philadelphia: Saunders, 1943;236.

Schindler R. Ein Vollig ungefahrliches, flexibles Gastroskop. *Munchener Wochenschr* 1932;79:1268–1269.

Schwarz K. Uber penetrierende magen und jejunalgeschwure. *Beitrage zur Klinischen Chirurgie* 1910;67:96–128.

Sippy BW. Gastric and duodenal ulcer. *JAMA* 1915;LXIV:1625–1630.

Spechler SJ, Goyol RK. The columnar-lined esophagus, intestinal metaplasia and Norman Barrett. *Gastroenterology* 1996;110:614–621.

Travers B. *Medico-Chirurgical Transactions* 1817; viii: 228–235.

Warren JR, Marshall BJ. Unidentified curved bacilli on gastric epithelium in active chronic gastritis. *Lancet* 1983;1:1273–1275.

Williams JG, Deakin M. *Classic Papers in Peptic Ulcer*. London: Science Press, 1988.

Willis T. *Pharmaceutice rationalis: sive diatrabe demedicorum; operationibus in humano corpore*. London: Hagae-Comitis, 1674.

Winkelstein A. Peptic esophagitis: a new clinical entity. *JAMA* 1935;104:906–909.

Warren JR. Unidentified curved bacilli on gastric epithelium in active chronic gastritis, *Lancet* 1983;1:1273 (Letter).

Wolf BS, Marshak RH, Som ML. Peptic ulcer and peptic ulcer of the esophagus. *Am J Roentgenol Radium Ther Nucl Med* 1958;79:741–759.

Wolf S, Wolff HG. Evidence on the genesis of peptic ulcer in man. *JAMA* 1942;120:670–675.

Zollinger RM, Ellison EH. Primary peptic ulcerations of the jejunum associated with islet cell tumors of the pancreas. *Ann Surg* 1955;142:709–723.

CHAPTER FIVE

Drossman DA, Li Z, Andruzzi E, et al. U.S. householder survey of functional gastrointestinal disorders: Prevalence, sociodemography and health impact. *Dig Dis Sci* 1993;38:1569–1580.

Fry J. Peptic ulcer: A profile. *Brit Med J* 1964;2:809–812.

Greibe J, Bugge P, Gjorup T, Lauritzen T, Bonnevie O, Wulff HR. Long-term prognosis of duodenal ulcer: Follow-up study and survey of doctors' estimates. BMJ 1977;2:1572–1574.

Jones R, Lydeard SE. Prevalence of symptoms of dyspepsia in the community. *Br Med J* 1989;298:30–32.

Langman MSJ., Carter DC, eds. *Peptic Ulcer Disease*. New York: Churchill Livingstone; 1985, Chapter 1:1–13.

Lindell G, Celebioglu F, Stael von Holstein C, Graffner H. On the natural history of peptic ulcer. *Scand J Gastroenterol* 1994;29:979–982.

Mayo WJ. A discussion on the surgical treatment of duodenal ulcer. *Brit Med J* 1906;ii:1299–1302.

Nebel OT, Fornes MF, Castell DO. Symptomatic gastroesophageal reflux: Incidence and precipitating factors. *Amer J Dig Dis* 1976;21:953–956.

Porro GB, Petrillo M. The natural history of ulcer disease: the influence of H_2 antagonist therapy. *Scand J Gastroenterol* 1986;21:46–52.

Schlemper RJ, van der Werf SD, Van den brouche JP, Biemond J, Lamers CB. Peptic ulcer, non-ulcer dyspepsia and irritable bowel syndrome in The Netherlands and Japan. *Scand J Gastroenterology* 1993;Suppl 200:33–41.

Thompson WG, Heaton KW. Functional bowel disorders in apparently healthy people. *Gastroenterology* 1980;79:283–288.

Thompson WG, Heaton KW. Heartburn and globus in apparently healthy people. *Can Med Assn J* 1982;126:46–48.

CHAPTER SIX

Goldschmiedt M, Feldman M. Gastric secretion in health and disease. In Sleisenger MH, Fordtran JS, eds. *Gastrointestinal Disease: Pathophysiology/Diagnosis/Treatment* (fifth edition). Philadelphia: W.B. Saunders, 1993;524–544.

Sachs G., Hersey SJ. *The Gastric Parietal Cell.* Oxford: Oxford Clinical Communications, 1994; p.7.

Schwarz, K. Ueber penetrierende Megen-und Jejunalgeschw re. *Beitrage zur Clinischer Chirurguire* 1910;67:96–128.

CHAPTER SEVEN

Allison MC, Howatson HG, Torrance CJ, Lee FD, Russell RI. Gastrointestinal damage associated with the use of antiinflammatory drugs. *New Engl J Med* 1992;327:749–754.

Bateman DN. NSAIDS: Time to reevaluate gut toxicity. *Lancet* 1994;343:1051–1052.

Carson JL, Strom BL, Morse ML, West SL, Soper KA, Stolley PD, Jones JK. The relative gastrointestinal toxicity of the nonsteroidal anti-inflammatory drugs. *Arch Intern Med* 1987;147:1054–1059.

Committee on Safety of Medicines. Non-steroidal anti-inflammatory drugs and serious gastrointestinal adverse effects. *Br Med J* 1986;392:1190–1191.

Griffen MR, Piper JM, Daugherty JR, Snowden M, Ray WA. Nonsteroidal anti-inflammatory drug use and increased risk for peptic ulcer disease in elderly persons. *Ann Intern Med* 1991;114:257–263.

Hayllar J, Bjarnason I. NSAIDs, Cox-2 inhibitors, and the gut. *Lancet* 1995;346:521–522.

Hogan DB, Campbell NRC, Crutcher RJ, Jennet P, Macleod N. Prescription of nonsteroidal anti-inflammatory drugs for elderly people in Alberta. *Can Med Assoc J* 1994;151:315–322.

Langman MJS. Treating ulcers in patients receiving NSAIDs. *Q J Med* 1989;73:1089–1091.

Langman MJS, Weil J, Wainwright P, Lawson DH, Rawlins MD, Logan RFA, Murphy M, Vessey MP, Collin-Jones DG. Risks of bleeding peptic ulcer associated with individual non-steroidal anti-inflammatory drugs. *Lancet* 1994;343:1075–1078.

Laporte J, Carne X, Vidal X, Moreno V, Juan J. Upper gastrointestinal bleeding in relation to previous use of analgesics and non-steroidal anti-inflammatory drugs. *Lancet* 1991;337:85–89.

Rodriquez LAG, Jick H. Risk of upper gastrointestinal bleeding and perforation associated with individual non-steroidal anti-inflammatory drugs. *Lancet* 1994;343:769–772.

Sarosiek J, Marcinkiewicz CZ, Parolisi S, Peura DA. Prostaglandin E2 content in residual gastric juice reflects endoscopic damage to the gastric mucosa after naproxen sodium administration. *Am J Gastroenterol* 1996;91:873–8.

Savage RL, Moller PW, Ballantyne CL, Wells JE. Variation in the risk of peptic ulcer complications with nonsteroidal antiinflammatory drug therapy. *Arthritis Rheum* 1996;36:84–90.

Shaffer E. The role of prostaglandins and cytoprotection in NSAID-induced gastropathy. *Can Therap* 1993(Oct);53–57.

Soll AH. Gastric, duodenal, and stress ulcer. In Sleisenger MH, Fordtran JS, eds. *Gastrointestinal Disease: Pathophysiology/Diagnosis/Treatment* (fifth edition). Philadelphia: W.B. Saunders, 1993;580–679.

Taha AS, Dahill S, Sturrock RD, Lee FD, Russell RI. Predicting NSAID related ulcers—Assessment of clinical and pathological risk factors and importance of differences in NSAIDs. *Gut* 1994;35:891–895.

Taha AS, Sturrock RD, Russell RI. Mucosal erosions in longterm non-steroidal antiinflammatory drug users: Predisposition to ulceration and relation to *Helicobacter pylori. Gut* 1995;36:334–336.

Taha AS, Hudson N, Hawkey CJ, Swannell EJ, Trye PN, Cottrell J, Mann SG, Simon TJ, Sturrock RD, Russell RI. Famotidine for the prevention of gastric and duodenal ulcers caused by nonsteroidal antiinflammatory drugs. *New Engl J Med* 1996;334:1435–9.

Van der Merwe CF. A different and physiological approach to manipulating the inflammatory response. *Eur J Gastroenterol Hepatol* 1993;5:433–436.

Walt RP, Wallace JR, Shorrock CR, Hudson N, Hawkey CJ, Porro GB, Lazzaroni M. Non-steroidal antiinflammatory drugs in the upper gastrointestinal tract. Review in depth. *Eur J Gastroenterol Hepatol* 1993;5:401–432.

CHAPTER EIGHT

Barbara L, Camilleri M, Corinaldesi R, Crean GP, Heading RC, Johnson AG, Malagelada JR, Stanghellini V, Weirbech M. Definition and investigation of dyspepsia. Consensus of an international working party. *Dig Dis Sci* 1989;34:1272–1276.

Cullen DJE, Collins BJ, Kristiansen KJ, Epis J, Warren JR, Surveyer I, Cullen KJ. When is *Helicobacter pylori* acquired? *Gut* 1993;34:1681–162.

Cutler AF, Havstad S, Ma CK, *et al.* Accuracy of invasive and noninvasive tests to diagnose *Helicobacter pylori* infection. *Gastroent* 1995;109:136–141.

Davis GR. Neoplasma of the stomach. In Sleisenger MH, Fordtran JS, eds. *Gastrointestinal Disease: Pathophysiology/Diagnosis/Treatment* (fifth edition). Philadelphia: WB Saunders, 1993; 763–791.

Dubos RJ. Man adapting: Quoted in *Familiar Medical Quotations*. Strauss MB. (ed.) Boston: Little Brown, 1968:241.

Goddard A, Logan R. One-week low-dose triple therapy: New standards for *Helicobacter pylori* treatment. *Eur J Gastroenterol Hepatol* 1995;7:1–3.

Harris A, Misiewicz JJ. Hitting *H pylori* for four. *Lancet* 1995;345:806–807.

Hawkey CJ. Eradication of *Helicobacter pylori* should be pivotal in managing peptic ulceration: Eradication largely prevents relapse. *Br Med J* 1994;309:1570–1571.

Hudson M, Brydon WG, Eastwood MA, Ferguson A, Palmer KR. Successful *Helicobacter pylori* eradication incorporating a one-week antibiotic regimen. *Aliment Pharmacol Therap* 1995;9:47–50.

Korman MG, Marks IN, Hunt RH, Axon A, Blazer MJ, McCarthy DM, Tytgat GNJ. *Helicobacter pylori*: A workshop review. *Eur J Gastroenterol Hepatol* 1994;5:953–967.

Langman MJS, Weil J, Wainwright P, Lawson DH, Rawlins MD, Logan RFA, Murphy M, Vessey MP, Collin-Jones DG. Risks of bleeding peptic ulcer associated with individual non-steroidal anti-inflammatory drugs. *Lancet* 1994;343:1075–1078.

Lebenz J, Stolte M, Ruhl GH, Becker T, Tillenberg B, Sollbohmer M, Borsch G. One-week low-dose triple therapy for the eradication of *Helicobacter pylori* infection. *Eur J Gastroenterol Hepatol* 1995;7:9–11.

Malaty HM, Engstrand L, Pedersen NL, Graham DY. *Helicobacter pylori* infection: genetic and environmental influences—a study of twins. *Ann Intern Med* 1994;120:982–985.

Mendall MA, Jazrawi RP, Marrero JM, Molineaux N, Levi J, Maxwell JD, Northfield TC. Serology for *Helicobater pylori* compared with symptom questionnaires in screening before direct access endoscopy. *Gut* 1995;36:330–333.

Moss S, Calem J. Acid secretion and sensitivity to gastrin in patients with duodenal ulcer: Effect of eradication of *Helicobacter pylori*. Gut 1993;34:888–892.

NIH Consensus Conference. *Helicobacter pylori* in peptic ulcer disease. *JAMA* 1994;272:65–68.

Nomura A, Stemmerman GM, Chyou P, Perez-Perez GI, Blaser MJ. *Helicobacter pylori* infection and the risk for duodenal and gastric ulceration. *Ann Intern Med* 1994;120:977–981.

Olbe L, Hamlet A, Dalenbach J, Fandriks L. A mechanism by which *Helicobacter pylori* infection of the antrum contributes to the development of duodenal ulcer. *Gastroent* 1996;110:1386–94.

Patel P, Mendall MA, Khulusi H, Molineaux N, Levy J, Maxwell JD, Northfield TC. Salivary antibodies to *Helicobacter pylori*: Screening dyspeptic patients before endoscopy. *Lancet* 1994;344:511–513.

Rabeneck L, Ransohoff DF. Is *Helicobacter pylori* a cause of duodenal ulcer? A methodologic critique of current evidence. *Am J Med* 1991;91:556–572.

Record CO. *Helicobacter pylori* is not the causative agent. *Br Med J* 1994;309:15711572.

Riccardi VM, Rotter JI. Familial *Helicobacter pylori* infection: Societal factors, human genetics and bacterial genetics. *Ann Intern Med* 1994;120:1043–1044.

Slomianski A, Schubert T, Cutler AF. ^{13}C urea breath test to confirm eradication of *Helicobacter pylori*. *Am J Gastroenterol* 1995;90:224–226.

Smoot DT. *Helicobacter pylori* diagnostic tests. Benefits, sensitivity, and specificity (Abstract). *Helicobacter pylori in Peptic Ulcer Disease.* National Institute of Health, Washington, D.C. Consensus development conference 1994;77–79.

Tytgat GNJ, Lee A, Graham DY, Dixon MF, Rokkas T. The role of infectious agents in peptic ulcer disease. *Gastroenterol Int* 1993;6:76–89.

Warren JR. Unidentified curved bacilli on gastric epithelium in chronic active gastritis. *Lancet* 1983;i:1273 (Letter).

Weinstein WM. Gastritis and gastropathies. In Sleisenger MH, Fordtran JS, eds. *Gastrointestinal Disease: Pathophysiology/Diagnosis/Management* (fifth edition). Philadelphia: W.B. Saunders, 1993; 545–571.

Zala G, Giezendenner S, Flury R, Wast J, Meyenberger C, Ammann R, Wirth HP. Omeprazole/amoxacillin: Impaired eradication of *Helicobacter pylori* by smoking but not by omeprazole pretreatment. *Schweiz Med Wochenschr* 1994;124:1398–1404.

CHAPTER NINE

Aird I, Bentall HH, Mehigan JA, Fraser Roberts JA. The blood groups in relation to peptic ulceration and carcinoma of colon, rectum, breast and bronchus. *Br Med J* 1954;2:315–321.

Alexander F. *Psychosomatic Medicine: Its Principles and Applications.* New York: W.W. Norton, 1950.

Beaumont W. Experiments and observations on the gastric juice and the physiology of digestion. Plattsburgh, New York: F.P. Allen, 1833.

Chey WD, Spybrook M, Carpenter S, Nostrant TT, Elta GH, Scheman, JM. Prolonged effect of omeprazole on the ^{14}C urea breath test. *Amer J Gastroenterology* 1996;91:89–92.

Gledhill T, Leidester RJ, Addis B, Lightfoot N, Barnard J, Viney N, Darkin D, Hunt RH. Epidemic achlorhydria. *Br Med J* 1985;290:1384–1386.

Hoetzel F. Quoted in *Samson Wright's Applied Physiology.* Maizels M, Jepson JP, eds. London: Oxford University Press; 1928; 787.

Khulusi S, Badue S, Patel P, Lloyd R, Marrero JR, Finfayson C, Mandall MA, Northfield TC. Pathogenesis of gastric metaplasia of the human duodenum: Role of *Helicobacter pylori*, gastric acid, and ulceration. *Gastroenterology* 1996;110:452–458.

Langman MJS, Doll R. ABO blood group and secretor status in relation to clinical characteristics of peptic ulcers. *Gut* 1965;6:270–273.

Levenstein S, Prantara C, Varvo V, Scribino ML, Berto E, Spinella S, Lanari G. Patterns of biologic and psychologic risk factors in duodenal ulcer patients. *J Clin Gastroenterol* 1995;21:110–117.

Mirsky A. Physiologic, psychologic and social determinants in the etiology of peptic ulcer. *Am J Dig Dis* 1958;3:285–313.

Slomiauski A, Schubert T, Cutler AF. [13]C urea breath test to confirm eradication of *Helicobacter pylori*. *Amer J Gastroenterology* 1995;90:224–226.

Soll AH. Gastric, duodenal, and stress ulcer. In Sleisenger MH, Fordtran JS, eds. *Gastrointestinal Disease: Pathophysiology/Diagnosis/Treatment* (fifth edition). Philadelphia: W.B. Saunders, 1993; 580–679.

Sontag S, Graham DY, Belsito A, Weiss J, Farley A, Grunt R, Cimetidine, cigarette smoking, and recurrence of duodenal ulcer. *New Engl J Med* 1984;311:689–693.

Thompson WG. *The Irritable Gut.* Baltimore: University Park Press, 1979.

Weiner H. From simplicity to complexity (1950–1990): The case of peptic ulceration—I. Human studies. *Psychosom Med* 1991;53:467–490.

Wolf S, Wolff HG. *Human Gastric Function.* New York: Oxford University Press, 1943.

CHAPTER TEN

Axon ATR, Bell GD, Jones RH, Quine MA, McCloy RF. Guidelines on appropriate indications for upper abdominal endoscopy. *Br Med J* 1995;310:853–856.

Bainton DG, Davies GT, Evans KT, Gravellel IH. Gallbladder disease. *New Engl J Med* 1976;294:1147–1149.

Bytzer P. Diagnosing dyspepsia: Any controversies left? *Gastroenterology* 1996;110:302–306.

Bytzer P, Hansen JM, Schlaffalitzky de Muckadell OB. Empirical H2-blocker therapy or prompt endoscopy in management of dyspepsia. *Lancet* 1994;343:811–816.

Barbara L, Sama C, Marselli Labate AM, Taroni F, Rusticali AG, Festi D, Sapio C, Roda E, Banterie C, Puci A. A population study on the prevalence of gallstone disease: the Sirmione study. *Hepatology* 1987;7:913–917.

Greenberg PD, Koch H, Cello JP. Clinical utility and cost effectiveness of *Helicobacter pylori* testing for patients with duodenal and gastric ulcers. *Amer J. Gastroenterol* 1996;91:228–232.

Deaver JB. Gastric neuroses. *Am J Med Sci* 1909;137:157–166.

Fendrick AM, Chernew ME, Hirth RA, Bloom BS. Alternative management strategies for patients with suspected ulcer disease. *Ann Int Med* 1995;123:260–268.

George R, Hellier MD, Kennedy HJ, Smits BJ. Definition and sub-typing of non-ulcer dyspepsia. *Gastroenterol Int* 1993;6:93–99.

Graham DY, Rabenec KL. Patients, payers, and paradigm shifts: What to do about *Helicobacter pylori. Amer J Gastroenterol* 1996;91:188–189.

Hungin APS, Thomas PR, Bramble MG, Corbett WA, Idle N, Contractor BR, Berridge DC, Cann G. What happens to patients following open access gastroscopy? An outcome study from general practice. *Brit J Gen Pract* 1994;44:519–521.

Hutchison R. *Lectures on Dyspepsia* (second edition). London: Edward Arnold, 1927.

Koch JP, Donaldson RM. A survey of food intolerances in hospitalized patients. *New Engl J Med* 1964;271:657–660.

Lindell G, Celebioglu F, Stael von Holstein C, Graffner H. On the natural history of peptic ulcer. *Scand J Gastroenterol* 1994;29:979–982.

Mendall MA, Jazrawi RP, Marrero JM, Molineaux N, Levi J, Maxwell JD, Northfield TC. Serology for *Helicobacter pylori* compared with symptom questionnaires in screening before direct access endoscopy. *Gut* 1995;36:330–333.

Moynihan B. A Hunterian lecture: Some problems of gastric and duodenal ulcer. *Br Med J* 1923;1:221–226.

Nansen JM, Bytzer P, Bondesen S, Schaffalitzky de Muckadell OB. Efficacy and outcome of an open access endoscopy service. *Dan Med Bull* 1993;38:388–391.

NIH Consensus Conference. *Helicobacter pylori* in peptic ulcer disease. *JAMA* 1994;272:65–68.

Nyren O, Lindberg G, Lindstrom E, Marke L, Seensalu R. Economic costs of functional dyspspsia. *Pharmacoeconomics* 1992;1:312–324.

Patel P, Mendall MA, Khulusi H, Molineaux N, Levy J, Maxwell JD, Northfield TC. Salivary antibodies to *Helicobacter pylori*: Screening dyspeptic patients before endoscopy. *Lancet* 1994;344:511–513.

Price WH. Gallbladder dyspepsia. *Br Med J* 1963;ii:138–141.

Silverstein MD, Petterson T, Talley NJ. Initial endoscopy or empiric therapy for dyspepsia: A toss-up. Gastroenterology 1996;110:72–83.

Spiro HM. Moynihan's disease? *New Engl J Med* 1974;291:567–569.

Talley NJ, Colin-Jones D, Koch KL, Koch M, Nyren O, Stanghellini V. Functional dyspepsia: A classification with guidelines for diagnosis and management. *Gastroenterol Int* 1991;4:145–160.

Talley NJ, Weaver AL, Tesmer DL, Zinsmeister AR. Lack of discriminant value of dyspspsia subgroups in patients referred for surgery. *Gastroenterology* 1993;105:1378–1386.

Tham TC, McLaughlin N, Hughes DF, Ferguson, Crosbie JJ, Madden M, Namnyet S, O'Connor FA. Possible role of *Helicobacter pylori* serology in reducing endoscopy workload. *Postgrad Med J* 1994;70:809–812.

Thompson WG. *The Irritable Gut.* Baltimore: University Park Press, 1979.

Thompson WG. Dyspepsia: Is a trial of therapy appropriate? *Can Med Assoc J* 1995;153:293–299.

CHAPTER ELEVEN

Abercrombie J. *Pathological and Practical Research on Diseases of the Stomach.* Edinburgh: 1830.

Crean GP, Holden RJ, Knill-Jones RP, Beattie AD, James WB, Majoribanks FM, Spiegelhalter DJ. A database on dyspepsia. *Gut* 1994;34:191–202.

Duggen JM. Is the aggressive management of peptic ulcer justified by the data? *J Clin Gastroenterol* 1993;17:109–116.

Priebe WM, DaCosta LR, Beck IT. Is epigastric tenderness a sign of peptic ulcer disease? *Gastroenterology* 1982;82:16–19.

Silverstein FE, Graham DY, *et al.* Misoprostol reduces serious gastrointestinal complications in patients with rheumatoid arthritis receiving nonsteroidal anti-inflammatory drugs. *Ann Intern Med* 1995;123:241–249.

Soll AH. Gastric, duodenol, and stress ulcer. In Sleisenger MH, Fordtran JS, eds. *Gastrointestinal Disease: Pathophysiology/Diagnosis/Treatment* (fifth edition). Philadelphia: W.B. Saunders, 1993; 580–679.

Walsh IH, Peterson WL. The treatment of *Helicobacter pylori* infection in the management of peptic ulcer disease. *New Engl J Med* 1995;333:984–989.

Walt RP. Drug therapy: Misoprostol for the treatment of peptic ulcer and antiinflammatory-drug-induced gastroduodenal ulceration. *New Engl J Med* 1992;327:1575–1580.

CHAPTER TWELVE

Ben-Menachem T, Fogel R, Patel RV, Touchette M, Zarowitz BJ, Hadzijahic N, Devine G, Vester J, Brasalier R. Prophylaxis for stress-related gastric hemorrhage in the medical intensive care unit. *Ann Intern Med* 1994;121:568–575.

Cook DJ, Fuller HD, Guyatt GH, Marshall JC, Leasa D, Hall R. Risk factors for gastrointestinal bleeding in critically ill patients. *New Engl J Med* 1994;330:377–381.

Driks MR, Craven DE, Celli BR, Manning M, Burke RA, Garvin GM, Kunches LM, Farber HW, Wedel SA, McCabe WR. Nosicomial pneumonia in intubated patients given sucralfate as compared with antacids or histamine type 2 blockers. *New Engl J Med* 1987;317:1376–1382.

Noseworthy TW, Shustack A, Johnston RG, Anderson BJ, Konopad E, Grace M. A randomized clinical trial comparing ranitidine and antacids in critically ill patients. *Crit Care Med* 1987;15:817–819.

Peterson WL. Prevention of upper gastrointestinal bleeding. *New Engl J Med* 1994;330:428–429.

Soll AH. Gastric, duodenal, and stress ulcer. In Sleisenger MH, Fordtran JS, eds. *Gastrointestinal Disease: Pathophysiology/Diagnosis/Treatment* (fifth edition). Philadelphia: W.B. Saunders, 1993;580–679.

Zollinger RM, Ellison EH. Primary peptic ulcers of the jejunum associated with islet cell tumors of the pancreas. *Ann Surg* 1955;142:709–723.

CHAPTER THIRTEEN

Graham DY. Ulcer complications and their nonoperative treatment. In Sleisenger MH, Fordtran JS, eds. *Gastrointestinal Disease: Pathophysiology/Diagnosis/Management* (fifth edition). Philadelphia: W.B. Saunders, 1993;698–712.

Longstreth JF. Epidemiology of hospitalization for acute upper gastrointestinal hemmorrhage: A population based study. *Am J Gastroenterol* 1995;90:206–210.

Longstreth GF, Feiterberg SP. Outpatient care of selected patients with acute nonvariceal upper gastrointestinal haemorrhage. *Lancet* 1995;345:108–11.

MacDonald JD. Son et lumicre? *Br Med J* 1973;2:676 (Letter).

Thomson ABR. Therapeutic options for patients bleeding with peptic ulcers. *Can J Gastroenterol* 1994;8:269–274.

CHAPTER FOURTEEN

Heine KJ, Mittal RK. Crural diaphragm and lower esophageal sphincter as antireflux barriers. *Viewpoints Dig Dis* 1991;23:1–6.

Jackson C. The diaphragmatic pinch-cock in so-called "Cardiospasm." *Laryngoscope* 1922;32:139–142.

Johnstone BT, Lewis SA, Love AHG. Psychological factors in gastro-esophageal reflux disease. *Gut* 1995;36:481–482.

Pope CE. Acid-reflux disorders. *New Engl J Med* 1994;331:656–660.

Shay SS, Conwell DL, Mehindru V, Hertz B. The effect of posture on gastroesophageal reflux event frequency and composition during fasting. *Am J Gastroenterol* 1996;91:54–60.

Shi G, Bruley des Varannes S, Scarpignato C, Le Rhun M, Galmiche JP. Reflux
symptoms in patients with normal oesophageal exposure to acid. *Gut*
1995;37:457–464.

Shoeman MN, Holloway RH. Integrity and characteristics of secondary oesophageal peristalsis in patients with gastro-oesophageal reflux disease. *Gut*
1995;36:499–504.

Thompson WG. *Gut Reactions*. New York: Plenum Press, 1989.

Trifan A, Shaker R, Ren J, Mittal RK, Saean K, Dua K, Kusano M. Inhibition of resting
lower esophageal sphincter pressure by pharyngeal water stimulation in humans. *Gastroenterology* 1995;108:441–446.

CHAPTER FIFTEEN

Feldman M, Barnett C. Relationships between acidity and osmolarity of popular
beverages and reported postprandial heartburn. *Gastroenterology*
1995;108:125–131.

Johnson NJ, Boyd EJ, Mills JG, Wood JR. Treatment of reflux esophagitis: A multicen-
tre trial to compare 150mg ranitidine bd with 300 mg ranitidine qds. *Aliment
Pharmacol Therap* 1989;3:259.

Johnstone BT, Lewis SA, Love AHG. Psychological factors in gastro-esophageal
reflux disease. *Gut* 1995;36:481–482.

Orlando RC. Esophageal epithelial defences. *Am J Gastroenterol* 1994;89:S48–452.

Pope CE. Acid-reflux disorders. *New Engl J Med* 1994;331:656–660.

Serosiek J, Scheurich CJ, Marcinkiewicz M, McCallum RW. Enhancement of salivary
esophagoprotection: rationale for a physiologic approach to gastroesophageal
reflux disease. Gastroent 1996;110:675–681.

Shi G, Bruley des Varannes S, Scarpignato C, Le Rhun M, Galmiche JP. Reflux
symptoms in patients with normal oesophageal exposure to acid. *Gut*
1995;37:457–464.

CHAPTER SIXTEEN

Freston JW. Omeprazole, hypergastrinaemia and gastric carcinoid tumours. *Ann
Intern Med* 1994;121:232–233.

Katz LC, Just R, Castell DO. Body position affects recumbant postprandial reflux. *J
Clin Gastroenterol* 1994;18:280–283.

Klinkenberg-Knol EC, Festen HPM, Jansen JBMJ, Lamers CBHW, Nelis F, Snel P,
Lukers A, Dekkers CPM, Havn N, Meuwissen SGM. Long-term treatment with
omeprazole for refractory reflux esophagitis: efficacy and safety. *Ann Intern Med*
1994;121:161–167.

McDonald-Haile J, Bradley LA, Bailey MA, Schan CA, Richter JE. Relaxation training reduces symptom reports and acid exposure in patients with gastroesophageal reflux disease. *Gastroenterology* 1994;107:61–69.

Nebel OT, Fornes MF, Castell DO. Symptomatic gastroesophageal reflux: incidence and precipitating factors. *Am J Dig Dis* 1976;21:953–956.

Pope CE. Acid-reflux disorders. *New Engl J Med* 1994;331:656–660.

Richter JE. Heartburn, dysphagia, odynophagia, and other esophageal symptoms. In Sleisenger MH, Fordtran JS, eds. *Gastrointestinal Disease: Pathophysiology/Diagnosis/Management* (fifth edition). Philadelphia: WB Saunders, 1993;331–340.

Shay SS, Conwell DL, Mehindru V, Hertz B. The effect of posture on gastroesophageal reflux event frequency and composition during fasting. *Am J Gastroenterol* 1996;91:54–60.

Thompson WG. *Gut Reactions*. New York: Plenum Press, 1989.

Thompson WG, Heaton KW. Heartburn and globus in apparently healthy people. *Can Med Assn J* 1982;126:46–48.

Tytgat GNJ. Long-term therapy for reflux esophagitis. *New Engl J Med* 1995;333:1148–1150.

Vigneri S, Termini R, Leandro G, Badalamenti S, Pantalena M, Savarino V, et al. A comparison of five maintenance therapies for reflux esophagitis. *New Engl J Med* 1995;333:1106–1110.

CHAPTER SEVENTEEN

Barrett NR. Chronic peptic ulcer of the esophagus and "esophagitis." *Br J Surg* 1950;37:175–182.

Earlam R, Cunha-Melo JR. Benign oesophageal strictures: Historical and technical aspects of dilatation. *Br J Surg* 1981;68:829–834.

Goddard A, Logan R. One-week low-dose triple therapy: new standards for *Helicobacter pylori* treatment. *Eur J Gastroenterol Hepatology* 1995;7:1–3.

Hameeteman W, Tytgat GNJ, Houthoff HJ, Van den Tweel JG. Barrett's esophagus: Development of dysplasia and adenocarcinoma. *Gastroenterology* 1989;96:1249–1256.

Kahrilas PJ, Hogan WJ. Gastroesophageal reflux disease. In Sleisenger MH, Fordtran JS, eds. *Gastrointestinal Disease: Pathophysiology/Diagnosis/Treatment* (fifth edition). Philadelphia: W.B. Saunders, 1993;378–401.

Pope CE. Acid-reflux disorders. *New Engl J Med* 1994;331:656–660.

Sampliner RE. Effect of up to 3 years of high-dose lansoprazole on Barrett's esophagus. *Am J Gastroenterol* 1994;89:1844–1848.

Smith PM, Kerr GD, Cockel R, Ross BA, Bate CM, Brown P. A comparison of omeprazole and ranitidine in the prevention of recurrence of benign esophageal stricture. *Gastroenterology* 1994;107:1312–1318.

Thompson WG. *Gut Reactions*. New York: Plenum Press, 1989.

Thompson WG. Pharmacotherapy of an ulcer in Barrett's esophagus: Carbonoxalone and cimetidine. *Gastroenterology* 1977;73:808–810.

Thompson WG, Heaton KW. Heartburn and globus in apparently healthy people. *Can Med Assn J* 1982;126:46–48.

Webb WA. Esophageal dilation: Personal experience with current instruments and techniques. *Am J Gastroenterol* 1988;83:471–475.

Schatzki R, Gary JE. Dysphagia due to a diaphragm-like localized narrowing in the lower esophagus. *Amer J Roent* 1953;70:911–913.

Schroeder PL, Filler SJ, Ramirez B, Lazarchick DA, Vaezi MF, Richter JE. Dental erosion and acid reflux disease. *Ann Intern Med* 1995;122:809–815.

CHAPTER EIGHTEEN

Agreus L, Engstrand L, Svardsudd K, Nyren O, Tibblin G. *Helicobacter pylori* seropositivity among Swedish adults with and without abdominal symptoms. A population-based epidemiologic study. *Scand J Gastroenterol* 1995;30:752–757.

Brummer P, Hakkinen I. X ray negative dyspepsia. *Acta Med Scand* 1959;165:329–332.

Calballero-Placencia AM, Muros-Navarro MC, Martin-Ruiz JL, Valenzuela-Barranco M, de los Reyes-Garcia MC, Casado-Caballero FJ, Rodriquez-Tellez M, Lopez-Manas JG. Dyspeptic symptoms and gastric emptying of solids in patients with functional dyspepsia. *Scand J Gastroenterol* 1995;30:745–751.

David D, Mertz H, Fefer L, Sytnik C, Raeen H, Niazi N, Kodner A, Mayer EA. Sleep and motor activity in patients with severe non-ulcer dyspepsia. *Gut* 1994;35:916–925.

Drossman DA, Li Z, Andruzzi E, Temple RD, Talley NJ, Thompson WG. U.S. householder survey of functional gastrointestinal disorders: Prevalence, sociodemography and health impact. *Dig Dis Sci* 1993;38:1560–1580

Drossman DA, Richter JE, Talley NJ, Thompson WG, Corrazziani E, Whitehead WE. *Functional Gastrointestinal Disorders.* Boston: Little, Brown, 1994.

George R, Hellier MD, Kennedy HJ, Smits BJ. Definition and sub-typing of non-ulcer dyspepsia. *Gastroenterol Int* 1993;6:93–99.

Gregory DW, Davies GT, Evans KT, Rhodes J. Natural history of patients with X ray negative dyspepsia in general practice. *Brit Med J* 1972;4:519–520.

Hutchison R. *Lectures on Dyspepsia* (second edition). London: Edward Arnold, 1927.

Lydeard S, Jones R. Factors affecting the decision to consult with dyspepsia: Comparison of consulters and non-consulters. *J Roy Coll Gen Pract* 1989;39:495–498.

McCarthy C, Patchett S, Collins RM, Beattie S, Keane C, O'Morain C. Long-term prospective study of *Helicobacter pylori* in nonulcer dyspepsia. *Dig Dis Sci* 1995;40:114–119.

Nyren O, Adami HO, Gustavsson S, Loof L. Excess sick-listing in nonulcer dyspepsia. *J Clin Gastroenterol* 1986;8:339–345.

Ryle JA. Chronic spasmodic afflictions of the colon and the diseases which they stimulate. *Lancet* 1928;ii:1115–1119.

Schlemper RJ, van der Werf SD, Vandenbrouche JP, Biemond I, Lamers CB. Nonulcer dyspepsia in a working Dutch population and *Helicobacter pylori*. Ulcer history as an explanation of an apparent association. *Arch Intern Med* 1995;155:82–87.

Sloth H, Jorgensen LS. Chronic non-organic upper abdominal pain diagnostic safety and prognosis of gastrointestinal and nongastrointestinal symptoms. A 5-to-7-year follow-up study. *Scand J Gastroenterol* 1988;23:1275–1280.

Spiro HM. Moynihan's Disease? The diagnosis of duodenal ulcer. *New Engl J Med* 1974;291:567–569.

Talley NJ, Colin-Jones D, Koch KL, Koch M, Nyren O, Stanghellini V. Functional dyspepsia: A classification with guidelines for diagnosis and management. *Gastroenterol Int* 1991;4:145–160.

Talley NJ, McNeil D, Hayden A, Colreavy C, Piper DW. Prognosis of chronic unexplained dyspepsia. A prospective study of potential predictor variables in patients with endoscopically diagnosed nonnuclear dyspepsia. *Gastroenterology* 1987;92:1060–1066.

Talley NJ, Weaver AL, Zinsmeister AR. Impact of functional dyspepsia on quality of life. *Dig Dis Sci* 1995;40:584–589.

Thompson WG. *Gut Reactions*. New York: Plenum Press, 1989.

Veldhuyzen van Zanten SJO, Malatjalian D, Tanton R. The effect of eradication on *Helicobacter pylori* on symptoms of nonulcer dyspepsia: a randomized, double-blind, placebo-controlled trial. *Gastroent* 1995;108:A250.

Veldhuyzen van Zanten SJO, Tytgat KM, Jalali S, Goodacre RL, Hunt RH. Can gastritis symptoms be evaluated in clinical trials? An overview of treatment of gastritis, nonulcer dyspepsia and Campylobacter-associated gastritis. *J Clin Gastroenterol* 1989;11:496–501.

Veldhuyzen van Zanten SJO, Cleary C, Talley NJ, Peterson TC, Nyren O, Bradley LA, Verlinden M, Tytgat NJT. Drug treatment of functional dyspepsia: A systematic analysis of trial methodology with recommendations for design of future trials. *Amer J Gastroent* 1996;91:660–673.

CHAPTER NINETEEN

Anderson KO, Dalton CB, Bradley LA, Richter JE. Stress induces alteration of esophageal pressures in healthy volunteers and non-cardiac chest pain patients. *Dig Dis Sci* 1989;34:83–91.

Clouse RE. Antidepressants for functional gastrointestinal symptoms. *Dig Dis Sci* 1994;39:2352–2363.

Clouse RE. Motor disorders. In Sleisenger MH, Fordtran JS, eds. *Gastrointestinal Disease: Pathysiology/Diagnosis/Treatment* (fifth edition). Philadelphia: WB Saunders, 1995;341–377.

Clouse RE, Lustman PJ. Psychiatric illness and contraction abnormalities of the esophagus. *New Engl J Med* 1983;309:1337–1342.

Ghillebert G, Janssens J, Vantrappen G, Nevens F, Piessens J. Ambulatory 24 hour intra-oesophageal pH and pressure recordings versus provocation tests in the diagnosis of chest pain of oesophageal origin. *Gut* 1990;31:738–744.

Patterson WG, Wang H, Vanner S. Increasing pain sensation to repeated esophageal balloon distension in patients with chest pain of undetermined etiology. *Dig Dis Sci* 1995;40:1325–1331.

Peters L, Maas L, Petty D, Dalton CB, Penner D, Wu WC, Castell DO, Richter JE. Spontaneous noncardiac chest pain. Evaluation by 24-hour ambulatory esophageal motility and pH monitoring. *Gastroenterology* 1988;94:878–886.

Richter JE. Heartburn, dysphagia, odynophagia, and other esophageal symptoms. In Sleisenger MH, Fordtran JS, eds. *Gastrointestinal Disease: Pathopyhsiology/Diagnosis/ Management* (fifth edition). Philadelphia: W.B. Saunders, 1993;331–340.

Richter JE, Barish CF, Castell DO. Abnormal sensory perception in patients with esophageal chest pain. *Gastroent* 1986;91:845–852.

Richter JE, Bradley LA, Castell DO. Esophageal chest pain: Current controversies in pathogenesis, diagnosis, and therapy. *Ann Intern Med* 1989;110:66–78.

Richter JE, Dalton CB, Bradley LA, Castell DO. Oral nifedipine in the treatment of noncardiac chest pain in patients with the nutcracker esophagus. *Gastroenterology* 1987;93:21–28.

Vantrappen G, Janssens J. What is irritable esophagus? *Gastroenterology* 1988;94:1092–1093.

Ward BW, Wu WC, Richter JE, Hackshaw BT, Castell DO. Long-term follow-up of symptomatic status of patients with noncardiac chest pain: Is diagnosis of esophageal etiology helpful? *Am J Gastroenterol* 1987;82:215–218.

Winters C, Artnak EJ, Benjamin SB, Castell DO. Esophageal bougienage in symptomatic patients with the nutcracker esophagus. *JAMA* 1984;252:363–366.

Young LD, Richter JE, Anderson KO, Bradley LA, Katz PO, McElveen L, Obrecht WF, Dalton C, Snyder RM. The effects of psychological and environmental stressors on peristaltic esophageal contractions in healthy volunteers. *Psychophysiology* 1987;24:132.

CHAPTER TWENTY

Alvarez WC. Hysterical type of non gaseous abdominal bloating. *Arch Intern Med* 1949;84:217–245.

Bright R. Hysterical distension of the bowels mistaken for an ovarian tumour—operation to attempt its removal. *Guy's Hosp Rep* 1838;3:257–258.

Drossman DA, Li Z, Andruzzi E, Temple RD, Talley NJ, Thompson WG. U.S. householder survey of functional gastrointestinal disorders: Prevalence, sociodemography and health impact. *Dig Dis Sci* 1993;38:1569–1580.

Fries JF. Intestinal gases in man. *Am J Physiol* 1906;16:468–474.

Hammer HF, Sheikh MS. Colonic gas excretion in carbohydrate malabsorption—effect of simethicone. *Eur J Gastroenterol Hepatol* 1991.

Hutchison R. *Lectures on Dyspepsia* (second edition). London: Edward Arnold; 1927.

Lasser RB, Levitt MD. The role of intestinal gas in functional abdominal pain. *New Engl J Med* 1975;293:524-526.

Levitt MD, Hirsch P, Fetzer A, Sheahan M, Levine AS. Hydrogen excretion after ingestion of complex carbohydrates. *Gastroenterol* 1987;92:383–389.

Maxton DG, Martin DF, Whorwell PJ, Godfrey M. Abdominal distension in female patients with irritable bowel syndrome: Exploration of possible mechanisms. *Gut* 1991;32:662–664.

Maxton DG, Whorwell PJ. Abdominal distension in irritable bowel syndrome: the patient's perception. *Eur J Gastroenterol Hepatol* 1992;4:241–243.

Strocchi A, Furne JK, Ellis CJ, Levitt MD. Competition for hydrogen by human faecal bacteria: Evidence for the predominance of methane producing bacteria. *Gut* 1991;32:1498–1501.

Sullivan SN. Functional abdominal bloating. *J Clin Gastroenterol* 1994;19:23–27.

Sullivan SN. Prospective study of unexplained visible abdominal bloating. *New Zealand Med J* 1994;107:428–430.

Thompson WG. *Gut Reactions*. New York: Plenum Press, 1989.

Thompson WG, Creed F, Drossman DA, Heaton KW, Mazzacca G. Functional bowel disorders and functional abdominal pain. *Gastroenterol Int* 1992;5:75–91.

CHAPTER TWENTY-ONE

Boyce HW. Tumors of the esophagus. In Sleisenger MH, Fordtran JS, eds. *Gastrointestinal Disease: Pathophysiology/Diagnosis/Treatment* (fifth edition). Philadelphia: W.B. Saunders, 1993;401–418.

Davis GR. Neoplasms of the stomach. In Sleisenger MH, Fordtran JS, eds. *Gastrointestinal Disease: Pathophysiology/Diagnosis/Treatment* (fifth edition). Philadelphia: W.B. Saunders, 1993;763–791.

Graham DY, Schwartz JT, Cain GD, Gyorkey F. Prospective evaluation of biopsy number in the diagnosis of esophageal and gastric carcinoma. *Gastroenterology* 1982;82:228.

Hussell T, Isaacson PG, Crabtree JE, Spencer J. The response of cells from low grade B-cell gastric lymphomas of mucosa-associated lymphoid tissue to *Helicobacter pylori. Lancet* 1993;342:571–574.

Moller H, Toftgaard C. Gastric cancer occurence in patients previously treated for peptic ulcer disease. *Eur J Gastroenterol Hepatol* 1994;6:1104–1110.

NIH Consensus Conference. *Helicobacter pylori* in peptic ulcer disease. *JAMA* 1994;272:65–68.

Stolte M, Eidt S. Healing MALT lymphomas by eradicating H pylori? *Lancet* 1993;342:568.

The Eurogast Study Group. An international association between *Helicobacter pylori* infection and gastric cancer. *Lancet* 1993;341:1359–1362.

Wotherspoon AC, Doglioni C, Diss TC, Pan L, Moschini A, deBoni M, Isaacson PG. Regression of primary low-grade B-cell gastric lymphoma of mucosa-associated lymphoid type after eradication of H pylori. *Lancet* 1993;342:575–577.

CHAPTER TWENTY-TWO

Fortran JS, Morowski SG, Richardson CT. In vivo and in vitro evaluation of liquid antacids. *New Engl J Med* 1973;288:923–928.

Graham DY, Smith JL, Patterson DJ. Why do apparently healthy people use antacid tablets? *Am J Gastroenterol* 1983;78:257–260.

MacCara ME, Nugent FJ, Garner JB. Acid neutralization capacity of Canadian antacid formulations. *Can Med Assn J* 1985;132:523–527.

Thompson WG. *The Irritable Gut*. Baltimore: University Park Press, 1979.

Thompson WG. *Gut Reactions*. New York: Plenum Press, 1989.

CHAPTER TWENTY-THREE

Dollery C, ed. *Therapeutic Drugs.* New York: Churchill Livingstone, 1991.

Bardhan KD. Can the H2 receptor antagonists change the history of duodenal ulcer disease? *Am J Gastroenterol* 1994;89:3–6.

DiPadova C, Roine R, Frezza M, Gentry RT, Baraona E, Leiber CS. Effects of ranitidine on blood alcohol levels after alcohol ingestion. Comparison with other H2-receptor antagonists. *JAMA* 1992;267:83–86.

El-Omar E, Bannerjee S, Wirz A, Penman I, Ardill JES, McColl KEL. Marked rebound acid hypersecretion after treatment with ranitidine. *Am J Gastroenterol* 1996;91:355–359.

Fraser AG, Hudson M, Sawyer AM, Mark SH, Smith MB, Sercombe J, Rosalki SB, Pounder RE. Ranitidine has no effect on postbreakfast ethanol levels. *Am J Gastroenterol* 1993;88:217–221.

Illingworth RN, Jarvie DR. Absence of toxicity in cimetidine overdose. *Brit Med J* 1979;1:453–454.

Jensen DM, Cheng S, Kovacs TOG, Randall G, Jensen ME, Reedy T. A controlled study of ranitidine for the prevention of recurrent hemorrhage after duodenal ulcer. *New Engl J Med* 1994;330:382–386.

Knapp AB, Maguire W, Karen G, Karmen A, Levitt B, Miura DS, Somberg DC. The cimetidine-lidocaine interaction. *Ann Intern Med* 1983;98:174–177.

Navab F, Steingrub J. Stress ulcer: is routine prophylaxis necessary? *Am J Gastroenterol* 1995;90:708–712.

Penston JC, Wormsley KG. Nine years of maintenance treatment with ranitidine in patients with duodenal ulcer disease. *Aliment Pharmacol Therap* 1992;6:629–645.

Raskin JB, White RH, Jaszewski R, Korsten MA, Schubert TT, Fort JG. Misoprostol and ranitidine in the prevention of NSAID-induced ulcers: a prospective, double-blind, multicenter study. *Am J Gastroenterol* 1996;91:223–227.

Reitberg DP, Bernhard H, Schentag JJ. Alteration in theophylline clearance and half life by cimetidine in normal volunteers. *Ann Intern Med* 1981;95:582–585.

Ryder SD, O'Reilly S, Miller RJ, Ross J, Jacyna MR, Levi AJ. Long term acid suppressing treatment in general practice. *Brit Med J* 1994;308:827–830.

Shamburek RD, Schubert ML. Control of gastric acid secretion. *Clinics Gastroenterol* 1992;21:527–550.

Silver BA, Bell WR. Cimetidine potentiation of the hypoprothrombinemic effect of warfarin. *Ann Intern Med* 1979;90:348–349.

Sontag S, Graham DY, Belsito A, Weiss J, Farley A, Grunt R. Cimetidine, cigarette smoking, and recurrence of duodenal ulcer. *New Engl J Med* 1984;311:689–693.

Susi D, Neri M, Ballone E, Mazzetti A, Cuccurullo F. Five-year maintenance treatment with ranitidine: Effects on the natural history of duodenal ulcer therapy. *Am J Gastroenterol* 1994;89:26–32.

CHAPTER TWENTY-FOUR

Bardhan KD, Morris P, Thompson M, Dhande DS, Hinchliffe RF, Jones RB, Daly MJ, Carroll NJ. Omeprazole in the treatment of erosive oesophagitis refractory to high dose cimetidine and ranitidine. *Gut* 1990;31:745–749.

Bate CM. Omeprazole 20 mg once-daily is more cost effective than ranitidine 150 bid. *Brit J Md Econ* 1993;6:81–90.

Chiba N, Wilkinson J, Hunt R. Symptom relief in erosive GERD: A meta-analysis (abstract). *Am J Gastroenterol* 1994;88:1484(abstract).

Colin-Jones DG. Acid suppression: how much is needed? Adjust it to suit the condition. *Brit Med J* 1990;301:564–565.

de Boer W, Driessen W, Jansz A, Tytgat G. Effect of acid suppression on efficacy of treatment for *Helicobacter pylori* infection. *Lancet* 1995;345:817–820.

Freston JW. Omeprazole, hypergastrinaemia and gastric carcinoid tumours. *Ann Intern Med* 1994;121:232–233.

Graham DY, McCullough A, Sklar M, Sontag SJ, Roufail WM, Stone R, Bishop RH, Gitlin N, Cagliola AJ, Berman RS, Humphries TJ. Omeprazole versus placebo induodenal ulcer healing: The United States experience. *Dig Dis Sci* 1990;35:66–72.

Harris A, Misiewicz JJ. Hitting *H pylori* for four. *Lancet* 1995;345:806–807.

Klinkenberg-Knol EC, Festen HPM, Jansen JBMJ, Lamers CBHW, Nelis F, Snel P, Lukers A, Dekkers CPM, Hauu N, Meuwissen SGM. Long-term treatment with omeprazole for refractory reflux esophagitis: Efficacy and safety. *Ann Intern Med* 1994;121:161–167.

Marcuard SF, Albernaz L, Khazanie PG. Omeprazole therapy causes malabsorption of cyanocobalamin (vitamin B12). *Ann Intern Med* 1994;120:211–215.

Marks RD, Richter JE, Rizzo J, Koehler RE, Spenney JG, Mills TA, Champion G. Omeprazole versus H2 antagonists in treating patients with peptic stricture and esophagitis. *Gastroenterology* 1994;106:907–915.

Sachs G, Hersey SJ. *The Gastric Parietal Cell.* Oxford: Oxford Clinical Communication, 1994.

CHAPTER TWENTY-FIVE

Algozzine GJ, Hill G, Scoggins WG, Marr MA. Sucralfate bezoar (letter). *New Engl J Med* 1983;309:1389.

Banergee S, El-Omar E, Mowat A, Ardill JES. Sucralfate supresses *Helicobacter pylori* infection and reduces acid secretion by 50% in patients with duodenal ulcer. *Gastroenterology* 1996;110:717–724.

Coste T, Raurureau J, Beaugrand M, Delas N, Glikmanas M, Gouffier E, Henry-Biahaud E, Latrive JP, Lanaus JP, Liebeskind M. Comparison of two sucralfate dosages presented in tablet form in duodenal ulcer healing. *Am J Med* 1987;83:86–90.

Kuipers EJ, Lundell R, Klinkenberg-Knol EC, Havu N, Festen HPM, Liedman B, Lamers CBHW, Jansen JBMJ, Dalemback J, Snel P, *et al.* Atrophic gastritis and *Helicobacter* infection in patients with reflux esophagitis treated with omeprazole or funcoplication. *New Engl J Med* 1996;334:1018–22.

Martin F, Farley A, Gagnon M, Bensemana D. Comparison of the healing capacities of sucralfate and cimetidine in the short-term treatment of duodenal ulcer: A double-blind randomized trial. *Gastroenterology* 1982;82:401–405.

Nagashima R. Development and characteristics of sucralfate. *J Clin Gastroenterol* 1981;3:103–110.

CHAPTER TWENTY-SIX

Euler USV. On the specific vasodilating and plain muscle stimulating substance from accessory genital glands in man and certain animals (prostaglandin and vasiglandin). J Physiol 1936;88:213–234.

Feldman M. Can gastroduodenal ulcers in NSAID users be prevented? *Ann Int Med* 1993;119:337–338.

Graham DY, White RH, Moreland LW, Schubert TT, Katz R, Jaszewski R, Tindall E, Triadafilopoulos G, Stromat SC, Teoh LS. Duodenal and gastric ulcer prevention with misoprostol in arthritis patients taking NSAIDS. *Ann Int Med* 1993;119:257–262.

Levine JS. Misoprostol and nonsteroidal anti-inflammatory drugs: a tale of effects, outcomes and costs. *Ann Intern Med* 1996;123:309–310.

Paakkari I. Epidemiological and financial aspects of the use of non-steroidal inflammatory analgesics. *Pharm Tox* 1994;75(suppl II):56–59.

Raskin JB, White RH, Jaszewski R, Korsten MA, Schubert TT, Fort JG. Misoprostol and ranitidine in the prevention of NSAID-induced ulcers: a prospective, double-blind, multicenter study. *Am J Gastroenterol* 1996;91:223–227.

Shaffer E. The role of prostaglandins and cytoprotection in NSAID-induced gastropathy. *Can Therap* 1993(Oct):53–57.

Silverstein FE, Graham DY, Senior JR, Davies HW, Struthers BJ, Bittman RM, Geis GS. Misoprostol reduces serious gastrointestinal complications in patients with rheumatoid arthritis receiving nonsteroidal anti-inflammatory drugs. *Ann Intern Med* 1995;123:241–249.

Sontag SJ, Schnell TG, Budiman-Mak E, Adelman K, Fleischmann R, Cohen S, Roth SH, Ipe D, Schwartz KE. Healing of NSAID-induced gastric ulcer with a synthetic prostaglandin analogue (Enprostyl)! *Am J Gastroenterol* 1994;89:1014–1020.

Wallace JL. Prostaglandins, NSAIDs, and cytoprotection. *Gastroenterol Clin North Am* 1992;21:631–641.

Walt RP. Drug therapy: Misoprostol for the treatment of peptic ulcer and antiinflammatory-drug-induced gastroduodenal ulceration. *New Engl J Med* 1992;327: 1575–1580.

Vane JR. Inhibition of prostaglandin synthesis as a mechanism of action for the aspirin-like drugs. *Nature* 1971;231:232–235.

CHAPTER TWENTY-SEVEN

Bazzoli F, Zagari RM, Fossi S, Pozzato P, Alampi G, Simoni P, Sottili S, Roda A, Roda E. Short term, low dose triple therapy for the eradication of *Helicobacter pylori*. *Eur J Gastroenterol Hepatol* 1994;6:773–777.

Bertoni G, Sassatelli R, Nigrisoli G, Tansini P, Bianchi G, Cella-Casa G, Bagni A, Bedogni G. Triple therapy with azithromycin, omeprazole, and amoxacillin is highly effective in the eradication of *Helicobacter pylori*: a controlled trial versus omeprazole and amoxacillin. *Am J Gastroenterol* 1996;91: 258–264.

DiMario F, Dal Bo N, Grassi SA, Rugge M, Cassaro M, Donisi PM. Azithromycin for the cure of *Helicobacter pylori* infection. *Am J Gastroenterol* 1996;91:264–267.

Dollery S, ed. *Therapeutic Drugs* Suppl I, 1992, Suppl II, 1994. London: Churchill Livingstone, 1991.

de Boer W, Driessen W, Jansz A, Tytgat G. Effect of acid suppression on efficacy of treatment for *Helicobacter pylori* infection. *Lancet* 1995;345:817–820.

El Assi MT, Genta RM, Karttunen TJ, Cole RA, Graham DY. Azithromycin triple therapy for *Helicobacter pylori* infection: Azithromycin, tetracycline, and bismuth. *Am J Gastroenterol* 1995;90:403–405.

Forne M, Viver JM, Espinos JC, Coll I, Tressera F, Garou J. Impact of colloidal bismuth subcitrate in the eradication rates of *Helicobacter pylori* infection-associated duodenal ulcer using a short regimen with omeprazole and clarithromycin: A randomized study. *Am J Gastroenterol* 1995;90:718–721.

Goddard A, Logan R. One-week low-dose triple therapy: New standards for *Helicobacter pylori* treatment. *Eur J Gastroenterol Hepatol* 1995;7:1–3.

Graham JR. *Helicobacter pylori*: Human pathogen or simply an opportunist? *Lancet* 1995;345:1095–1097.

Harris A, Misiewicz JJ. Hitting *H Pylori* for four. *Lancet* 1995;806–807.

Hosking SW, Ling TK, Yung MY, Cheng A, Chung SCS, Leung JWC, Li AKC. Randomized controlled trial of *Helicobacter pylori* in patients with duodenal ulcer. *Brit Med J* 1992;305:502–504.

Hudson M, Brydon WG, Eastwood MA, Ferguson A, Palmer KR. Successful *Helicobacter pylori* eradication incorporating a one-week antibiotic regimen. *Aliment Pharmacol Therap* 1995;9:47–50.

Labenz J, Borsch G. Toward an optimal treatment of *Heliopbacter pylori*-positive peptic ulcers. *Am J Gastroenterol* 1995;90:692–694.

NIH Consensus Conference. *Helicobacter pylori* in peptic ulcer disease *JAMA* 1994;272:65–68.

Sung JJY, Chung S, Ling TKW, Yung MY, Leung UKS, Ng EKW, Li MKK, Cheng AFB, Li AKC. Antibacterial treatment of gastric ulcers. *New Engl J Med* 1995;332:139–142.

Shaheen M, Grimm IS. Fulminant hepatic failure associated with clarithromycin. *Am J Gastroenterol* 1996;91:394–395.

Vakil N, Fennerty MB. Cost-effectiveness of treatment regimens for the eradication of *Helicobacter pylori* in duodenal ulcer. *Am J Gastroenterol* 1996;91:238–245.

Walsh JH, Peterson WL. The treatment of *Helicobacter pylori* infection in the management of peptic ulcer disease. *New Engl J Med* 1995;333:984–989.

Zala G, Giezendanner S, Flury R, Wust J, Mayenberger C, Ammann R, Wirth HP. Omeprazole/amoxacillin: Impaired eradication of *Helicobacter pylori* by smoking but not by omeprazole pretreatment. *Schweiz Med Wochenschr* 1994; 124:1398–1404.

CHAPTER TWENTY-EIGHT

Dollery S, ed. *Therapeutic Drugs*. Suppl I, 1992, Suppl II, 1994. London: Churchill Livingstone, 1991.

Camilleri M. Appraisal of medium- and long-term treatment of gastroparesis and chronic intestinal dysmotility. *Am J Gastroenterol* 1994;89:1769–1774.

Malagalada JR. Diabetic gastroparesis in perspective. *Gastroenterology* 1994;107:581–582.

Peeters TL. Erythromycin and other macrolides as prokinetic agents. *Gastroenterology* 1993;105:1886–1899.

Quigley EMM. Gastroesophageal reflux disease: The roles of motility in pathophysiology and therapy. *Am J Gastroenterol* 1993;88:1649–1651.

Reynolds JC, Putnam PE. Prokinetic agents. *Gastroenterol Clin North Am* 1992;21:567–596.

Richter JE, Long JF. Cisapride for gastroesophageal reflux disease: A placebo-controlled, double blind study. *Am J Gastroenterol* 1995;90:423–450.

Talley NJ. Drug treatment of functional dyspepsia. *Scand J Gastroenterol* (suppl 182)1991;26:47–60.

CHAPTER TWENTY-NINE

Thirlby RC, ed. *Postsurgical Syndromes.* Philadelphia: W.B. Saunders, 1994.

Hocking MP, Vogel SB. *Woodward's Postgastrectomy Syndromes.* Philadelphia: W.B. Saunders, 1991.

Low DE. Management of the problem patient after antireflux surgery. *Gastroenterol Clin North Am* 1994;23:371–389.

Moller H, Toftgaard C. Gastric cancer occurence in patients previously treated for peptic ulcer disease. *Eur J Gastroenterol Hepatol* 1994;6:1104–1110.

CHAPTER THIRTY

Brody H. The lie that heals: The ethics of giving placebos. *Ann Intern Med* 1982;97:112–118.

Chaput de Saintonge DM, Herxheimer A. Harnessing placebo effects in health care. *Lancet* 1994;344:995–998.

Gotzsche PC. Is there logic in the placebo? *Lancet* 1994;344:925–926.

Johnson AG. Surgery as a placebo. *Lancet* 1994;344:1140–1143.

Lance P, Wastell C, Schiller KF. A controlled trial of cimetidine for the treatment of nonulcer dyspepsia. *J Clin Gastroenterol* 1986;8:414–418.

Lind J. Stewart CP, Guthrie D, eds. *A Treatise of the Scurvey.* Edinburgh: University Press, 1953.

Nyren O, Adami HO, Bates S, Bergstrom R, Gustavsson S, Loof L, Nyberg A. Absence of therapeutic benefit from antacids or cimetidine in non-ulcer dypepsia. *New Engl J Med* 1986;314:339–343.

Thomas KB. General practice consultations: is there any point in being positive? *Br Med J* 1987;294:1200–1202.

Thomas KB. The placebo in general practice. *Lancet* 1994;344:1066–1067.

Veldhuyzen van Zanten SJO, Tytgat KMAJ, Pollack PT, Goldie G, Goodacre RL, Riddell RH, Hunt RH. Can severity of symptoms be used as an outcome measure in trials of non-ulcer dyspepsia and *Helicobacter pylori* associated gastritis? *J Clin Epidemiol* 1993;46:273–279.

Index